Not in the Pink

Tina Martel

Layout Define Design

Editor Barbara Scott

Copy Editor Jody Farrell

ISBN 978-0-9939548-0-1 (softcover)
978-0-9939548-1-8 (hardcover)

www.tinamartel.com
www.notinthepink.ca

Printed and bound in Canada by

Houghton Boston
709 - 43rd Street East
Saskatoon, SK
S7K 0V7

This project was completed with the generous support
of the following individuals and organizations:

Maggie and Fraser Pajak

Alberta Foundation for the Arts

DEFINE DESIGN

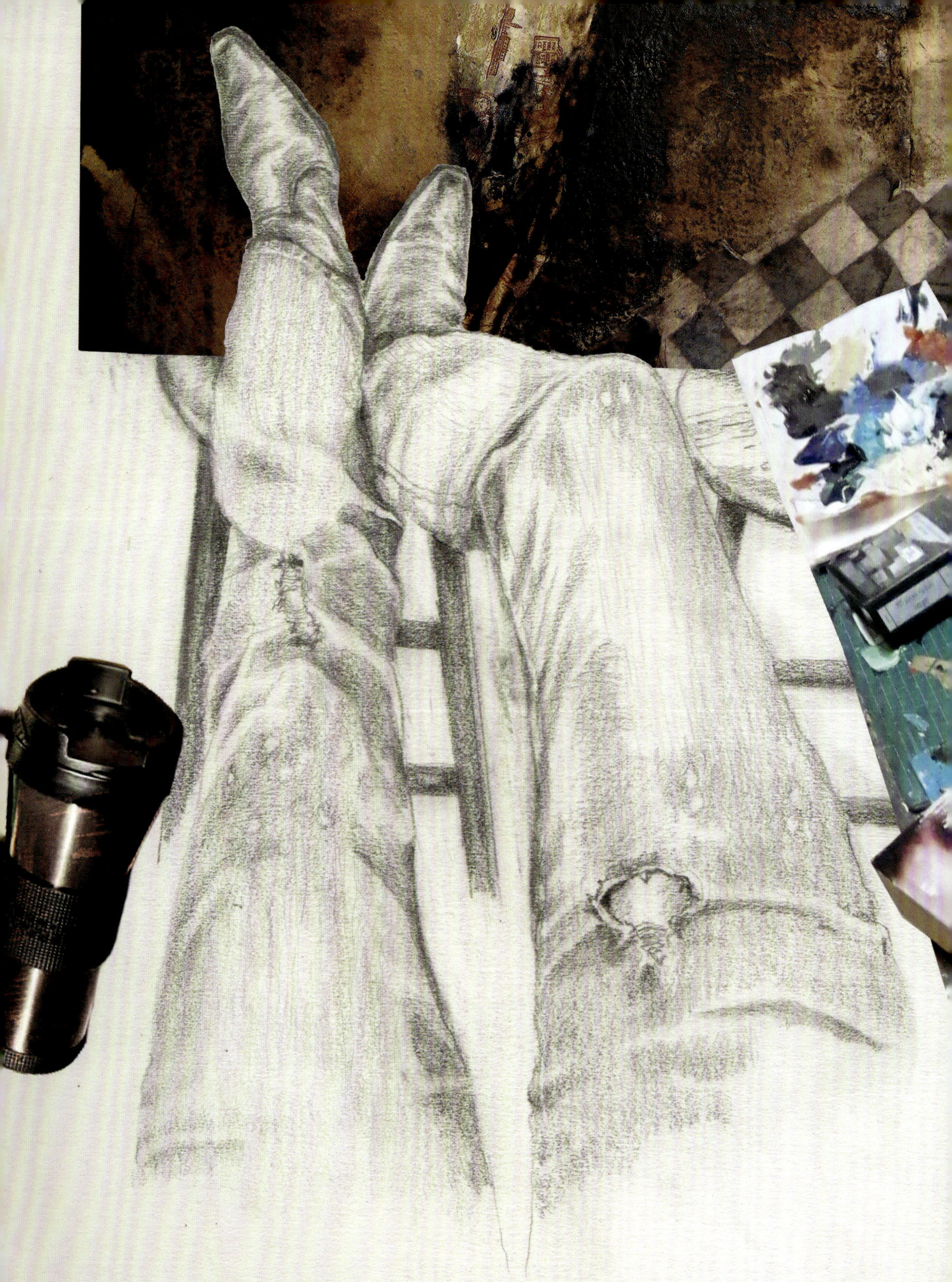

the artist

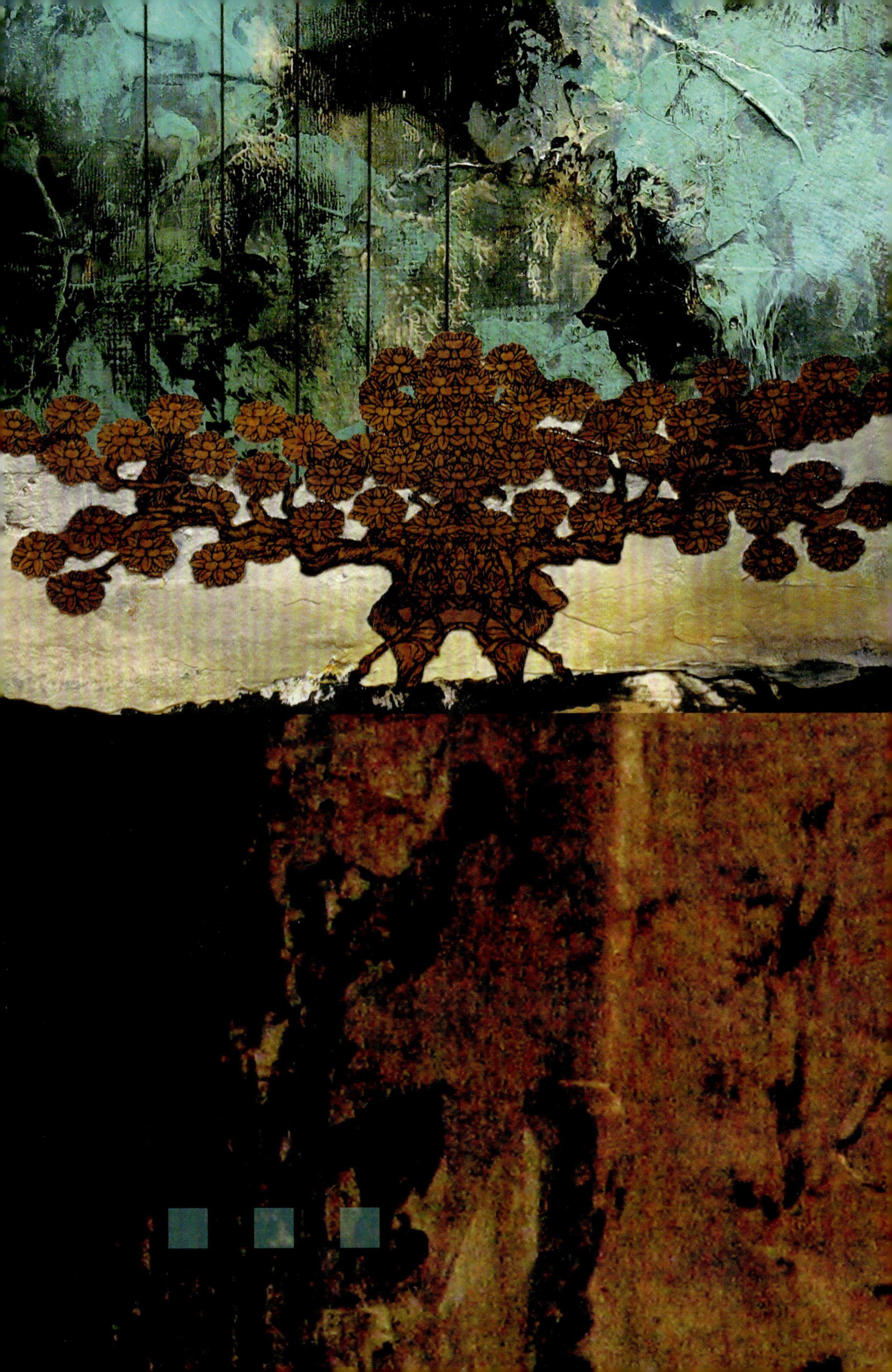

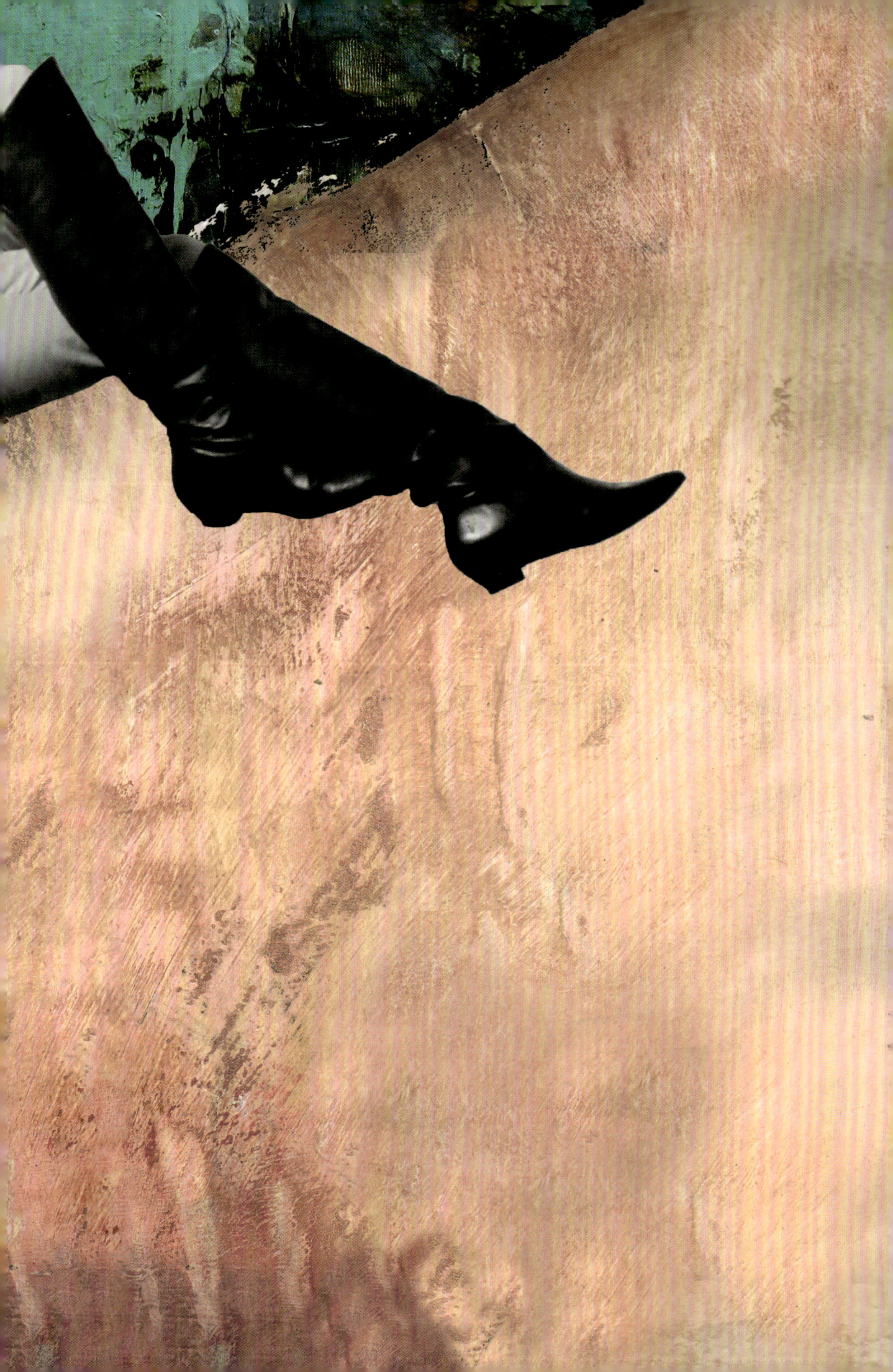

diagnosis

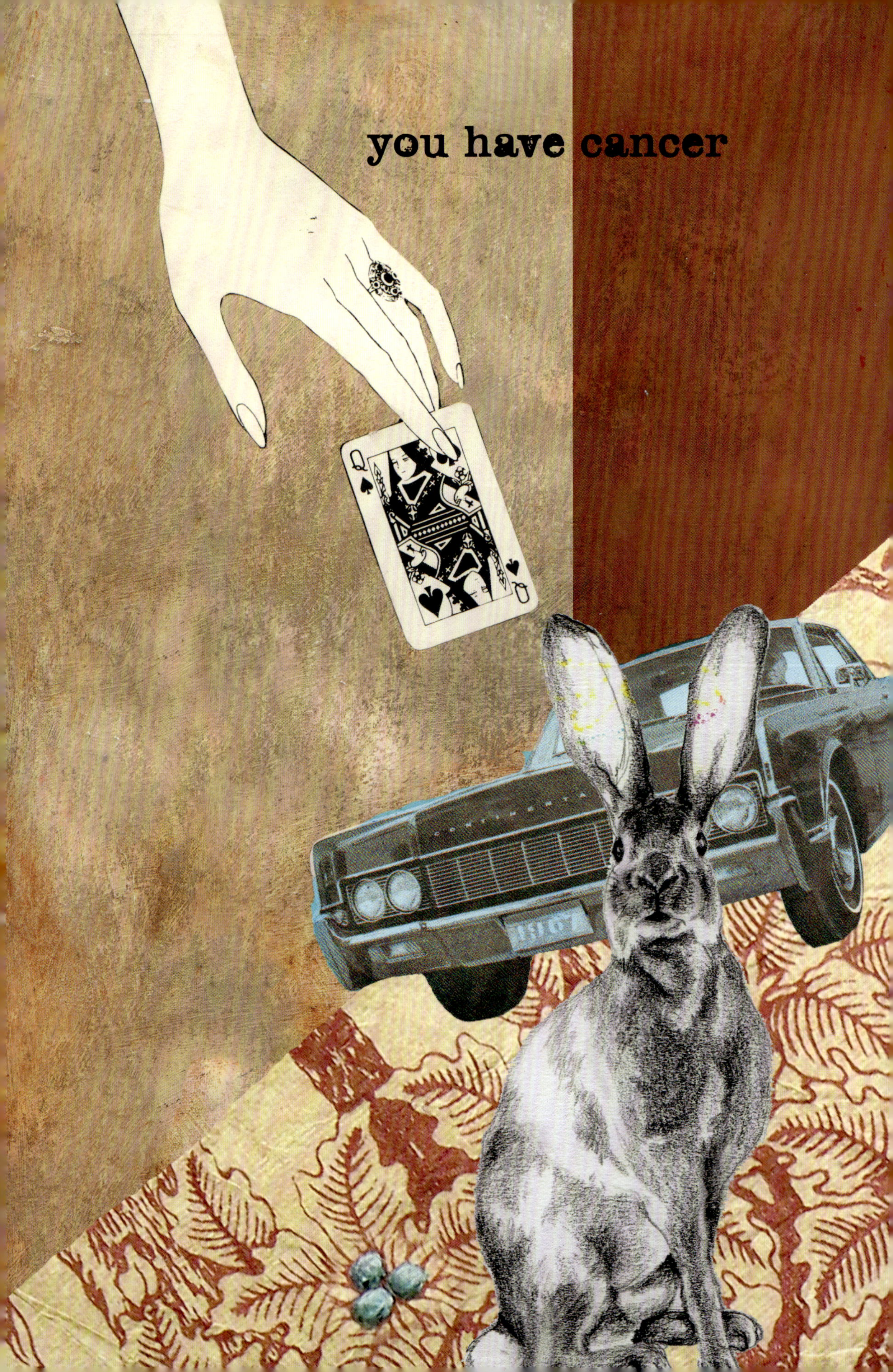
you have cancer

Before I can even sit down my family doctor says: "The biopsy has come back. You have breast cancer."

He says: "This is not my area. The Cancer Centre will call you."

All I can think is, shouldn't he give me a pamphlet or something?

As I leave he says, "Don't go on the Internet."

I sweep into the waiting room where my husband, Doug, is sitting patiently in a chair. Waiting. Through my numbness I remember that I am supposed to be at a reception. The college I work for has visiting dignitaries and they are waiting for me to start the speeches. When I slipped out for my test results I am fairly certain I told them I'd be right back. How long will they wait?

How much longer will I have to wait?

I have already been waiting for what seems like forever. Four months ago I found a lump. I have had a few over the years. I experience minor anxiety. I have them checked. They prove to be nothing.

This one is different. From its first appearance I know it. Deep in that part of you that knows when things are off centre. I make the appointment. And wait. During that time Mr. Lump and I become quite close. Sometimes he wakes me in the night because he aches. There is a dangerous myth: if it hurts, it is not cancer. Don't believe it. Over the next several months, I learn this is the first of many myths.

This time, after the usual mammogram and ultrasound, the doctor wants a biopsy. A core needle biopsy. It is less intrusive, he says. I remind myself of that when the radiologist comes at me with the needle. I use the term "needle" loosely. In art school I once put a nail from a pneumatic nail gun through my hand while I was making stretcher frames, attaching myself to the frame and giving an entirely new meaning to the artist becoming one with the work. This gun is only slightly less frightening: spring loaded and firing needles at least six millimetres in diameter, it takes core samples – five or six of them – about the size of a grain of rice.

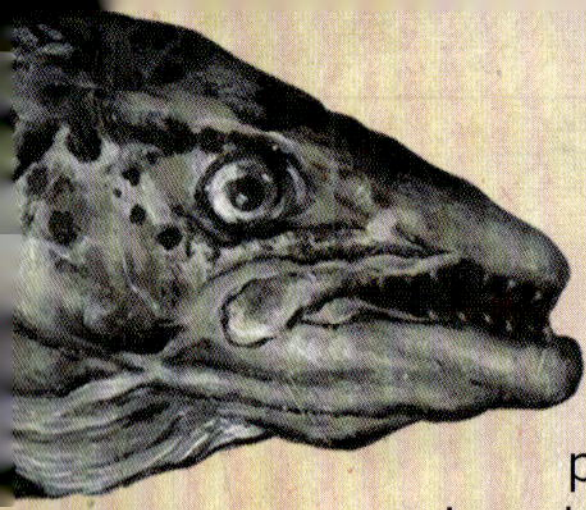

After the first two samples I say I don't think I have enough anesthetic. I am not frozen and each small pinch they promised is a full blown punch to my breast. After the third, I am backed up on the table, on all fours, scrambling as far away as possible. It is a standoff. I may even be hissing. I threaten the radiologist: come near me again and I will rip your arms off and beat you to death with them. He eyes me warily and it occurs to me I have slipped into wild-eyed lunatic territory.

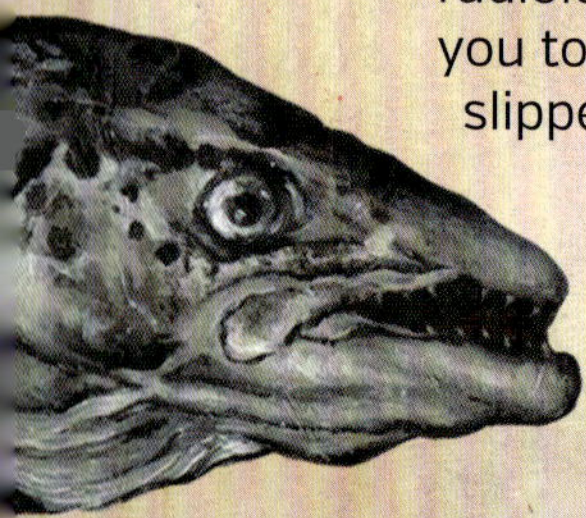

It takes only a few minutes to refreeze and there is mild discomfort as they finish.

That was several weeks ago and now I am in the parking lot breaking the news. Although Doug came with me to the appointment I did not think to have him in the room. It will be the last time either of us makes that mistake.

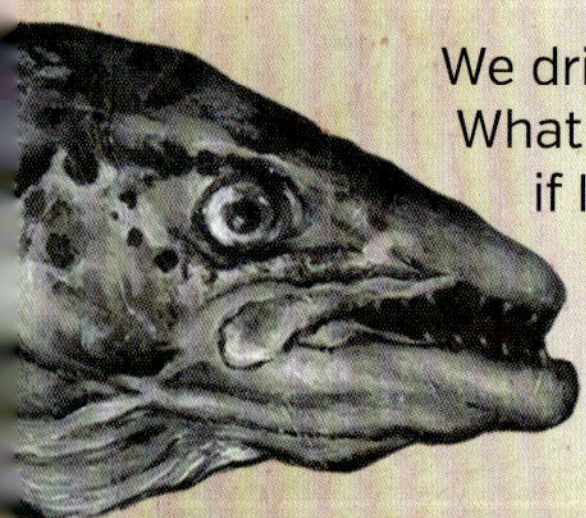

We drive home and I abandon the idea of returning to the reception. What would I do there? Shake hands. Smile. Tell everyone I am sorry if I seem a little distracted. I have just been diagnosed with breast cancer. Doug settles me on the couch with a blanket. My colleague and good friend Laura calls frantic with worry as soon as she gets home from the reception. Only when she tells me she covered for me do I realize I didn't let anyone know I wasn't coming back. And for the first time I have to say the words to someone other than Doug: I have cancer. Laura is angrier than I am. I don't really believe it. This must be happening to someone else because I am certain I am at the reception doing my job.

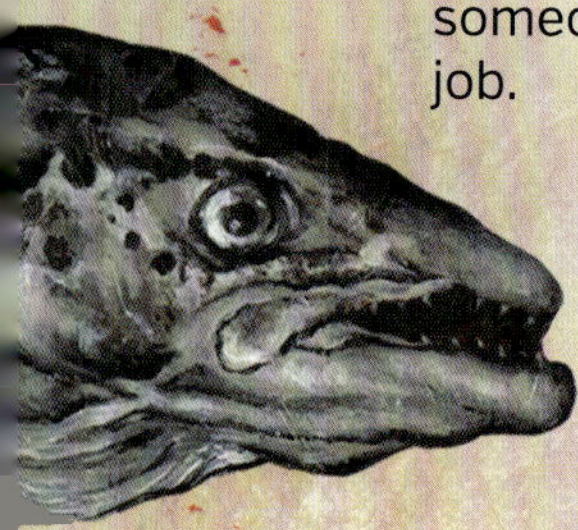

The next day I am back in the studio teaching my drawing class, remarking about the quality of this line or that shadow, about adding this or that element. I sit on the floor with the students and talk about art and being an artist. I have split myself into two people. One has cancer. One is here in this room. I can't reconcile the two versions.

I compare it to being hit by a truck. You are walking along, whistling a jaunty tune. Never mind that I can't whistle. Never could. My one aborted attempt to teach my pet cockatiel to wolf whistle sent my mother into gales of laughter. Suddenly you are staring at a huge grill plate, your face frozen like Wile E Coyote's just before the truck flattens him. Poor Wile E Coyote. His expression, week after week, of surprise, pain, then resignation. Nothing ever worked out the way he planned. You are waiting for the resignation to kick in. You don't even have a plan. And you should have one. Why don't you?

Another sleepless night. I roll over in the bed vainly attempting to find a position that gives me at least a modicum of comfort: on my stomach, my hand hanging a few inches off the floor. For the first time in countless years, the gap under the bed holds no fear for me. The monster that lives there has abandoned his long-held post. There is no chance he might grab my hand in the night. He now resides on top of the bed. And he's brought his friend, the closet monster. They both perch silently. Eyes glowing balefully. We watch each other. I have always known monsters were real.

N o w t h e y s i m p l y g o b y o t h e r n a m e s.

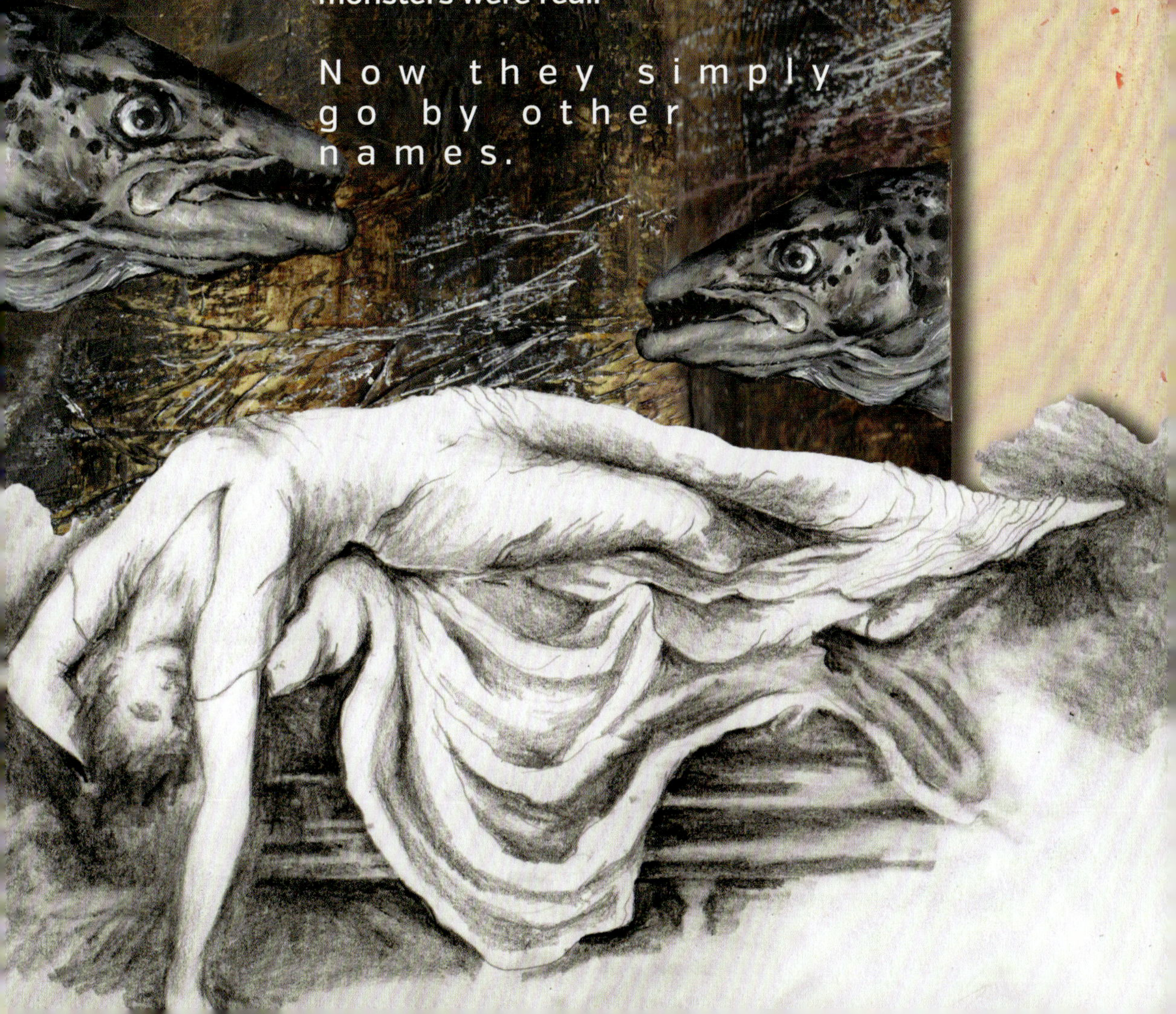

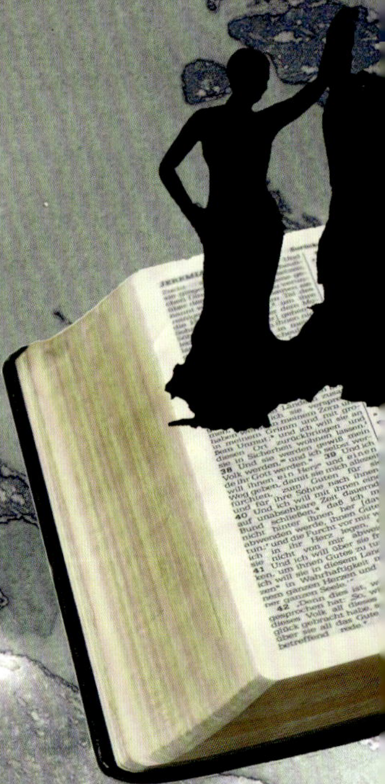

On the upcoming weekend, I am supposed to be performing with my tribal belly dance troop. We have been planning and practicing for months in preparation for our first major outdoor festival. Despite the recent developments, I decide to go. On the drive, we discuss costumes, life, books and movies. I wonder what would happen if I blurt out my news. I am not famous for my restraint. Usually the words tumble out and lie there, worms out of a can. I am unusually quiet, but no one mentions it. In the evening, I beg off from going to a concert and head to the hotel. At a bookstore down the street I stock up on books about cancer, wondering fleetingly how I'll get such a stack home without anyone asking what I am reading.

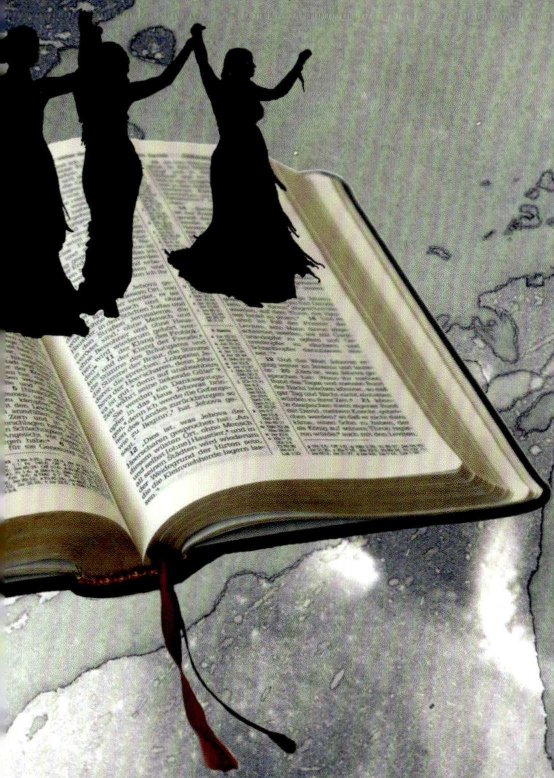

Mr. Lump and I make it through the performance with minor flaws, which privately I blame on him. I have a momentary blank when we exit in a carefully prepared strategy. I forget where the stairs are and lead us to the edge of the stage and a four foot drop. Later, when I see pictures, I appear happy and relaxed, but remain hidden behind my sunglasses. This could be the last time I ever dance with these women. My mortality hits me in the face like the shovel in a bad slapstick. It's not really funny but you have to laugh.

My family has a history of inappropriate humour. When my father died at 56, my brother Jeff and I accompanied my mother to the funeral home. We were choosing a casket when the director was called away. Jeff took the opportunity to try a few out for size to be sure Dad would fit.

At the gravesite

while the casket was being lowered into the ground,

my sister's two and a half year old boy asked

Mom, HOW IS gRANDPA

GOING tO GEt OUt?

He had been told his grandfather was going to heaven and, with a child's clarity of vision, foresaw a problem. I could tell from my mother's shaking shoulders that she was laughing and crying simultaneously and I squeezed her hand. We were on the same page. Laughter is our uneasy way of dealing with whatever unanswerable questions life throws at us.

I phone my mother with the news and she offers to call my sister and my brother. I know I am a weakling for ducking this responsibility, but the words don't want to surface. They bubble deep within me like slow boiling oil. There is still the problem of telling friends, the people at work. One of the books I read suggested wearing a t-shirt that sports the slogan "I have cancer." You don't have to say anything just flash the message at opportune times. It is one of the best ideas I have heard. As it is, I send a few emails and gradually the word spreads.

Days later and still no word from the Cancer Centre. I have a million questions and a doctor who is unlikely to be any more forthcoming than he was before. Defiantly, I turn to the Internet and read obsessively. It is monstrous that provided with no information I should be a good girl and wait until someone hits the right button and enters me into the system. It occurs to me I am not going to be a good patient. A more apt term is "impatient." I don't know how to have cancer. But soon enough I become familiar with these terms: mastectomy, lumpectomy, sentinel node biopsy.

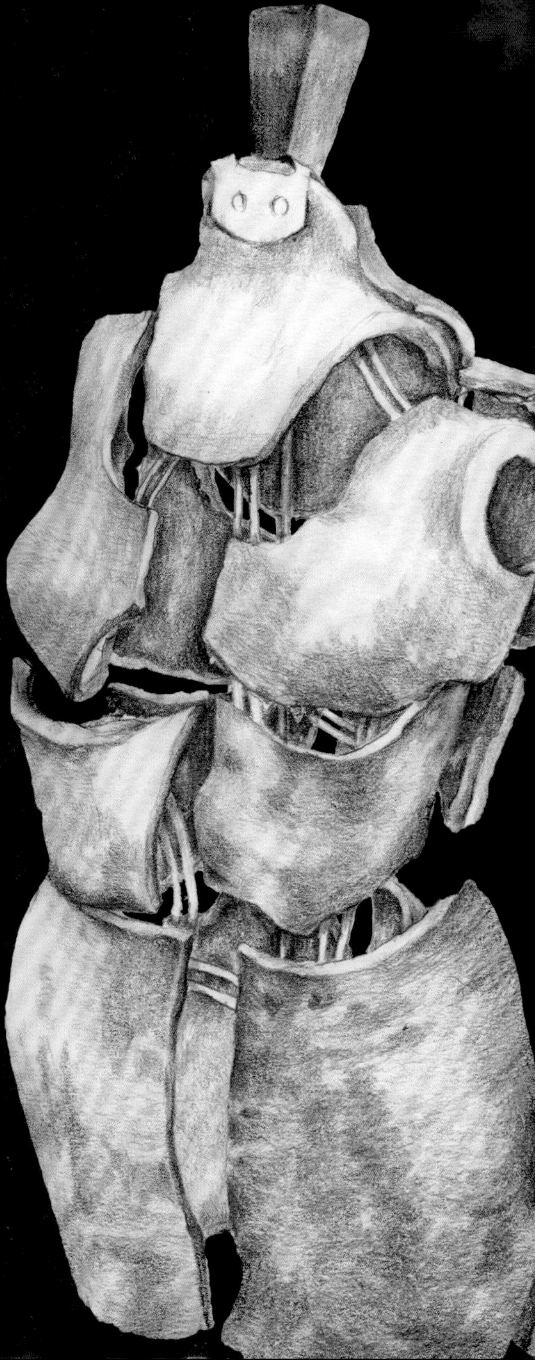

After another week passes, I call the Centre. The patient navigator is only in three days a week and I have missed her. I have to wait. There is that word again.

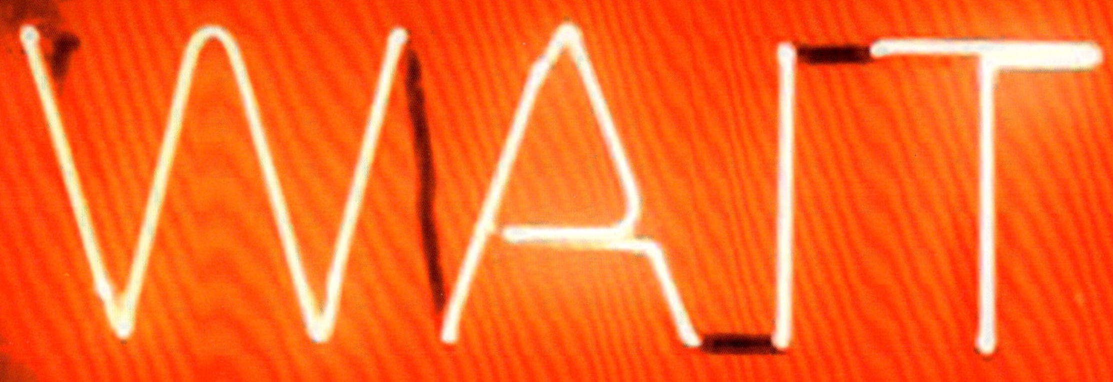

Only this time it is bigger and glows.

I tell my sister Trudy how frustrated I am. Her youngest daughter, a medical student, is just finishing a rotation with a top breast surgeon. She tells him her aunt has been diagnosed with breast cancer and has been offered little or no support. Would he be kind enough to answer some questions? This happens on Friday. By Tuesday I am in Dr. S's office, accompanied by Doug and my load of Catholic guilt over the possibility I have jumped a queue. He is charming and warm. I feel as if I have rejoined the human race. One piece of sage advice he offers to assuage my guilt: "If someone puts a hand out to help you right now, take it." I cling with all of my strength to the hand he offers.

Dr. S spends an hour or more with Doug and me, answering every question I can think of and some I hadn't. I need to make a decision. All of my reading prepared me for the question but not what my answer would be. Mastectomy or lumpectomy? My mother was diagnosed with breast cancer thirty years ago, a time when women had no choice. You did what they told you. And they removed everything: breast, lymph nodes, muscle.

mastectomy | maˈstektəmē |
noun (pl. mastectomies)
a surgical operation to remove a breast.

lumpectomy | ləmˈpektəmē|
noun (pl. lumpectomies)
a surgical operation in which a lump is removed from the breast, typically when cancer is present but has not spread.

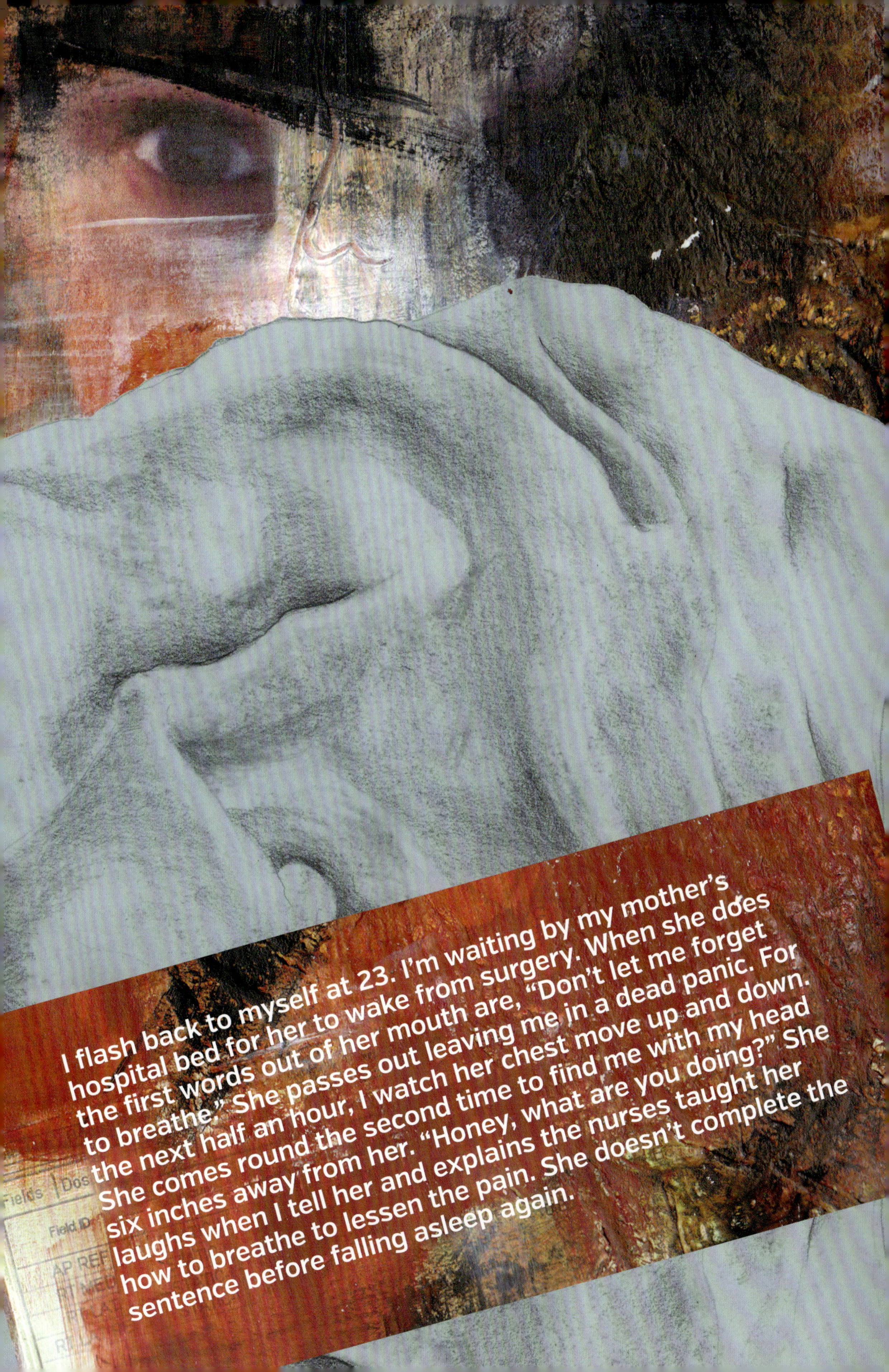

I flash back to myself at 23. I'm waiting by my mother's hospital bed for her to wake from surgery. When she does the first words out of her mouth are, "Don't let me forget to breathe." She passes out leaving me in a dead panic. For the next half an hour, I watch her chest move up and down. She comes round the second time to find me with my head six inches away from her. "Honey, what are you doing?" She laughs when I tell her and explains the nurses taught her how to breathe to lessen the pain. She doesn't complete the sentence before falling asleep again.

Now, at age 54, I inform Dr. S that I am not finished with my breasts. I am still using them. I ask what any woman would: If I were your wife, what would you recommend? He is cagey and waits for my decision before he answers that given my circumstances, it is what he would have told her do.

My lumpectomy surgery is scheduled for a week away. The truck that I was hit with morphs into a semi trailer that I am being dragged under. I realize I have to inform the powers that be at work. My hope that I can disappear for a few days and reappear healed is dashed. Now the semi is dragging me into a huge lake and I am struggling to keep my head above water while I gulp huge draughts of reality.

I can't
b r e a t h e

My longtime friend, Maggie, arrives from the coast. She has always been there for me. Her words, "You need a girl." It is true. I do need her. She accompanies me to my appointment with Human Resources to discuss my options. In the meeting the words skim off

my skin and swirl around the room

Back home, Maggie and I ensconce ourselves on the couch to talk, laugh and cry. After cleaning out my closet, we shop for pajamas, because she is horrified by the state of my sleeping wardrobe: an old worn t-shirt that I have always assumed blithely states I am mature and fabulous. Maggie buys me three pairs of Hugh Hefners and curtly informs me: "No friend of mine is going to lounge around for the next three months looking like a refugee." It is a little ironic that I will be wearing nightclothes named after a man who sexualizes women for a living while I am having part of my breast removed. But I love my new clothes and feel very cosmopolitan. She spends four days with me and I adjust to the idea of people knowing what is happening.

After researching alternative health solutions, I have switched to a raw food diet to prepare my immune system for surgery. Doug has been dutifully chopping, dicing, blending and drying. I warn Maggie, a diehard meat eater, before she visits. She claims she will have whatever we are having. She survives until lunchtime and I order sushi for her. I stick to my diet of seeds and nuts. I walk every day. My health is impressive for a woman

who might not make it.

I work until two days before my surgery. On the last afternoon, I forget to display my parking pass and am issued a ticket. I stuff it into the pocket of the driver's side of the car. I am not sure I ever pay it.

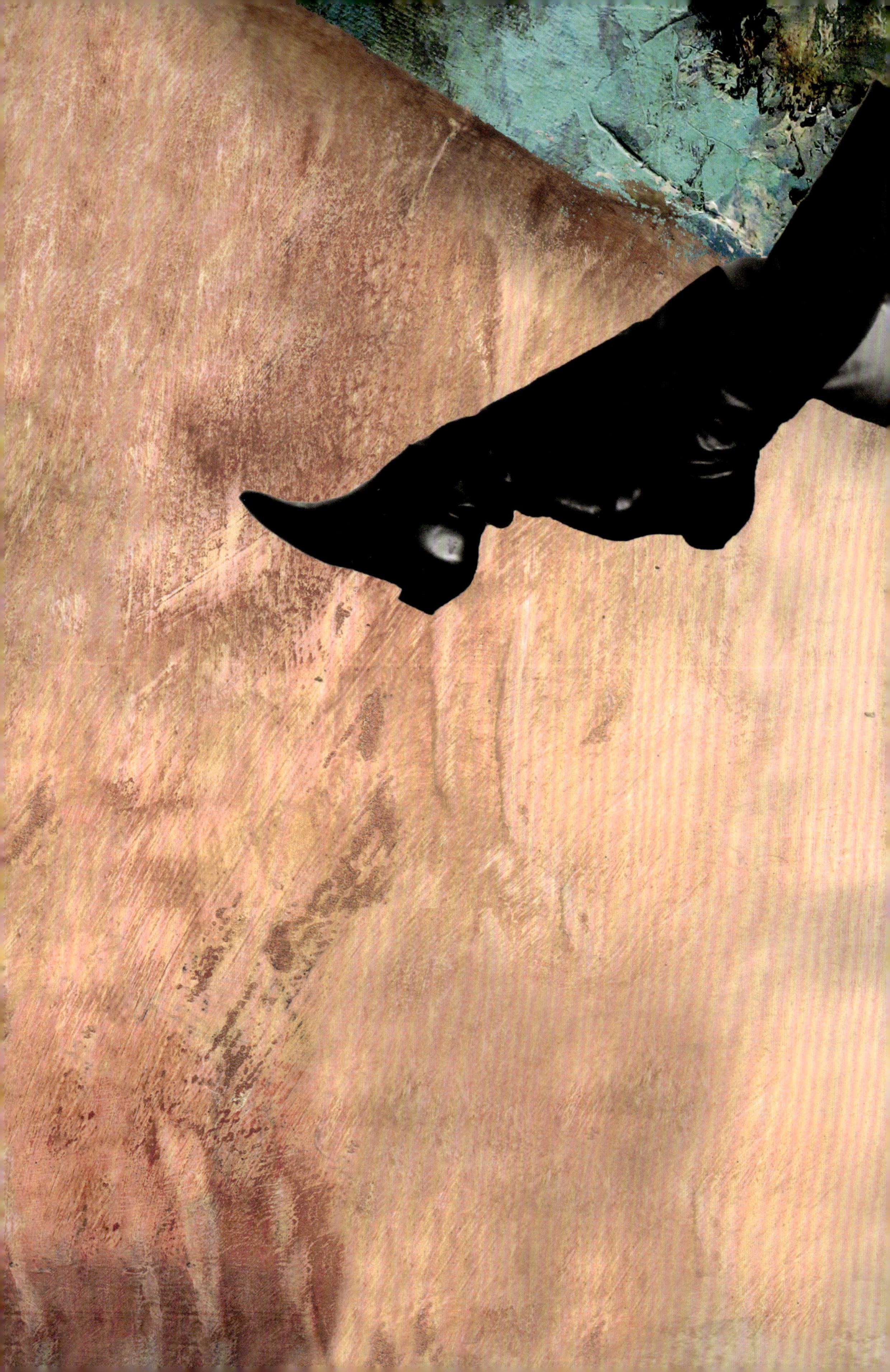

surgery

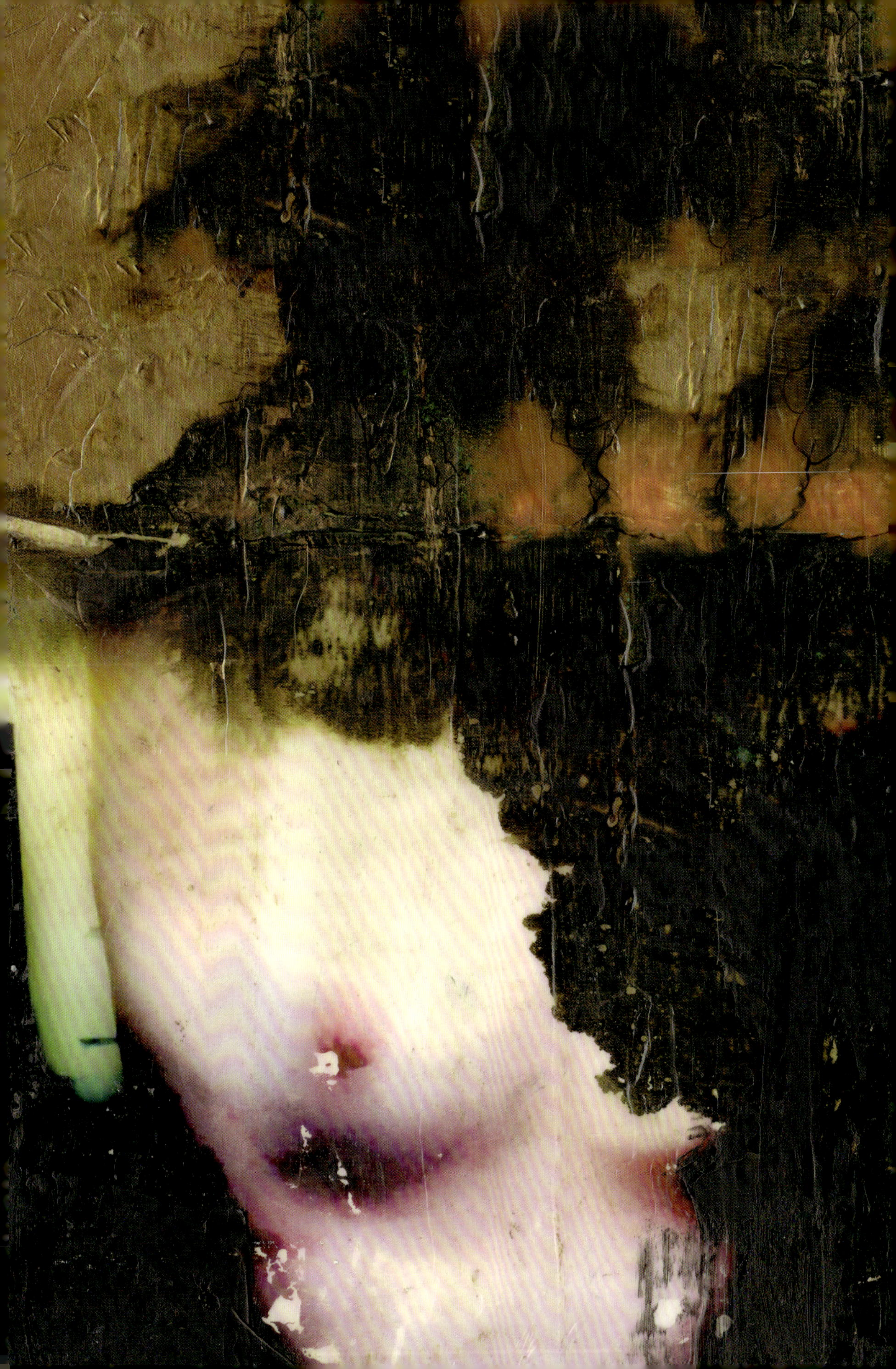

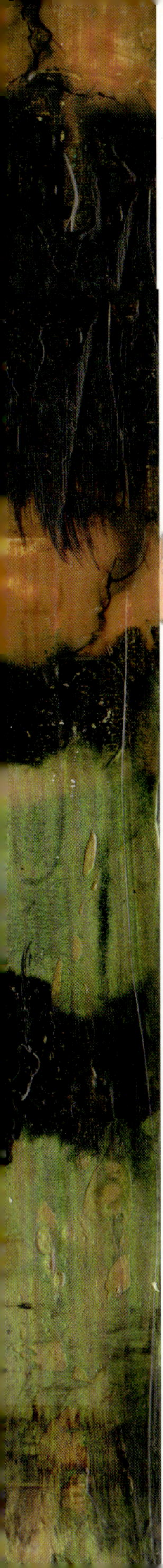

It is surgery day.
Seven o'clock in
the morning: no food, no
water and no sleep. Throw in a
meeting and it would be my version
of hell. My hospital experiences are
limited and I am extremely leery. There
is a young woman in the waiting room of
the day ward beside herself with worry and
perversely I feel calmer after I see her.

Prior to surgery, I will be injected with a blue, radioactive dye. It is supposed to travel along my lymph nodes and assist in indicating the position of the sentinel node which will then be removed and sent for a biopsy. If it tests positive further nodes will be removed. In the meantime I am on the gurney waiting. And answering a number of routine questions: Is there a possibility I am pregnant? Sure. There is also a possibility that I could rise off the table and start levitating. It is slim, but it is there. How long have I been in menopause? I am not. I catch the quick glance to the chart. Yes. I am the oldest living non-menopausal woman in the world. Probably one of the reasons I am in this predicament.

The needle with the dye is inserted through my nipple. It hurts, but my new standard for pain level is its comparison to the needle core biopsy. This doesn't even come close. I am warned that I could be blue when I wake up.

The nurse attempts to insert an IV. My veins are not cooperative. They are narrow. They roll. Come at them with a needle and they run. The staff are applying hot blankets to my arm, trying to get at least one vein to oblige. I am told next time to request an IV immediately upon arrival because the veins constrict the longer you go without water. Next time?

I wait in a quiet room. Do I need anything for anxiety? Yes, please allow me to keep my husband with me. He holds my hand while I am wheeled down to pre-op flat on my back and thinking how ridiculous this is when I could have walked. I watch the ceiling tiles flash by. The orderly says, "Do you want to take the elevator or the stairs?" It is probably a joke he has used hundreds of times. Still, I appreciate the attempt at humour.

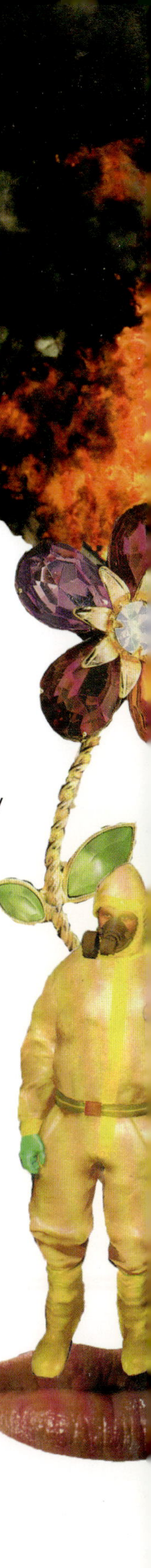

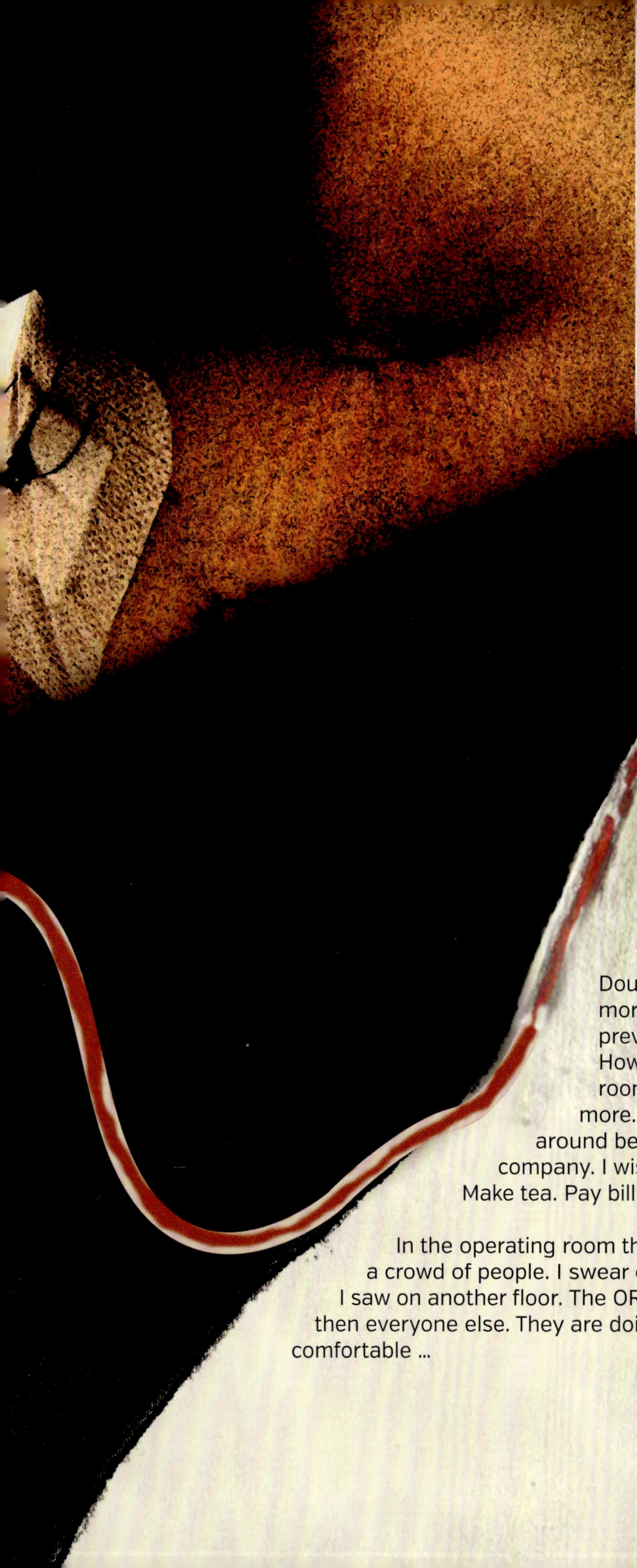

In pre-op I am asked: "What is your name? Can you spell it? When is your birthday?" Since my arrival I have answered these questions at least a dozen times. Is it a common occurrence for people to sneak in for operations? I picture a group of unruly teenagers, chewing gum, jostling each other slightly: What do you want to do today? Want to go to the hospital and see if we can have something

removed?

Doug finally has to leave. He is pale, more than a little frightened. His previous partner Janet died of cancer. How many times did he sit in waiting rooms with her? And here he is once more. My old friend, Guilt, shuffles around behind me. Sits with me. Keeps me company. I wish I could teach it to be useful. Make tea. Pay bills. Cure cancer? It is a bit catlike.

In the operating room there is a lot of equipment and a crowd of people. I swear one of them is the janitor that I saw on another floor. The OR nurse introduces herself and then everyone else. They are doing their best to make me feel comfortable ...

I wake up. Where am I? "The recovery room," someone says, "Go back to sleep." Ten minutes later I am still awake. Can I leave? When can I see my husband? A hint of irritation in the voice this time: "Go back to sleep." After another ten minutes, when it is obvious that I am not going to obey, I am sent to the day ward. I have a drain in my right arm. I have had lymph nodes removed. Translation: the cancer has spread. I don't want to look; I am afraid they have removed my whole breast. Finally I peak under the covers. My entire chest is covered with surgical gauze. My breasts are not that big. They could both be gone for all I know. An arrow on my chest points to my right breast. It is labelled "rt brst". Was there some confusion? My right, your right ...

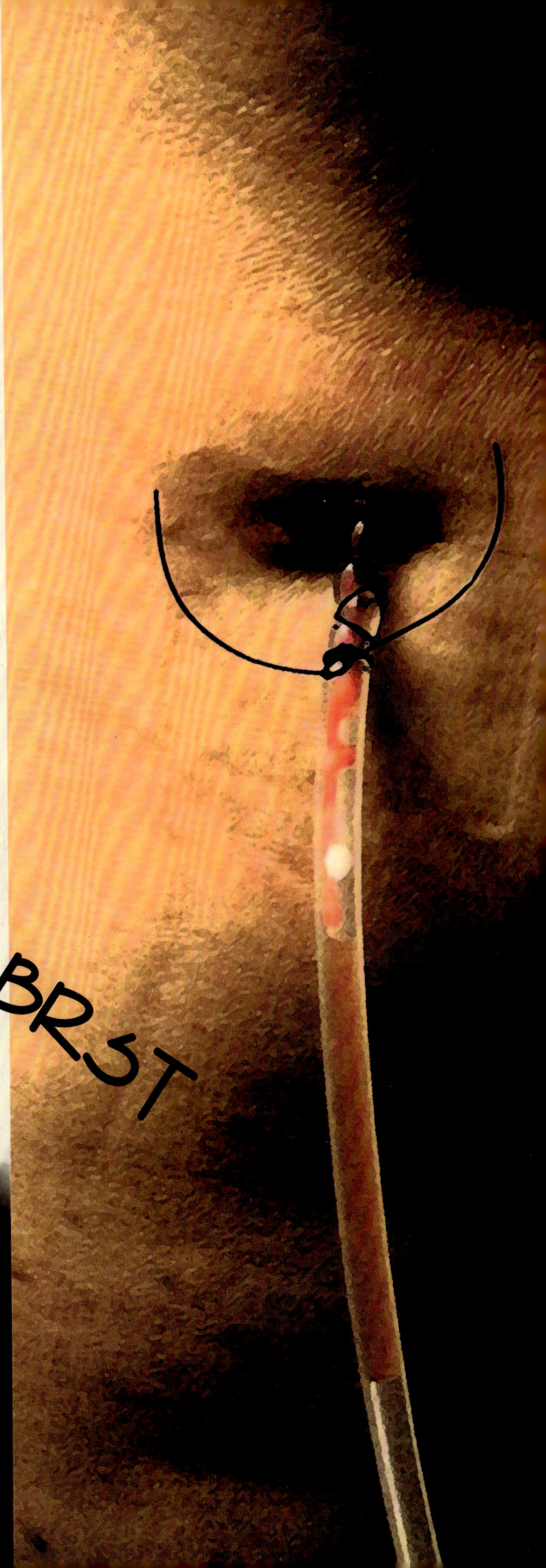

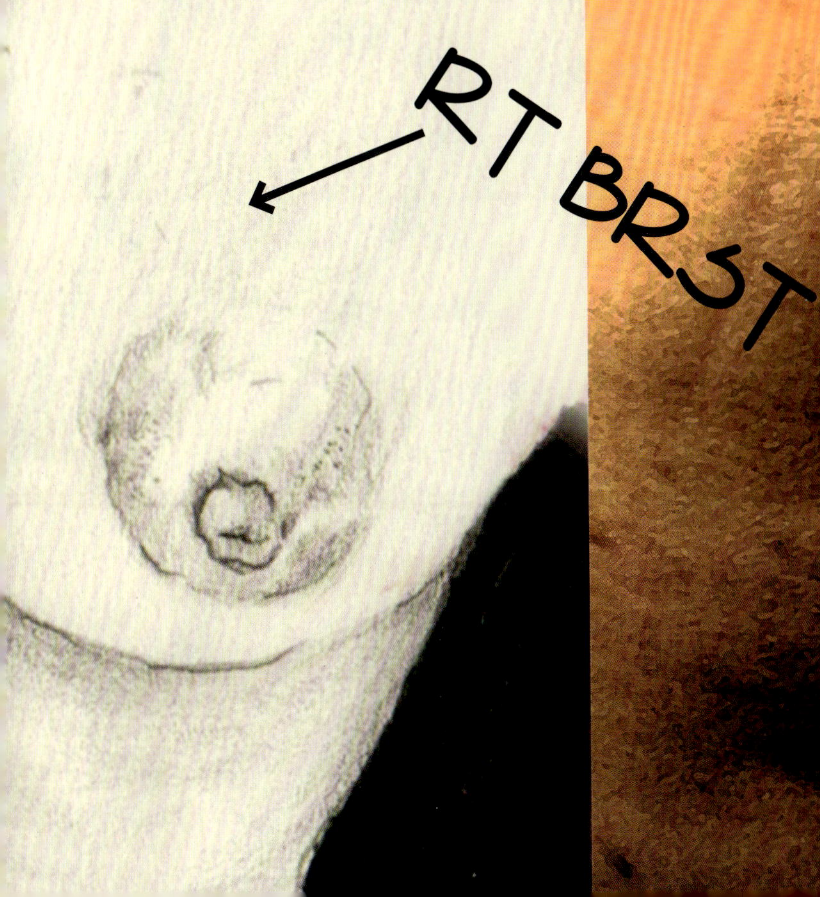

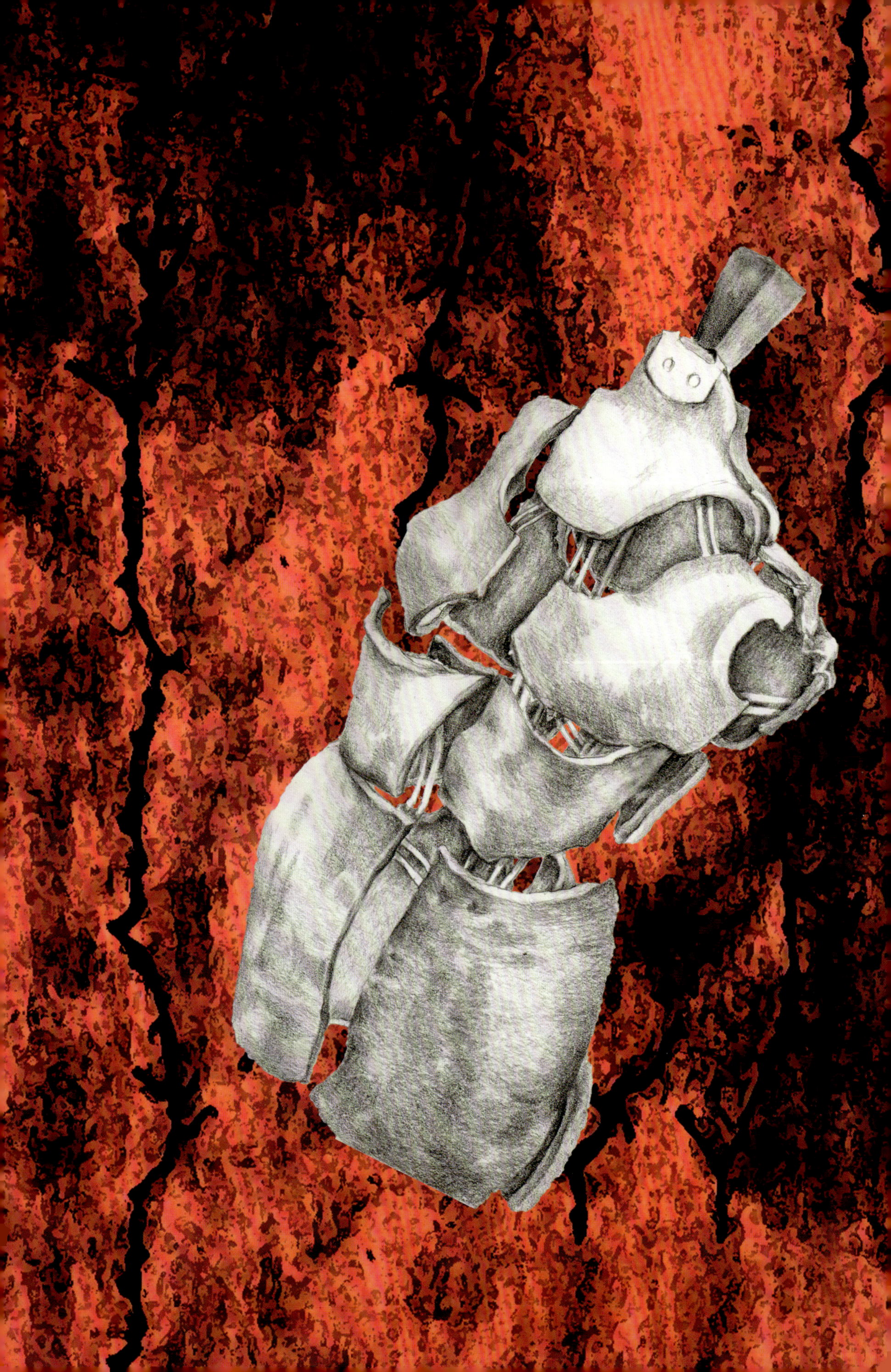

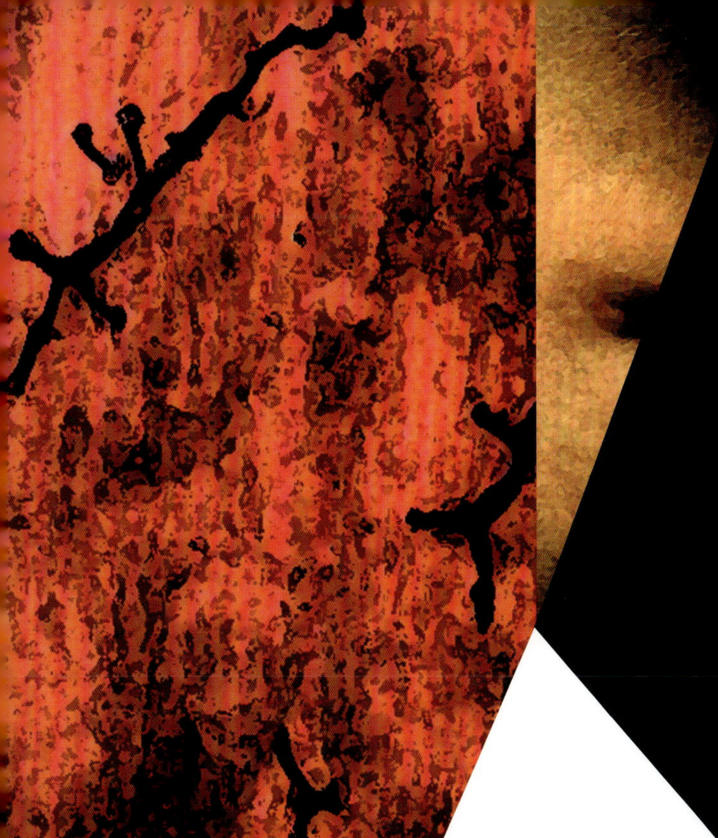

Doug is beside me. Anxious. I ask him about the drain, but before he can answer, my surgeon arrives. The lymph nodes have been removed. All of them. The sentinel node biopsy tested positive. Dr. S had to scrape back very close to the chest wall to get any stray cells that might be outside the tumour. Until the pathology reports come back, he won't know if those cells are also positive.

My mom and my sister arrive. I will become very familiar with the stricken look on the faces of people I love. I would do anything to remove it.

I have dutifully read all the pamphlets I was given so I know I need to move. I rotate my feet and try to sit up. The truth is I am kind of twitchy and not good at being still. Slowly and with the assistance of both Doug and my mother, I do two circles around the ward before returning to bed. By evening I am alternating between walking and sitting in a chair. Doug brings me a smoothie of raw vegetables and a shot of wheat grass. I won't eat the hospital food. If you can call it food. The same might be said about wheat grass.

The nurses keep coming by to offer me morphine. I pass, soliciting a comment about not needing to be brave, but the pain is not that bad. In the evening someone arrives to give me a blood thinner to prevent clots. Aren't blood clots caused by inactivity? I was up two hours after the operation. I refuse, she looks confused, and I am instantly sorry for her. Give it to someone else I say. Doug, trying to defuse the situation, offers to take it.

I spend a restless night in the hospital. Try to read. Try to sleep. My roommate rings constantly for painkillers. The nurses are getting short with her. With more exasperation than compassion I suggest they give her my morphine.

I wake at 6:00 a.m. to find several people standing around my bed, all holding clipboards. A doctor. A gaggle of interns. Is it alright if they have a look? I am tempted to say no but my niece is an intern and I wouldn't be here if it weren't for her. The least I can do is be cooperative. My breasts have been looked at so often lately it is no longer a big deal.

I wait eagerly to be released. As soon as my surgeon gives the go ahead I am out of bed like a shot. Dressed. As I walk by the reception desk in my jaunty red coat the nurses greet me with a chorus of "Love the coat!" and "Hope we never see you again!" I echo the sentiment. I have to exit the hospital in a wheelchair. In the elevator I suggest to Doug that we change places but he doesn't bite.

Because I have opted for surgery in Edmonton we are staying with my sister. When we pull up to her home I decide to go for a walk and I cautiously inch my way down a path in the adjacent park. It takes forever and I have a glimpse of what old age might be. Can't say I like it. But I hope I live to see it.

The drain in my arm consists of plastic tubing with a flexible bulb on the end to collect the bright red fluid seeping from the surgical wound. It is connected with a pin to the inside of my clothing. Every few hours it has to be emptied and the liquid measurements noted down. When the fluid diminishes to a certain level the drain can be removed. The tube tends to get blocked and when it does I have to

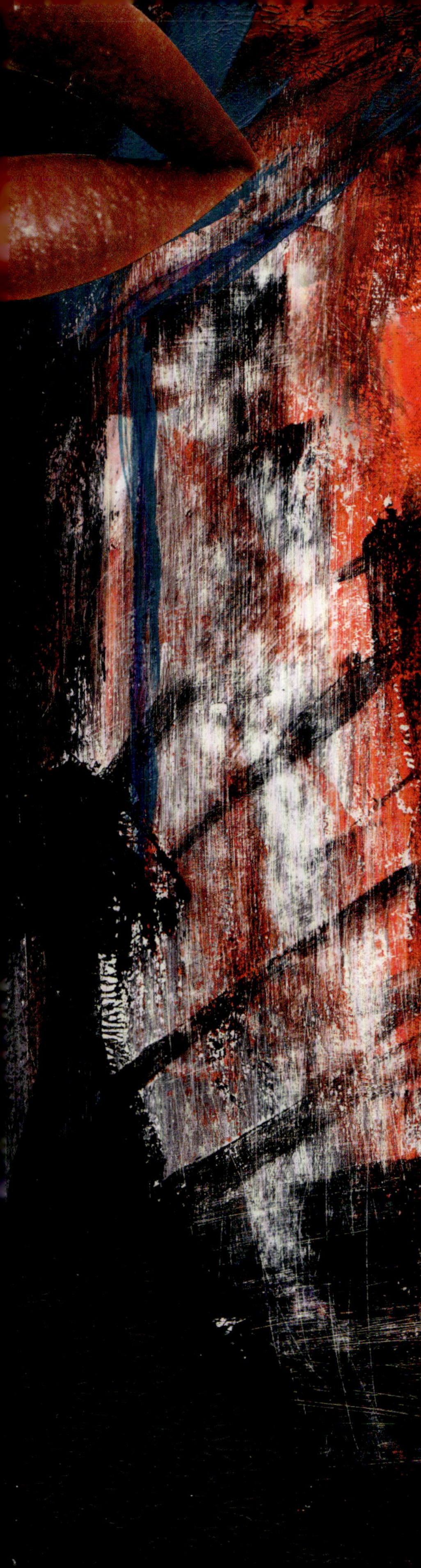

ask Doug to milk my drain. It sounds like code for something far more provocative. I know marriage is a partnership but honestly who signs up for this? Twenty-four hours after surgery I am allowed to have a shower. Naked, I have nothing to pin the tube to so Doug stands in the shower with me and holds it. I am trying not to laugh. Or maybe cry. It takes us three days to figure out I can drape it around my neck.

When the dressing comes off my nipple and the site where the tumour was are a bright robin's egg blue. It will go away. Maybe. Probably. Apparently it doesn't happen very often. This is something I will hear a lot. I learn not to trust these words.

Three days after surgery, the home care nurse comes by to check on how I am coping. I reach into the cupboard for teabags and the teapot. As I pour, she studies her notes. "When did you have surgery?" She looks startled, I seem to be healing incredibly quickly. I tell her I have been walking every day, following my raw food diet. As for pain, it is mostly centred around where the tube is inserted into my arm. I have been given a prescription for Tylenol 3s, which I haven't filled as I am taking a homeopathic painkiller and it is handling the pain adequately. As she leaves she smiles and says she just might have to check into the raw food diet.

A week later I am back in the surgeon's office so he can remove the drain, which by this time I thoroughly detest. I have been tempted to yank it out myself. Or better yet, as the surgeon is my sister's neighbour, maybe I could pop over and he could do it from home. Not all of my ideas are good ones. Dr. S pulls out at least twelve inches of tubing from my arm. It explains the discomfort.

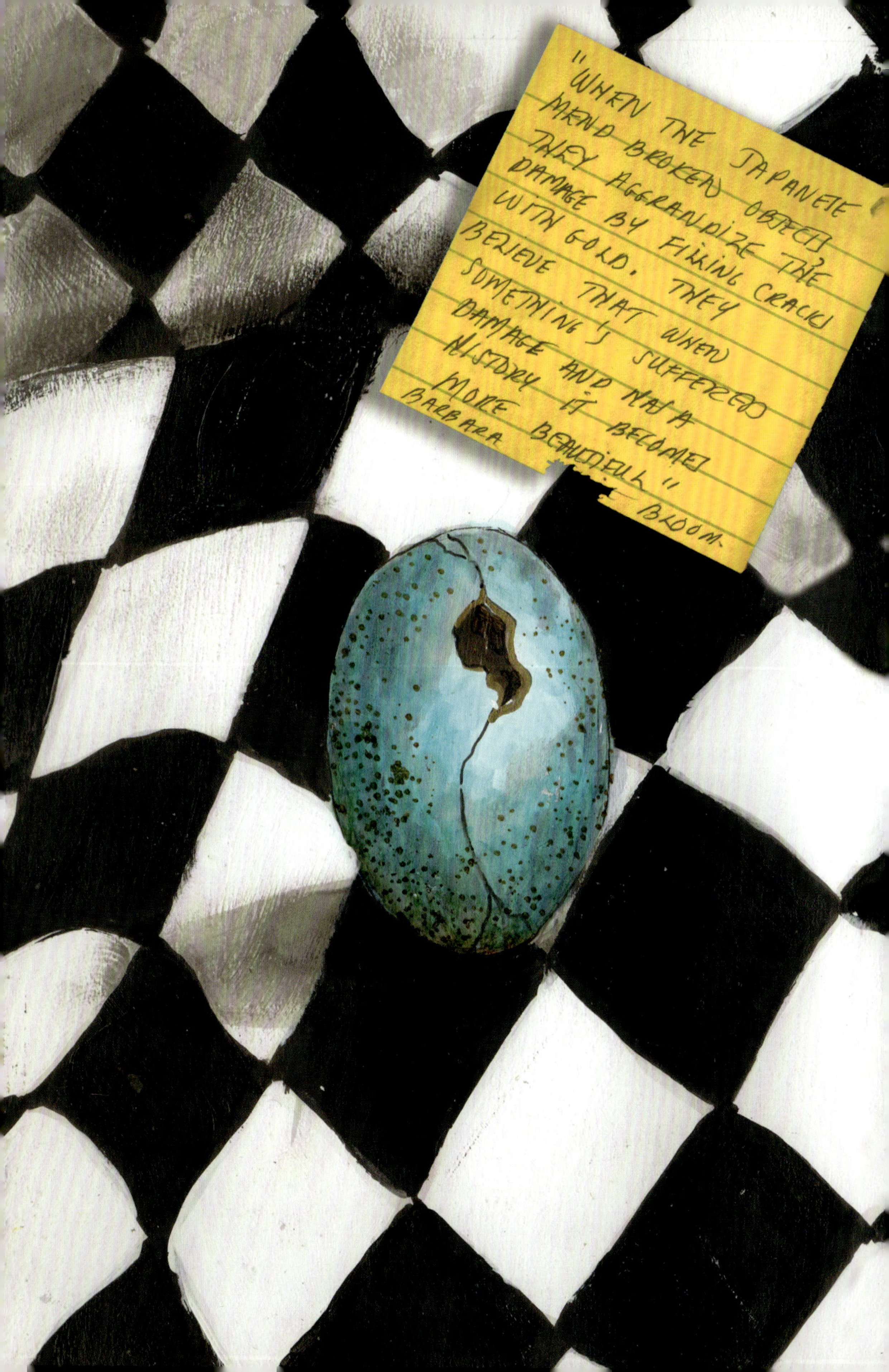
"WHEN THE JAPANESE
MEND BROKEN OBJECTS,
THEY AGGRANDIZE THE
DAMAGE BY FILLING CRACKS
WITH GOLD. THEY
BELIEVE THAT WHEN
SOMETHING'S SUFFERED
DAMAGE AND HAS A
HISTORY IT BECOMES
MORE BEAUTIFUL"
BARBARA BLOOM.

Then he gives me the bad news. Because the margins around the tumour are not clear, I have to return for another surgery. As for the lymph nodes, cancer was only found in the one that was biopsied, but because all of the lymph nodes from my right side were removed, I am at a lifetime risk for lymphedema, a swelling in the arm that happens when lymphatic fluids build up and the body can't drain them. I have to be very careful with that arm: no cuts, no burns, no needles. Even hangnails can be a risk. I am accident prone, and, it has been suggested, a bit of a klutz. As an artist I work with my hands. I build, paint, cut, staple, use hot wax ...it is my right arm. I am not holding out a lot of hope for remaining injury free.

I have been diagnosed with Stage Two B cancer. The B status is determined by the size of the tumour and the spread to the lymph node. It also means my survival rate is lower, the statistics stating anywhere between 75% and 86%. Three out of four. It is far more frightening in those terms.

Also frightening is the news that because of the nodal involvement, chemotherapy is definitely part of the treatment. My hope of having surgery followed by radiation and returning to work by January only slightly the worse for wear is rapidly receding.

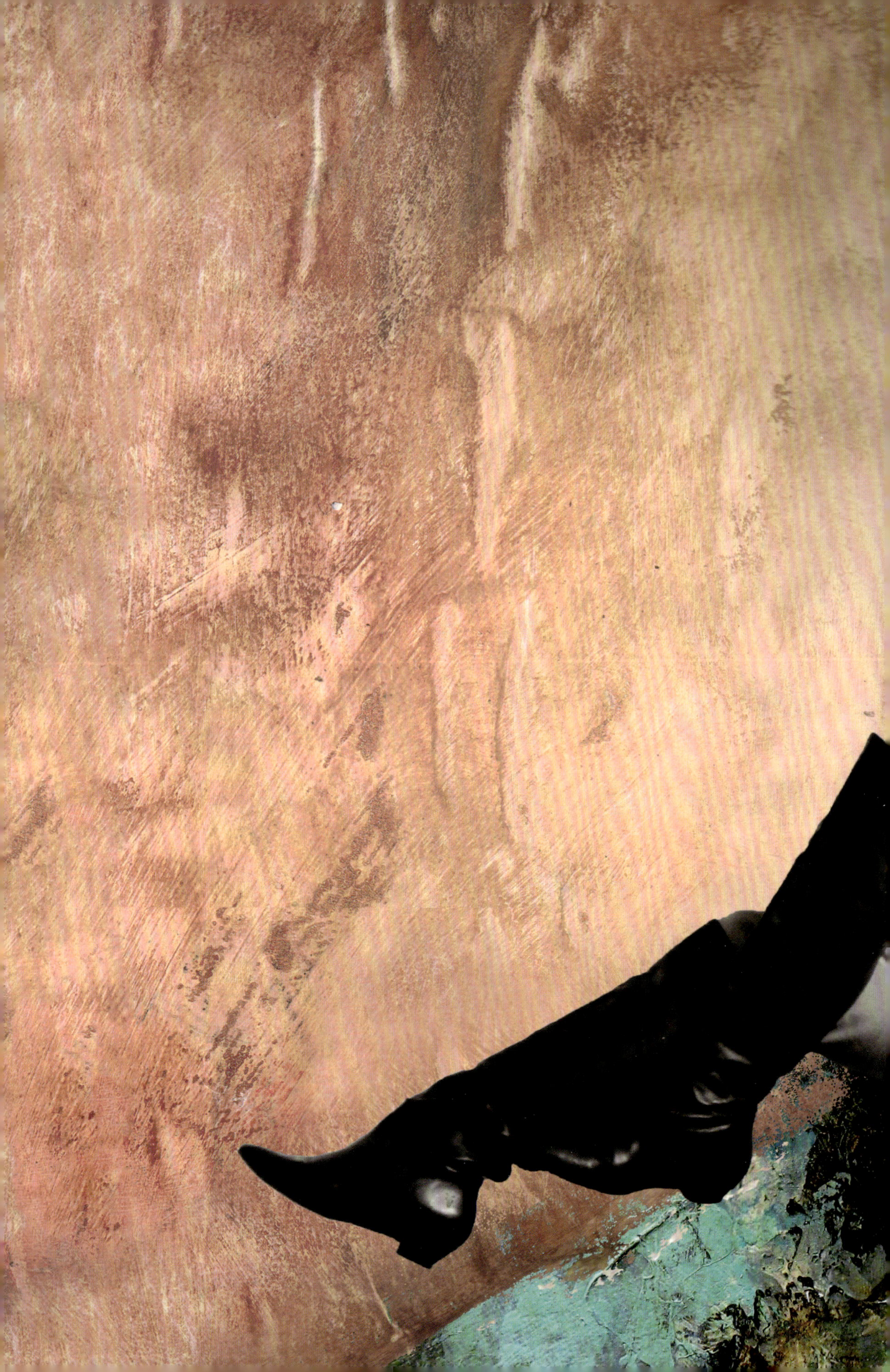

surgery redux

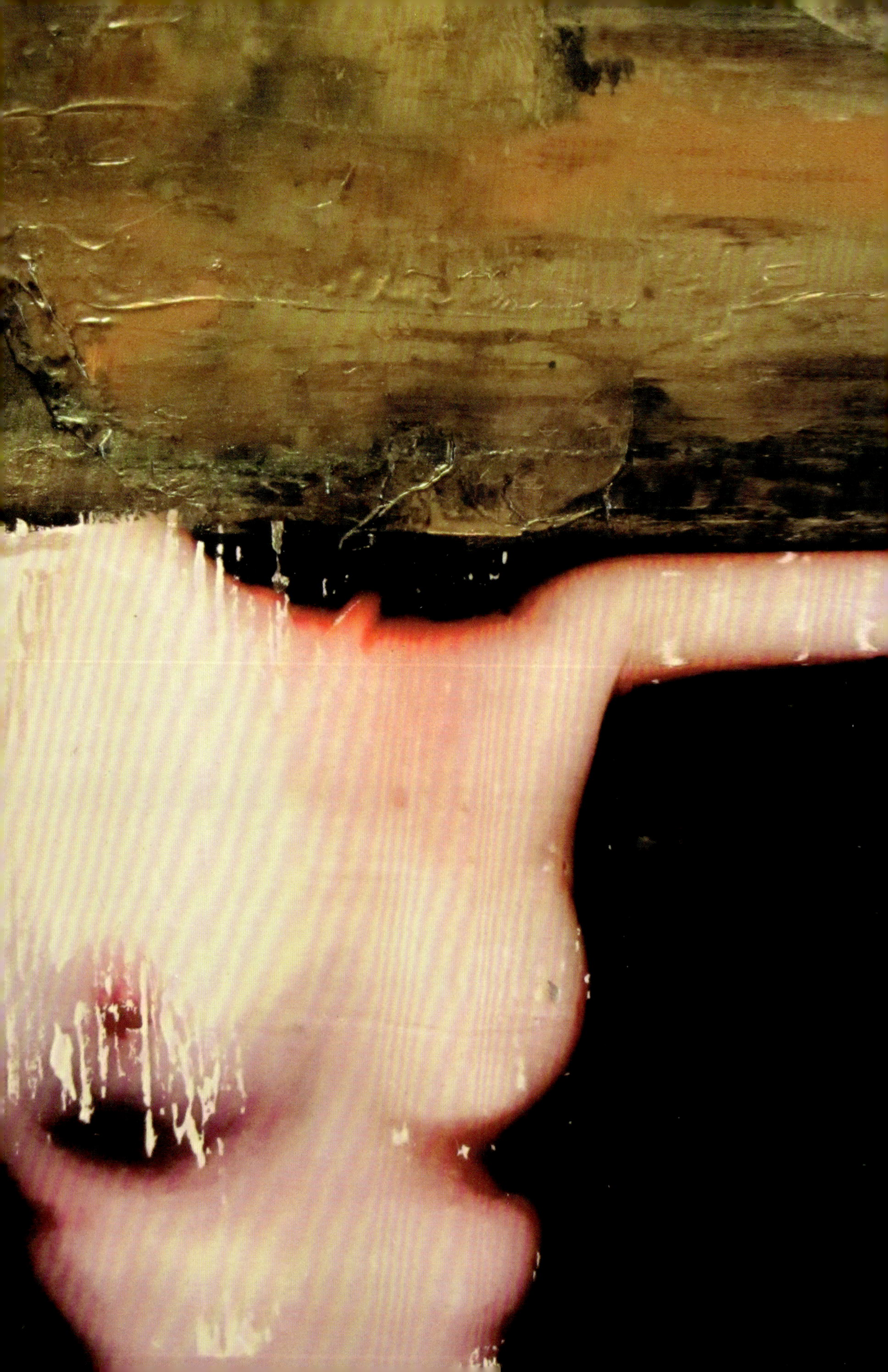

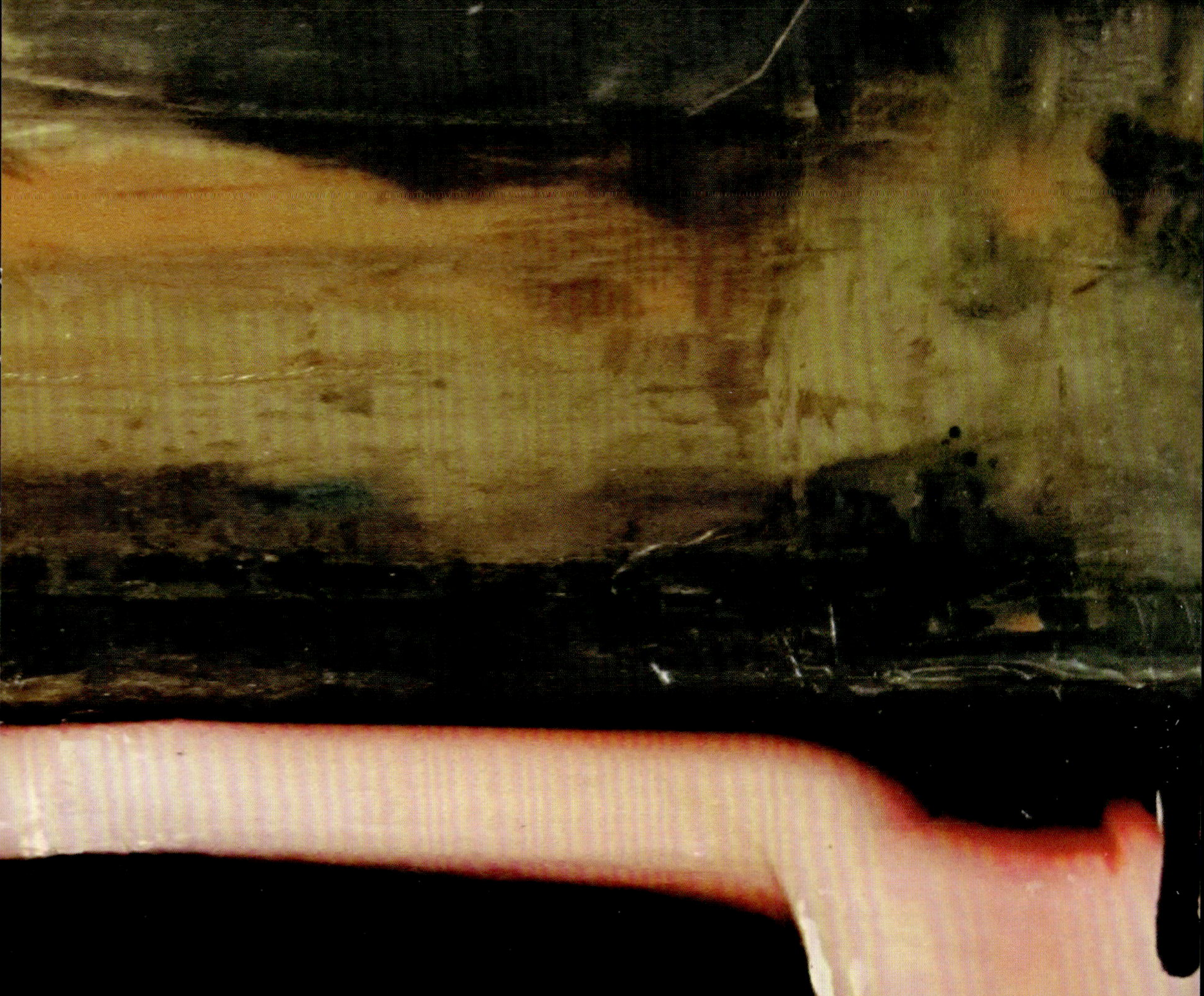

While waiting for my second surgery I start investigating chemotherapy. I am seriously considering alternative treatments because it seems to me that the strategy of Western medicine is simply to throw everything the doctors can at you and see what sticks. In my opinion this only works when testing spaghetti for doneness. And even then you have all that mess on the wall to clean up.

My mother fears I will eschew conventional treatment and opt for something obscure like Siberian pine sap crushed by virgins and applied as a compress by the full moon. But really, even if I could find the sap, it's hard to find virgins in my age group. The closest I could get would be a couple of recently divorced friends who never cared much for sex.

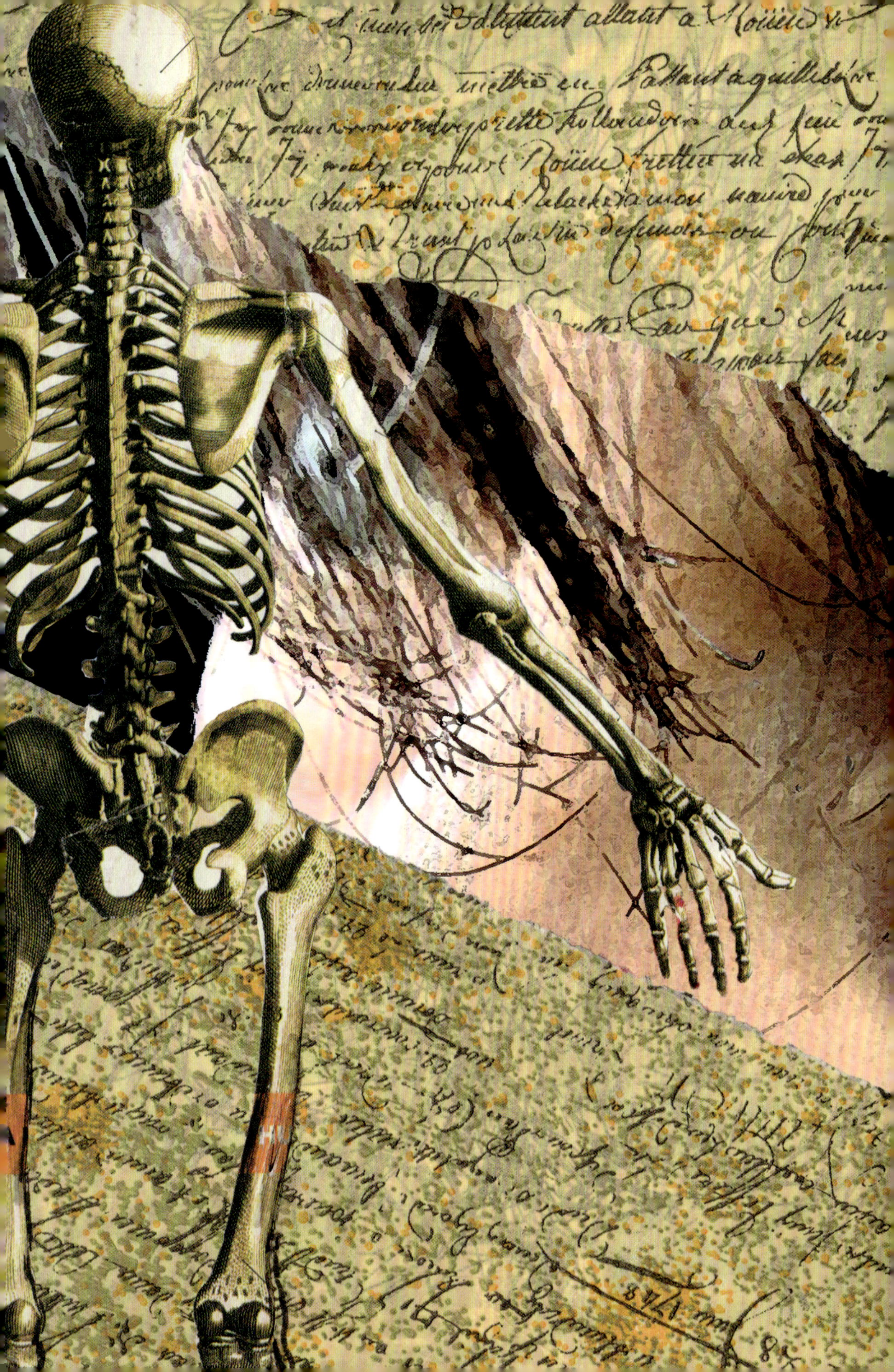

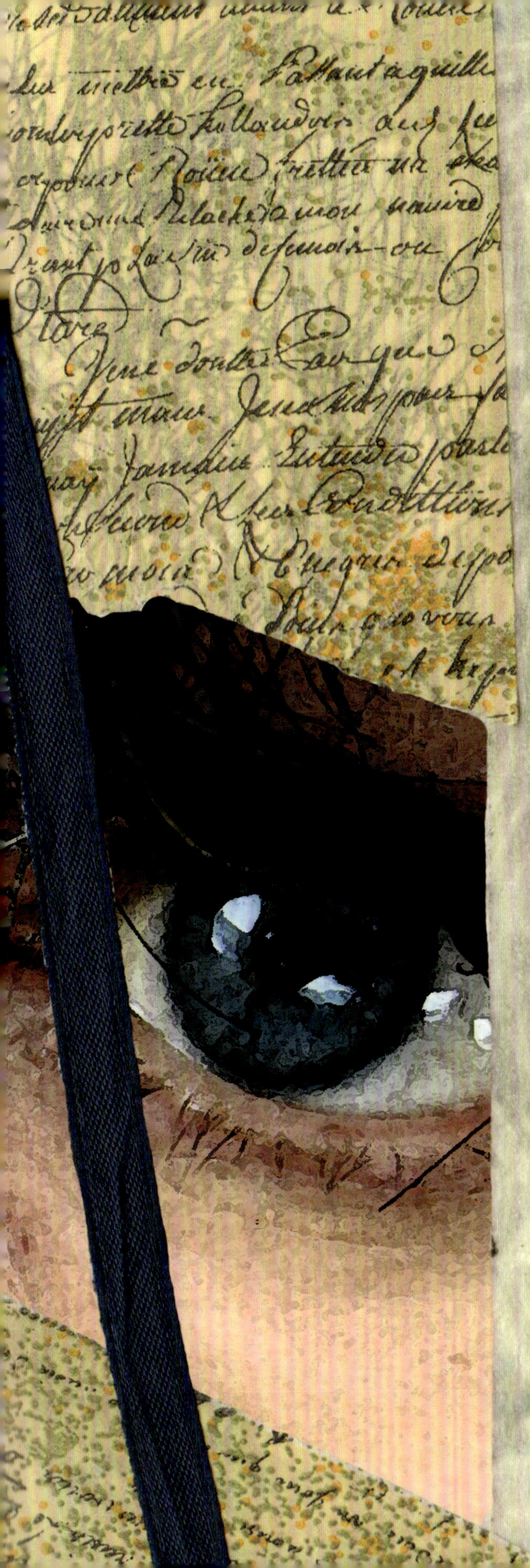

I submit to the routine examinations that follow a breast cancer diagnosis. A chest x-ray, an abdominal ultrasound and a bone scan. In preparation for my bone scan, I am injected with yet more radioactive dye. The technician confides that the pictures look good. Does she mean the quality of the image? My stunning bone structure? Her prowess with the technology? No. She is informing me there is nothing in my bones. Quietly. Because she is not supposed to. It takes a few minutes to realize what she has said and a weight lifts. Thank you.

The x-ray has similar non-results. However the ultrasound has picked up a growth of indeterminate origin on my liver. Given the circumstances it warrants further investigation. I am booked for a CAT scan.

On the day of the scan I read the waiver: You may have a metal taste in your mouth. Be slightly nauseous. Vomit. Break out in hives. Feel like you just wet yourself. Don't allow any of the radioactive dye to leak onto your skin. Your tongue may swell. If you are having trouble breathing let us know immediately. There is a 1 in 70,000 chance you might have serious life threatening complications and a 1 in 200,000 chance you could die. I wonder what number they are at today? If it is around 199,998, maybe I should wait ...

Seeing my apprehension they suggest I watch the video before going in. It reinforces the information but ends on an odd note: I have a better chance of dying on the highway between Edmonton and Calgary than during the scan. "Now that you've seen the video," the nurse asks, "do you feel more confident?" My answer: I don't want to be driving down Highway 2 anytime soon. I am greeted with a blank stare. Apparently, no one on staff has watched the video.

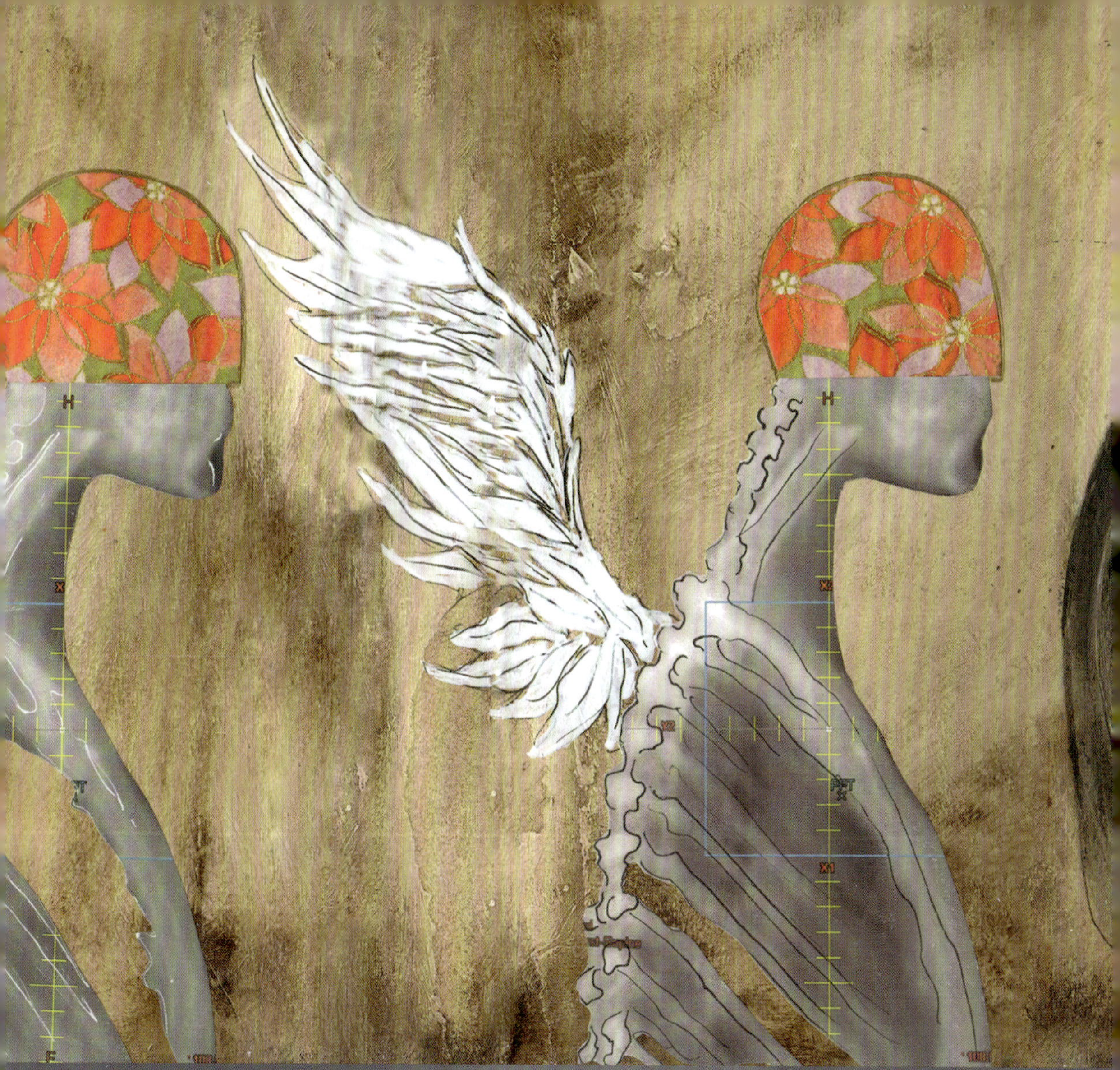

The technician fits me with an IV that injects the dye, tells me to put both hands over my head and hold very still while the machine does its scan. I tell her I can't raise my hand above shoulder level much less hold it there. She seems put out. "How long ago did you have surgery?" Two weeks. If it is possible, she looks even more put out. I slide into the machine feeling judged for my immobility.

Emerging from the scanner, I try to push myself off the table and realize I am stuck. The table is too narrow, one arm has an IV and the other won't take my weight. The technician reaches to help but I have had enough. I raise myself up on pure adrenaline and stomach muscles. Now she is apologetic. I give her my patented head-in-the-air, back ramrod straight, take-no-prisoners walk out the door. I am getting very good at it.

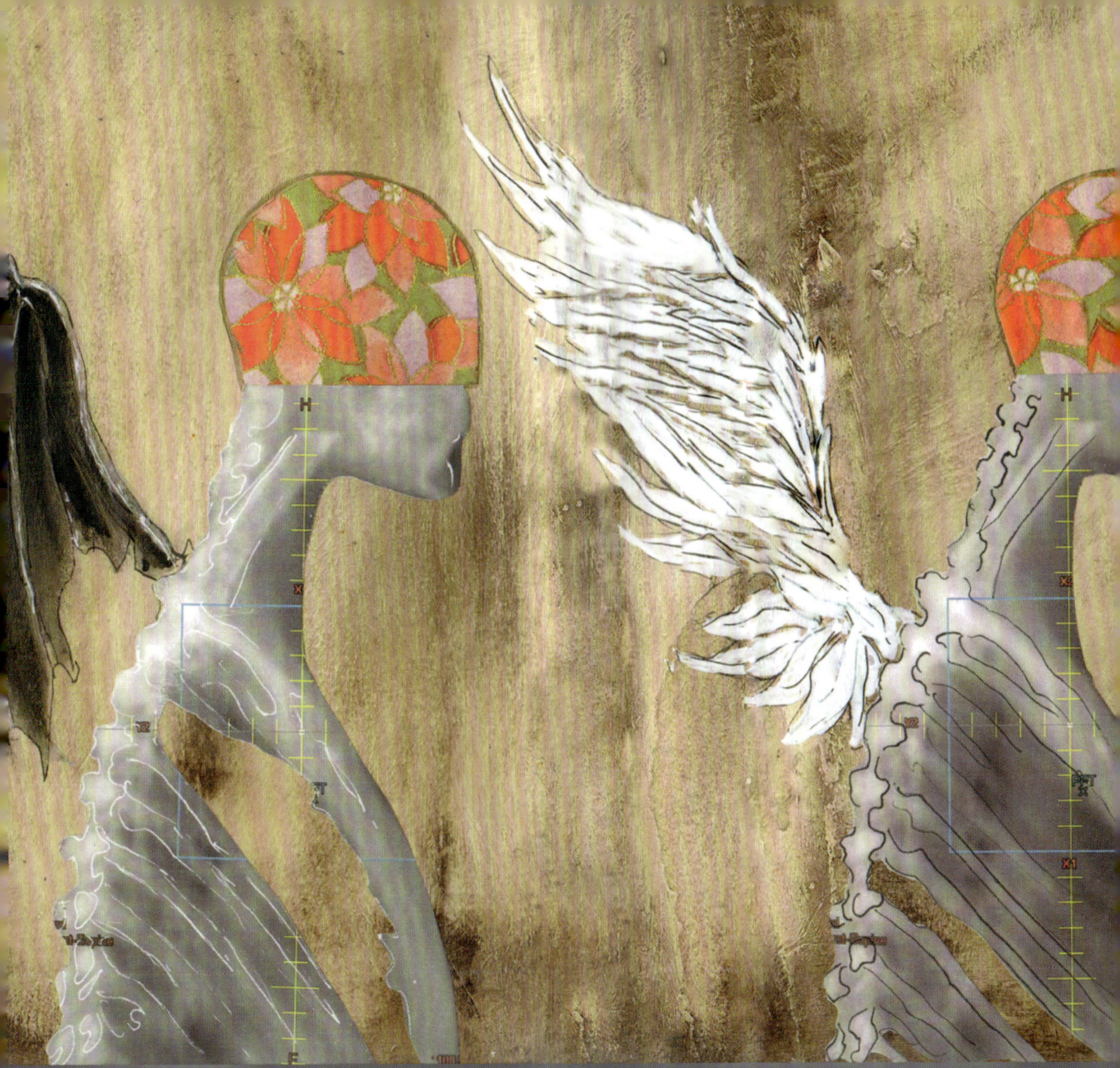

At least the results are good. The liver anomaly proves to be a hemangioma: a benign mass, present in about 20% of the population, not normally discovered unless there is a search for something else. Oddly, it is very rare in people who do drink heavily. After years of worrying about friends who consume a much higher amount of alcohol than I do, I'm the one who ends up with the liver growth. The irony is not lost on me and I circulate an email telling everyone to drink as much as they want.

I want it all to stop: no more ripping pieces out of me, no more shooting me up with radioactive dye, no more x-rays. Already I am convinced I glow slightly in the dark. If this continues I may no longer require a night light.

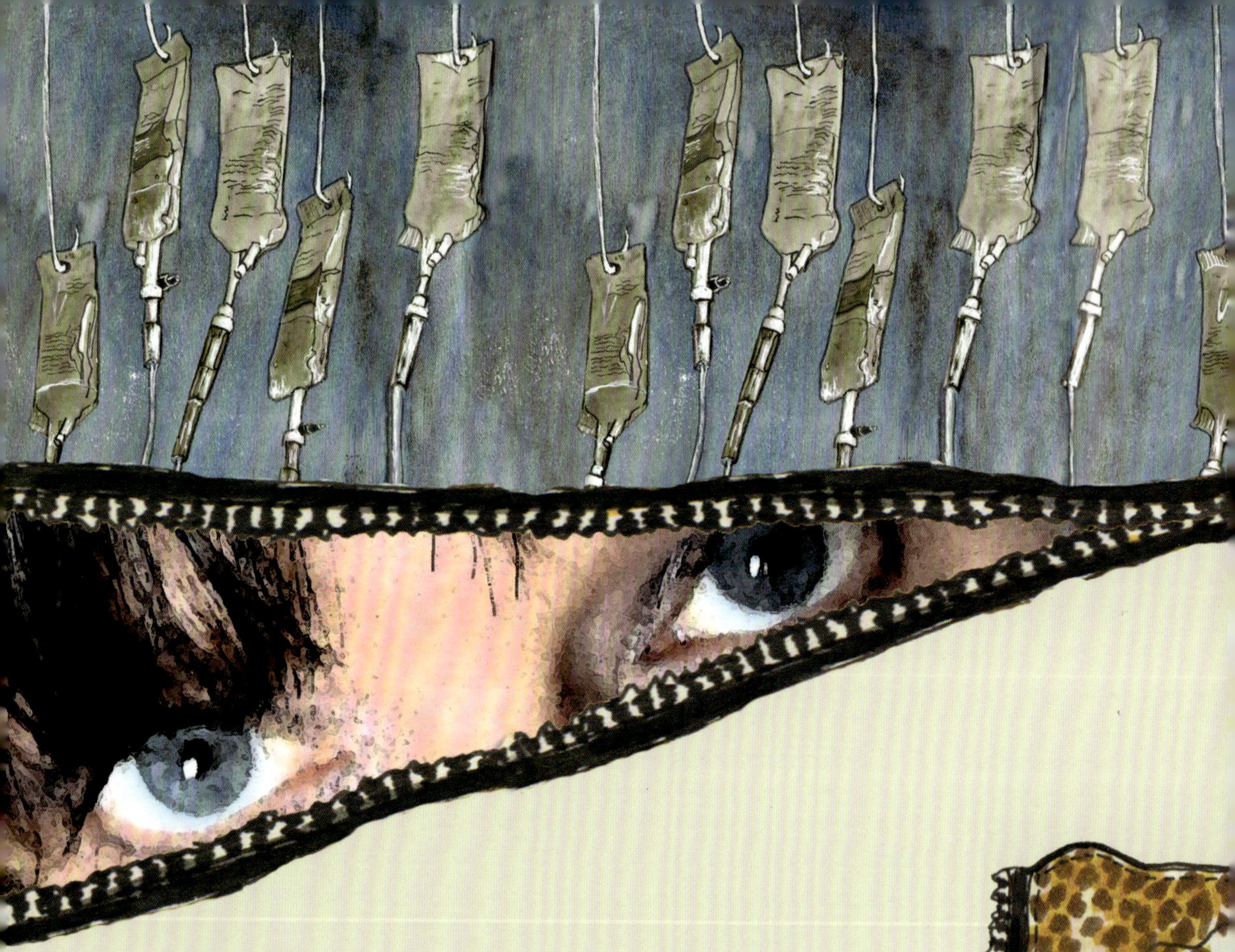

I return to the surgical day ward and following the previous advice ask for my IV to be inserted as soon as I get there. No one listens and a couple of hours pass while I dehydrate. I suggest they heat up blankets to wrap around my arm. That doesn't happen either. The result: the nurse tries three times with increasing frustration to get a needle into my recalcitrant veins. Finally, she wraps a warm blanket round my arm and a second nurse takes over with the same result. There is a conference. Maybe they are drawing straws. They decide to leave it to the surgeon and I am sent once again to pre-op, Doug in tow.

The anesthesiologist is extremely unhappy with me. "Why don't you have an IV?" Like I had a choice and opted against it. In the OR, the nurse says, "Wait a minute. You were just here. I remember your eyes." Is it possible for me to have a punch card so the next one is free? I ask. She laughs. "Do you know what you are doing here?" I am tempted to say, You mean you don't? Along with my name and my birth date, now I have to tell you what to do? Instead, I inform her I am in for a second surgery to remove more tissue from around the site of the tumour. She appears satisfied. I am not entirely comfortable with drifting off this time.

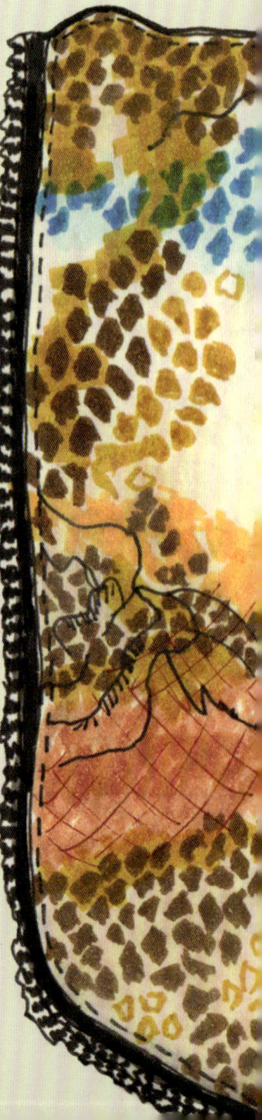

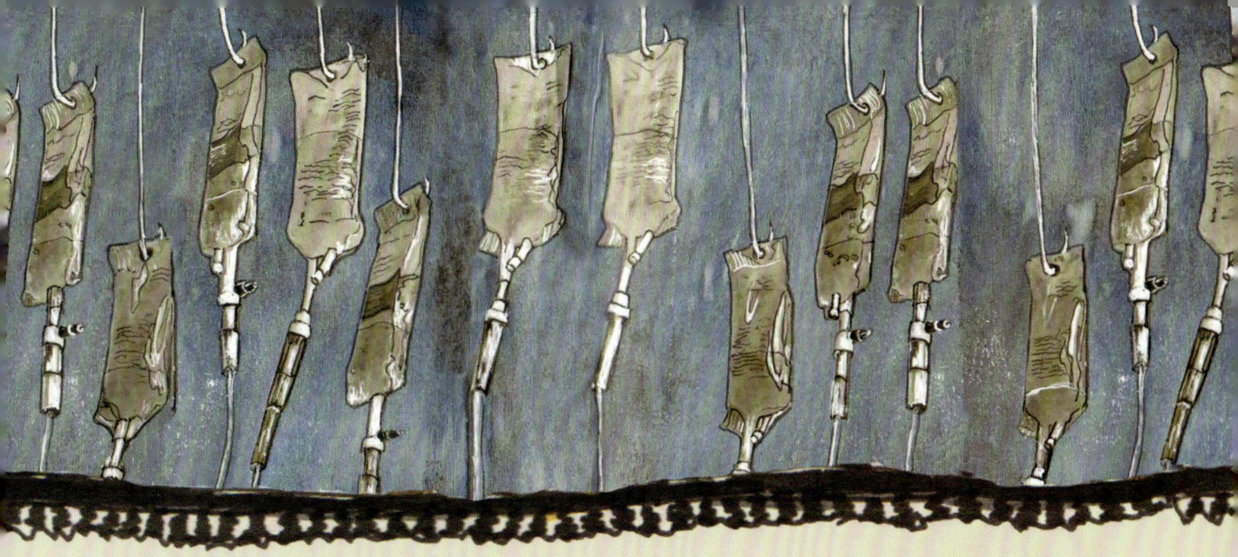

I wake up in the day room again. The nurse comes around with morphine telling me sternly it would be in my best interest to take it. This is the second surgery in a few weeks and it will hurt more. Because I am out of energy I relent. When I am released after a few hours I dress slowly, like I'm swimming through soup. I seem to have misplaced my socks. I wonder if someone has taken them but that seems unlikely since they were tucked into an expensive pair of Italian leather boots.

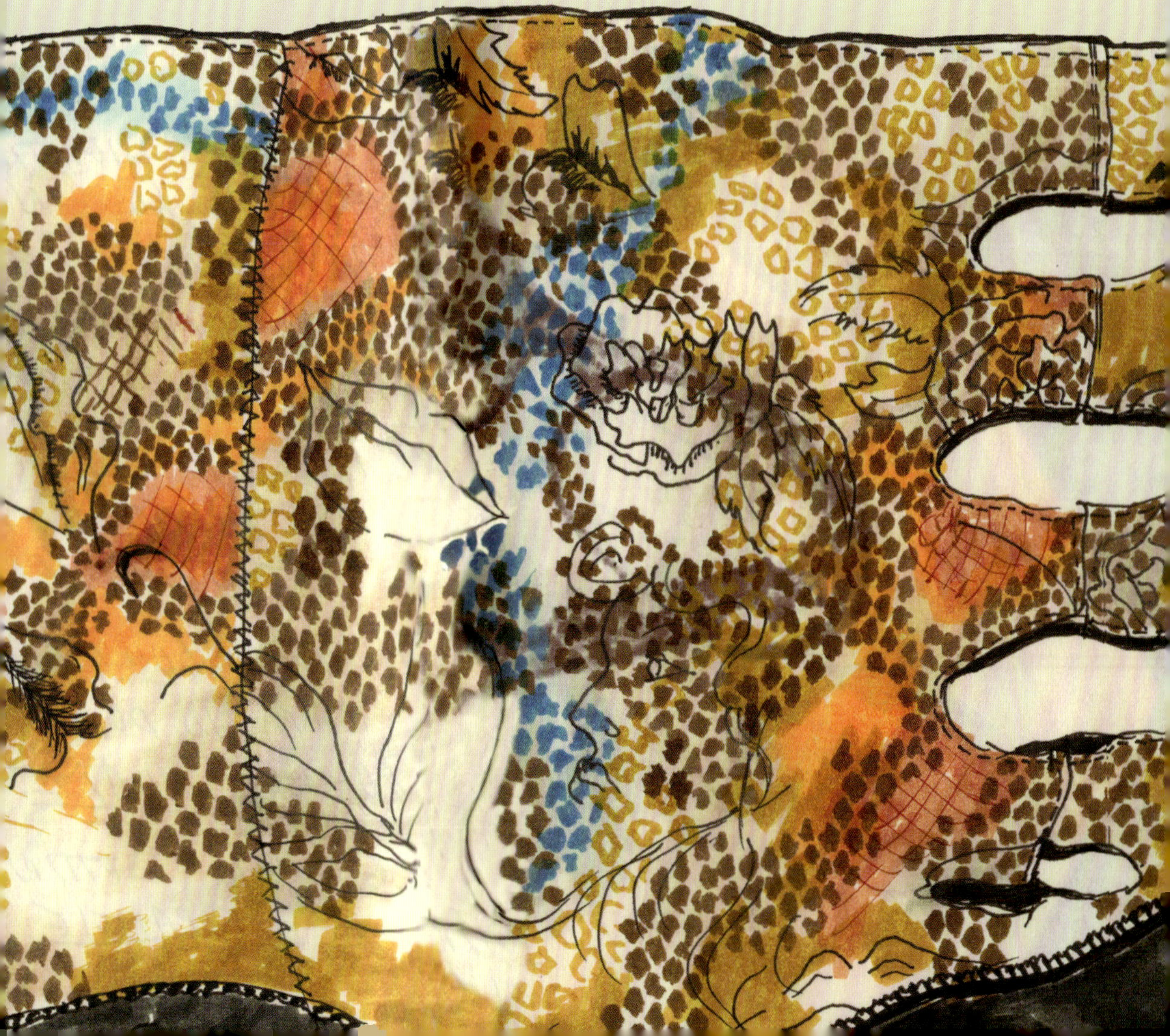

Perhaps I forgot to wear the socks.

Still, as I slide my bare feet into my boots I can't shake the vision of my socks being used on the ward for an after hours puppet show. At least they have gone to good use.

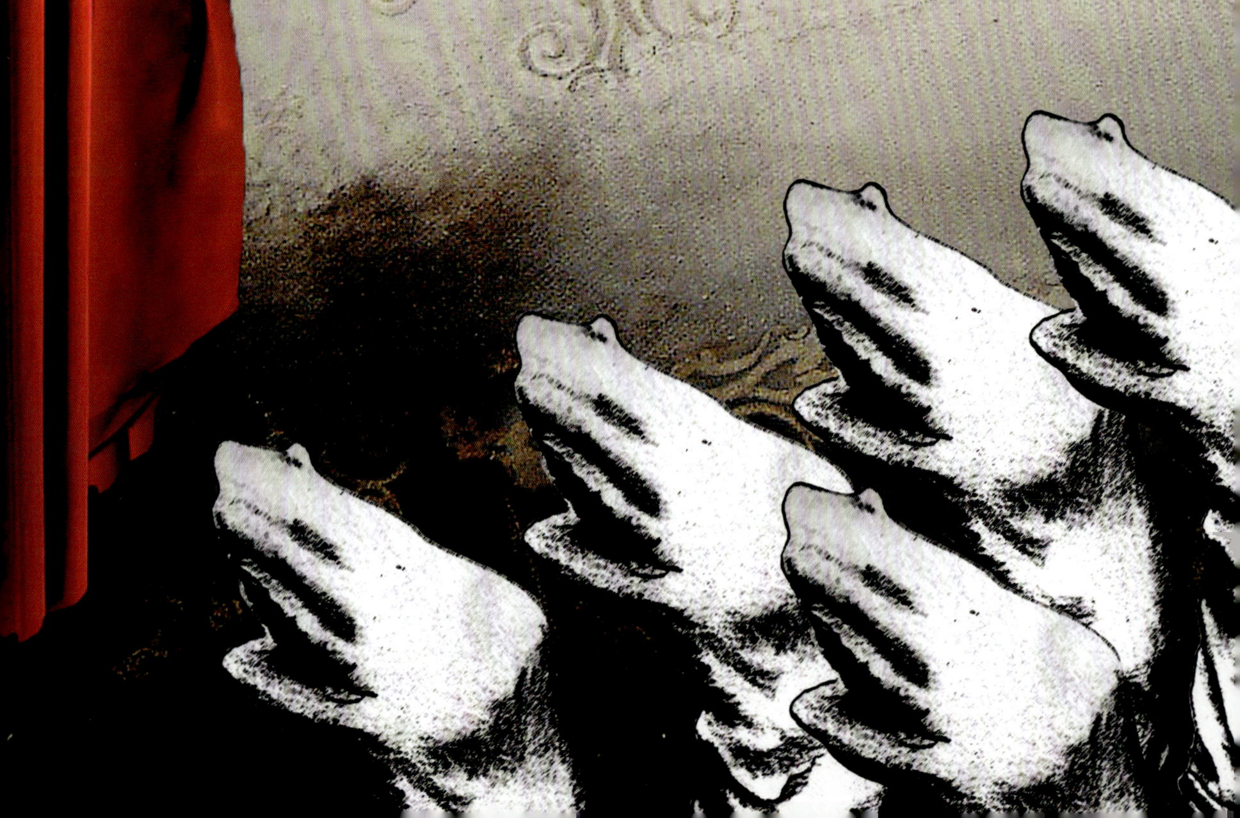

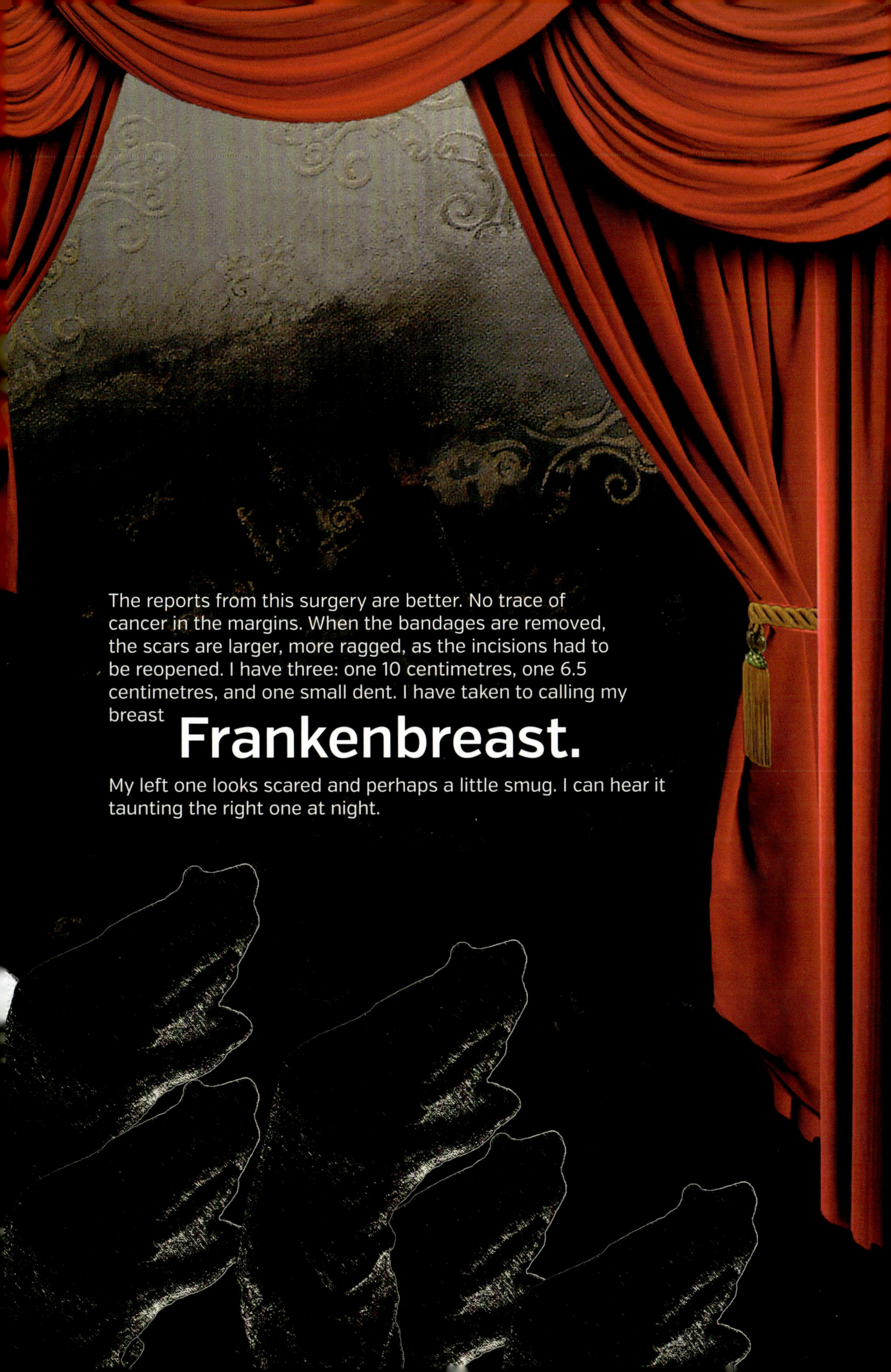

The reports from this surgery are better. No trace of cancer in the margins. When the bandages are removed, the scars are larger, more ragged, as the incisions had to be reopened. I have three: one 10 centimetres, one 6.5 centimetres, and one small dent. I have taken to calling my breast

Frankenbreast.

My left one looks scared and perhaps a little smug. I can hear it taunting the right one at night.

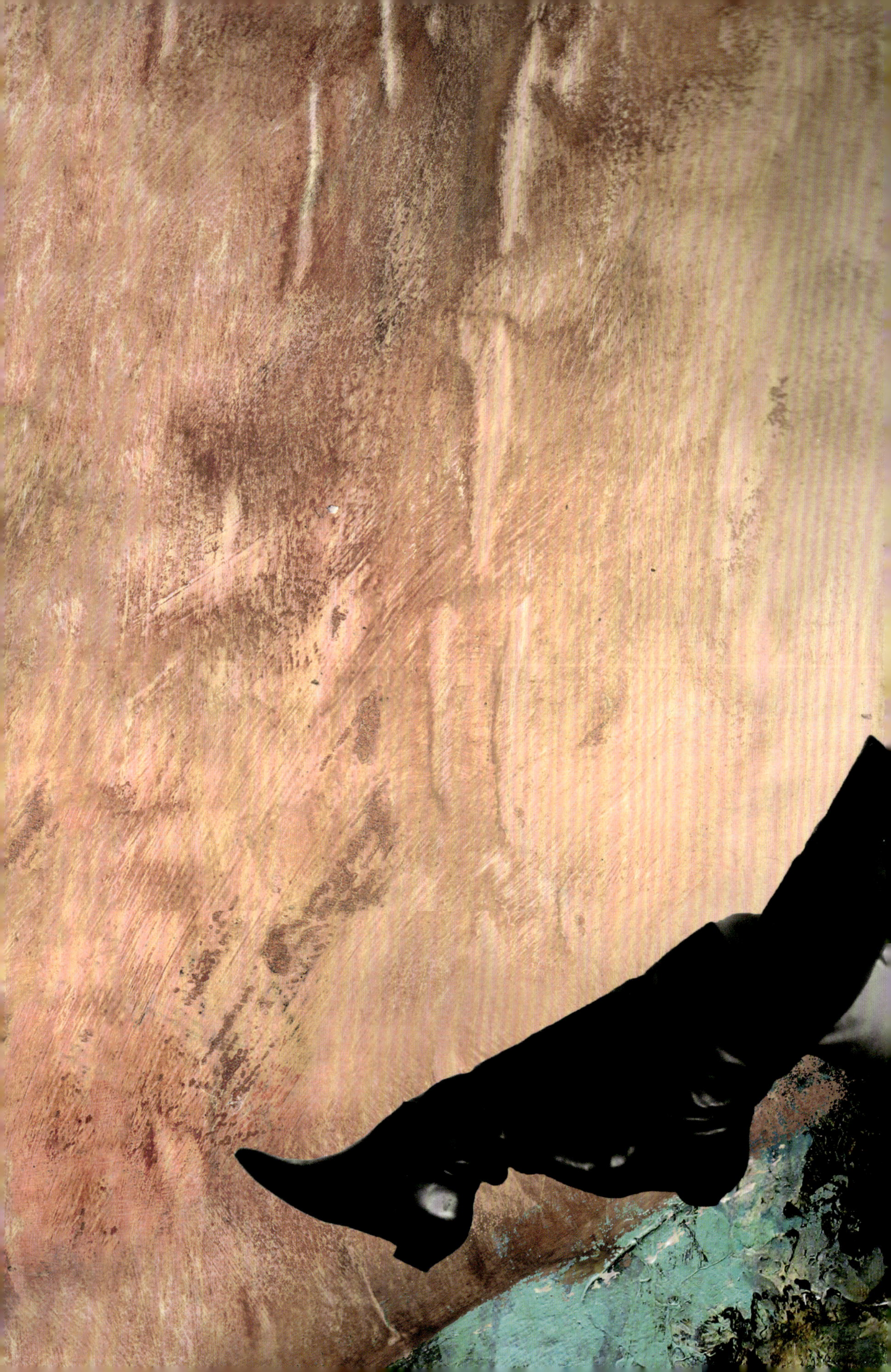

interlude

On my return home I call the Cancer Centre. Given the length of time it took to book previous appointments I am nervous about the expediency of treatment locally and ask to be sent to a larger location. They set up an appointment with an oncologist in Calgary. But when I call, the assistant treats me as though I haven't even considered the difficulties of having my treatment away from home. One of the things you notice when you get cancer is that people treat you like a child. Yes I know their centre is several hours from my home. Yes treatment will go on for months. Yes it would be more comfortable to be in my own bed. But who is she to assume that I won't have arranged for a place to live? Resources? A support circle? In the end my appointments with both an oncologist and a radiation oncologist are set for November. I also make one with a homeopath.

For the next six weeks I am in a little cocoon – hoping to emerge shortly as a butterfly, far more apt to become a large night flying moth. I continue walking. I faithfully perform my physiotherapy exercises according to the sheet provided by the operation prep team at the hospital. I am surprised by the level of difficulty and pain as I attempt to regain a full range of motion in my arm. I restart my belly dance classes and execute movements with only one arm. The result is awkward and graceless. Still, it is motion and it is healthy for me. Emotionally. Physically.

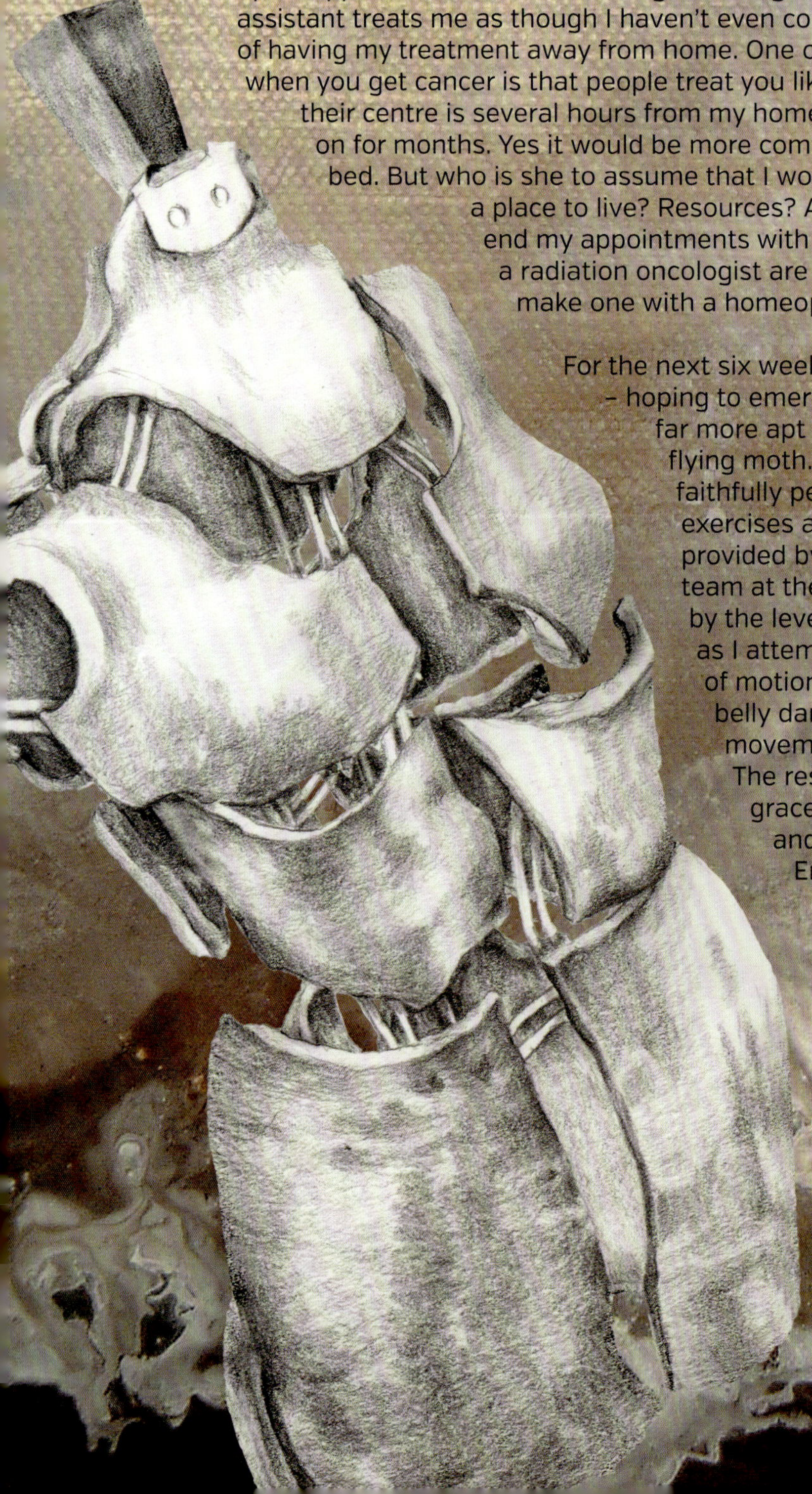

I notice a tendency to hunch forward when I am in public as if protecting my right breast from further harm. Sleep is a challenge. I am a side sleeper and both sides are painful for me. I lie on my back and stare at the ceiling. Count sheep. I can't decide if I wake at 4:00 in the morning because I am worried or if being uncomfortable wakes me and so I might as well worry. As my friend Marjan says with her typical Dutch shrug, "Six of these, six of those." What she means, of course, is "six of one and half dozen of another" but I prefer her version.

More poetic

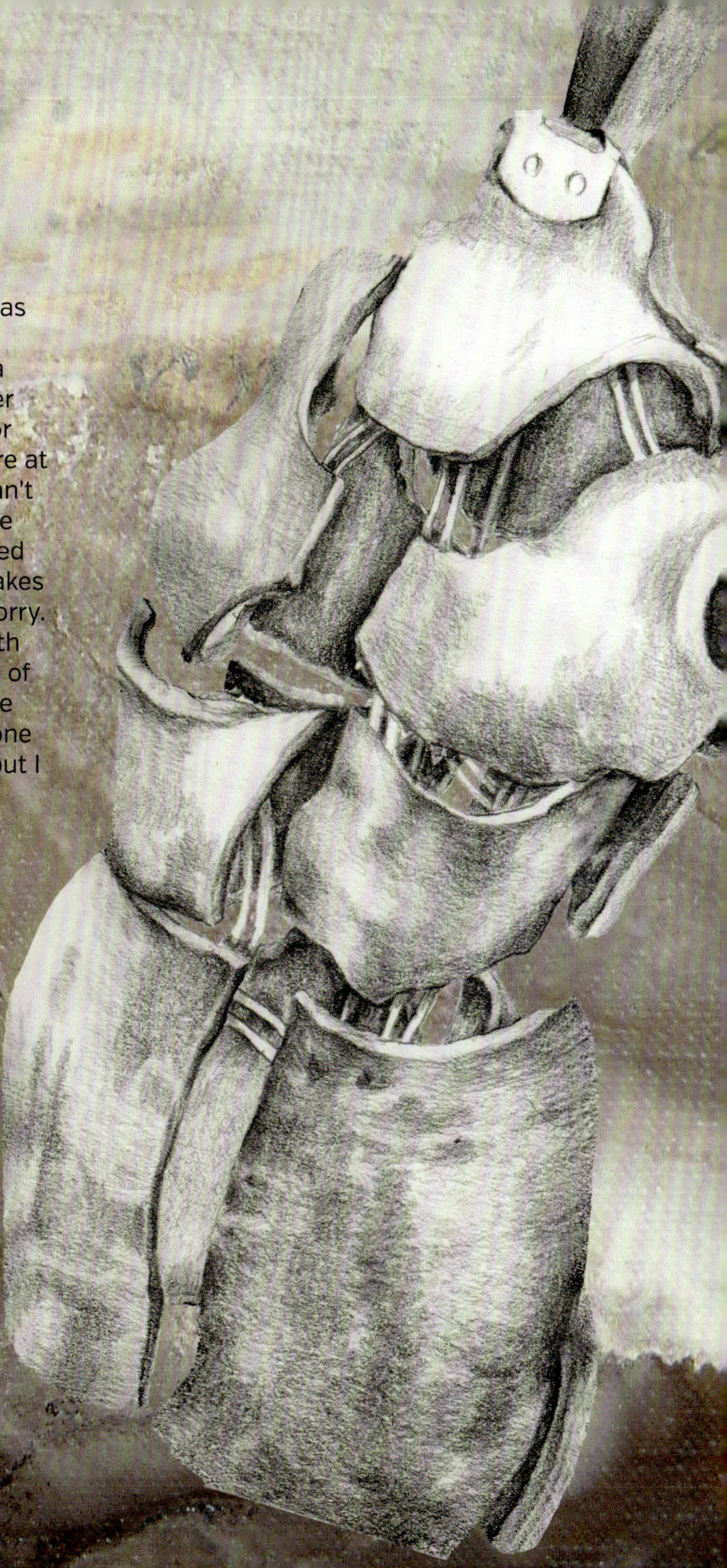

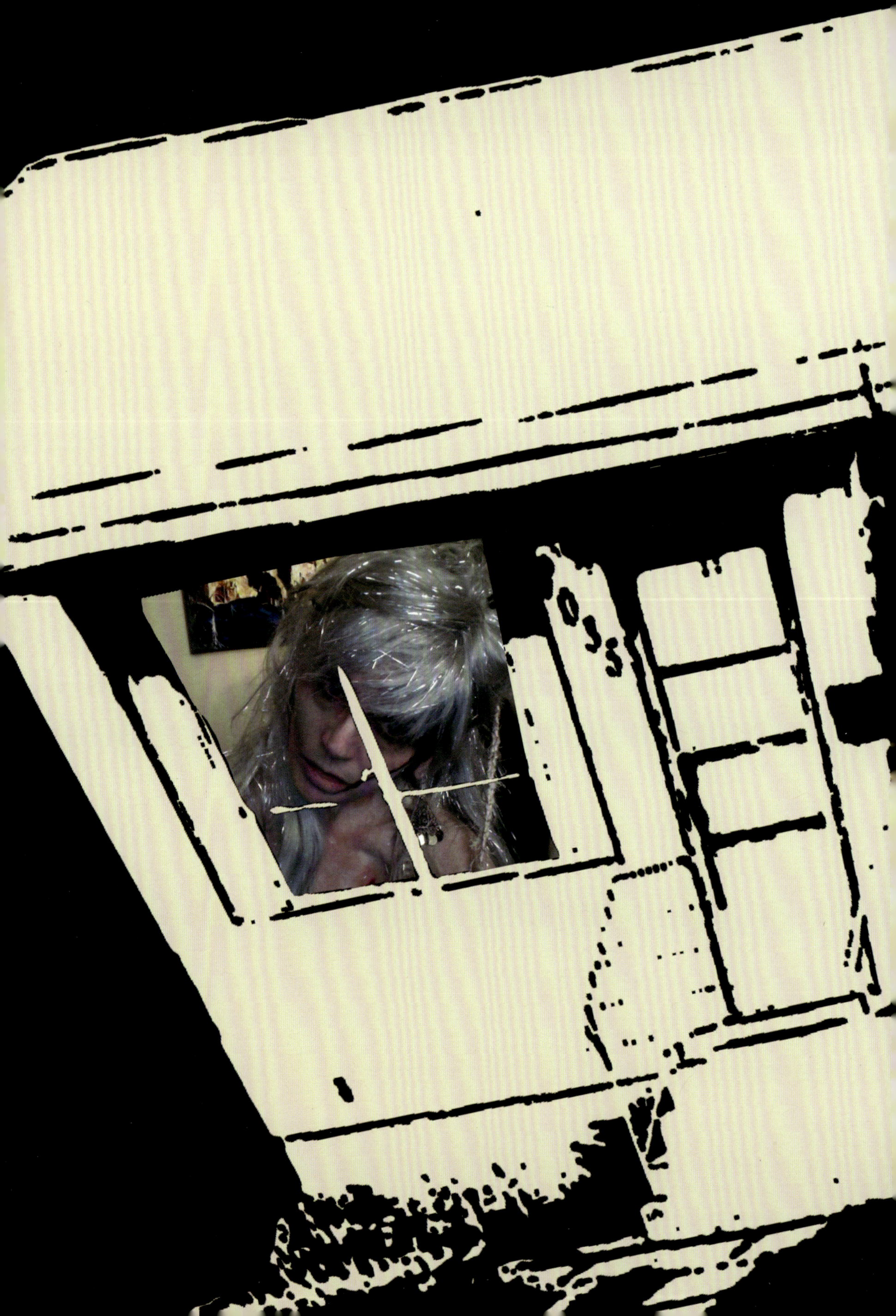

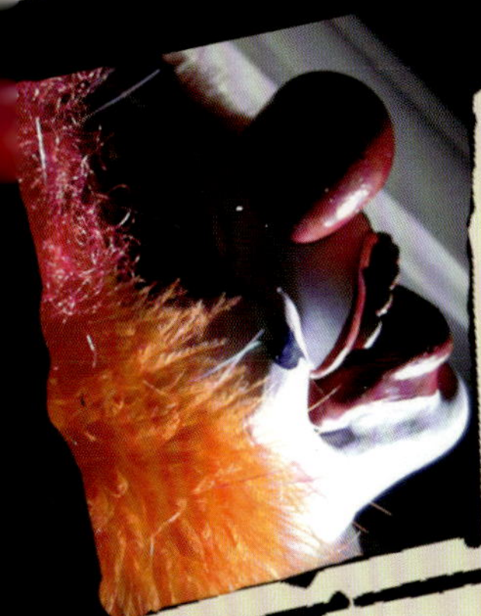

Halloween arrives. I dress up as a zombie belly dancer, place temporary tattoos of huge scars all over my chest in tongue-in-cheek homage to my newly scarred body. I hang a sign around my neck that says "Will dance for brains." Doug dons a terrifying clown mask. He stands in the darkened window of the spare room with a flashlight which he turns on when anyone walks up to the house. We blast "The Monster Mash" and "Spooky" on the stereo. Laughter is healing. The next day I rearrange the spice drawer. I am less sure of the healing benefits of cleaning.

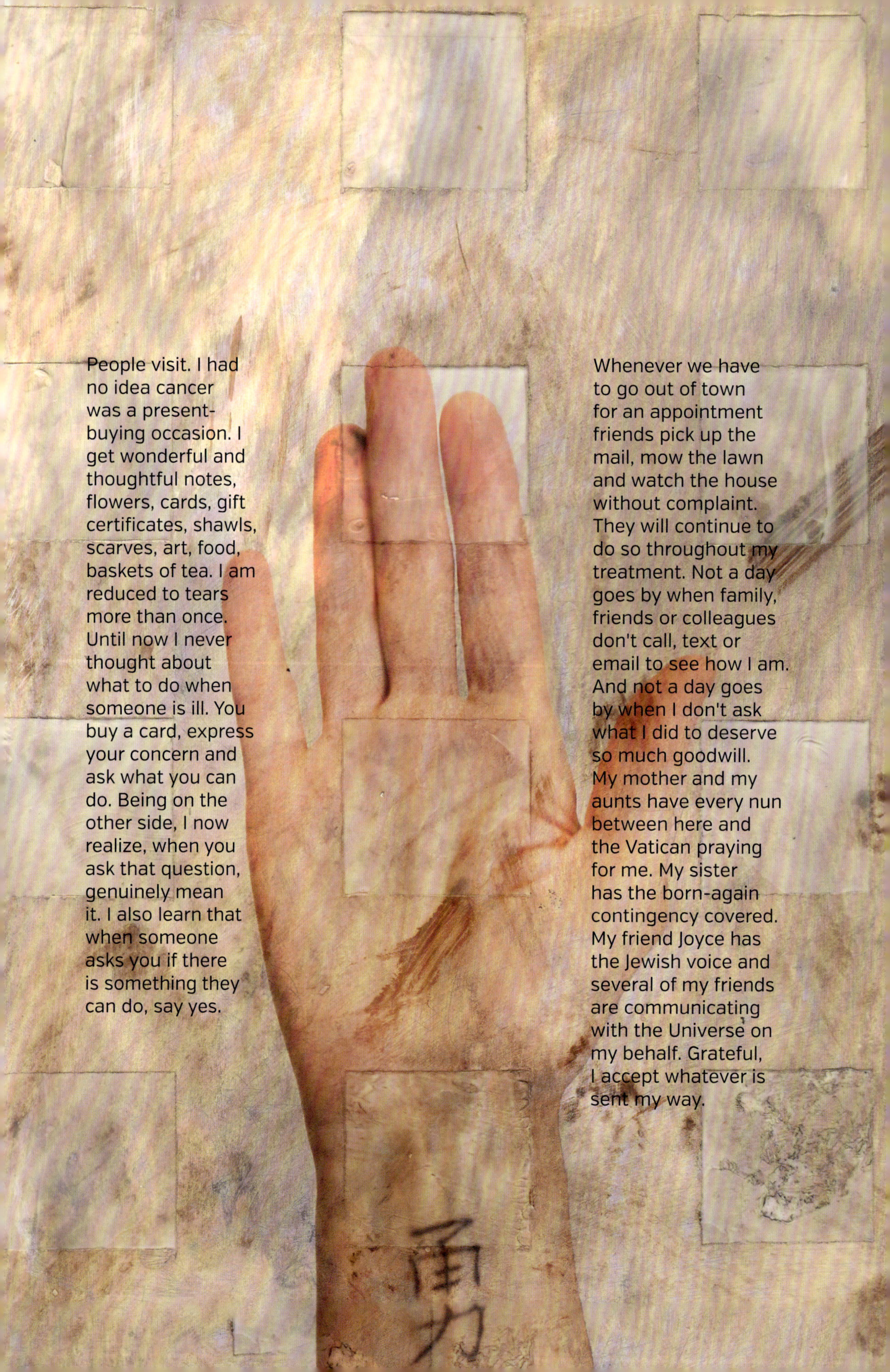

People visit. I had no idea cancer was a present-buying occasion. I get wonderful and thoughtful notes, flowers, cards, gift certificates, shawls, scarves, art, food, baskets of tea. I am reduced to tears more than once. Until now I never thought about what to do when someone is ill. You buy a card, express your concern and ask what you can do. Being on the other side, I now realize, when you ask that question, genuinely mean it. I also learn that when someone asks you if there is something they can do, say yes.

Whenever we have to go out of town for an appointment friends pick up the mail, mow the lawn and watch the house without complaint. They will continue to do so throughout my treatment. Not a day goes by when family, friends or colleagues don't call, text or email to see how I am. And not a day goes by when I don't ask what I did to deserve so much goodwill. My mother and my aunts have every nun between here and the Vatican praying for me. My sister has the born-again contingency covered. My friend Joyce has the Jewish voice and several of my friends are communicating with the Universe on my behalf. Grateful, I accept whatever is sent my way.

I decide to get a tattoo that reflects this fight but since tattooing is frowned on with my soon-to-be compromised immune system I settle for buying temporary ones. I find a design online that claims to be the Chinese symbol for courage. The minimum order is 500, more than I will ever need. After making sure the design doesn't mean "You stupid white girl" I order 1000. I take to applying it in a variety of places: the back of my neck, my arm, most frequently on the inside of my right wrist. And on Doug's. I hope it will remind us both in the coming months to endeavour to be brave.

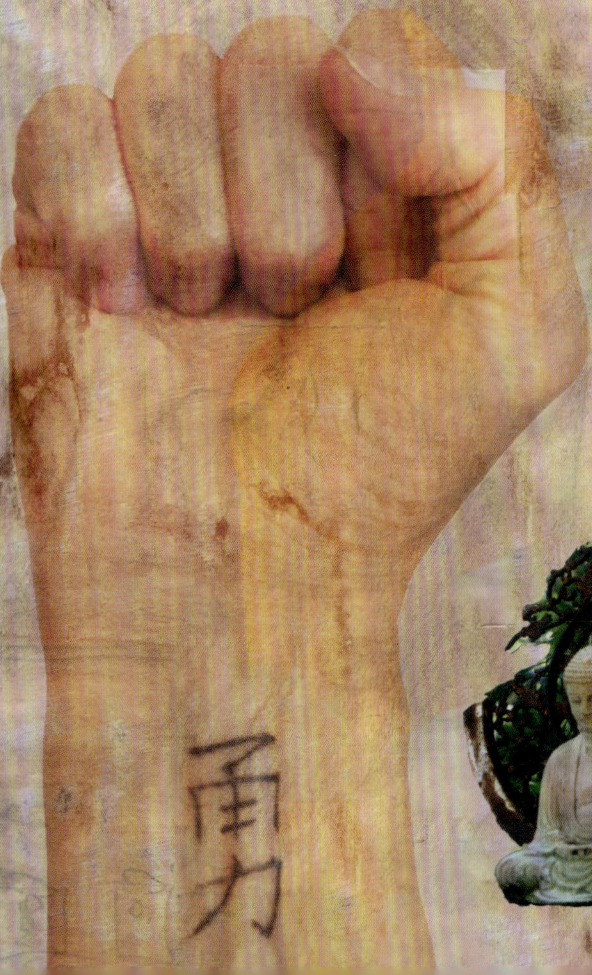

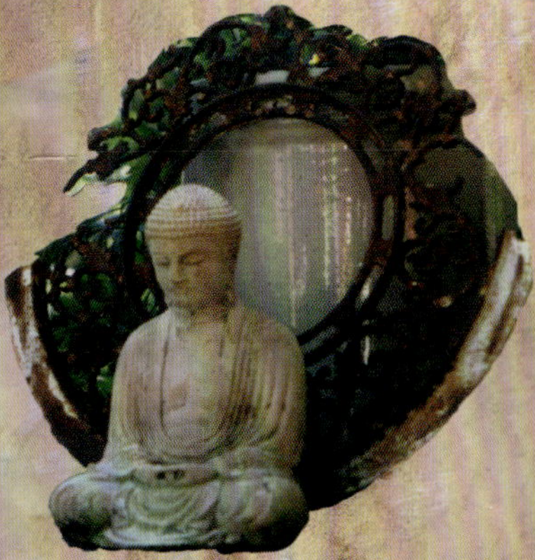

On the web I continue to find useful bits and pieces: Hats. Head scarves. Eyebrows that can be glued on. I am convinced I will not need them; I am equally determined to be the most well-prepared cancer patient ever. When the eyebrows arrive they seem a little pathetic in their box. Marginalized. I shove them in a drawer ... at the back. Why do they seem more disturbing than the fake eyelashes?

I discover that the long-term benefits I was counting on to see me through this challenge financially are nowhere near adequate. What is available to me through my workplace can only be described as paltry. To add insult to injury, if I had only put off my cancer a few more weeks I could have had a new and more lucrative benefit plan. In my initial discussion with Human Resources I was not informed of any of this. I am angry. In addition to everything else I now have extreme monetary worries. The Academic Staff Association, the organization responsible for negotiating our contracts, as well as senior administration all fight for me to no avail.

I spend long hours in the studio painting, a calming occupation for me right now. The work that is developing contains a lot of water imagery which according to some dream interpretations indicates change. What can I say? Things have changed. Immersed in my work I arrive at what should have been an obvious solution. I will have an art sale in my home. I've never done this on a large scale before but I know people always seem fascinated by artists' studios. I am caught up in planning and organizing. It takes my mind off the uncertainties that lie before me which is not easy given the amount of trauma I am coping with. The sale is a huge success. Grateful for the support, I wonder how others who don't have these options manage.

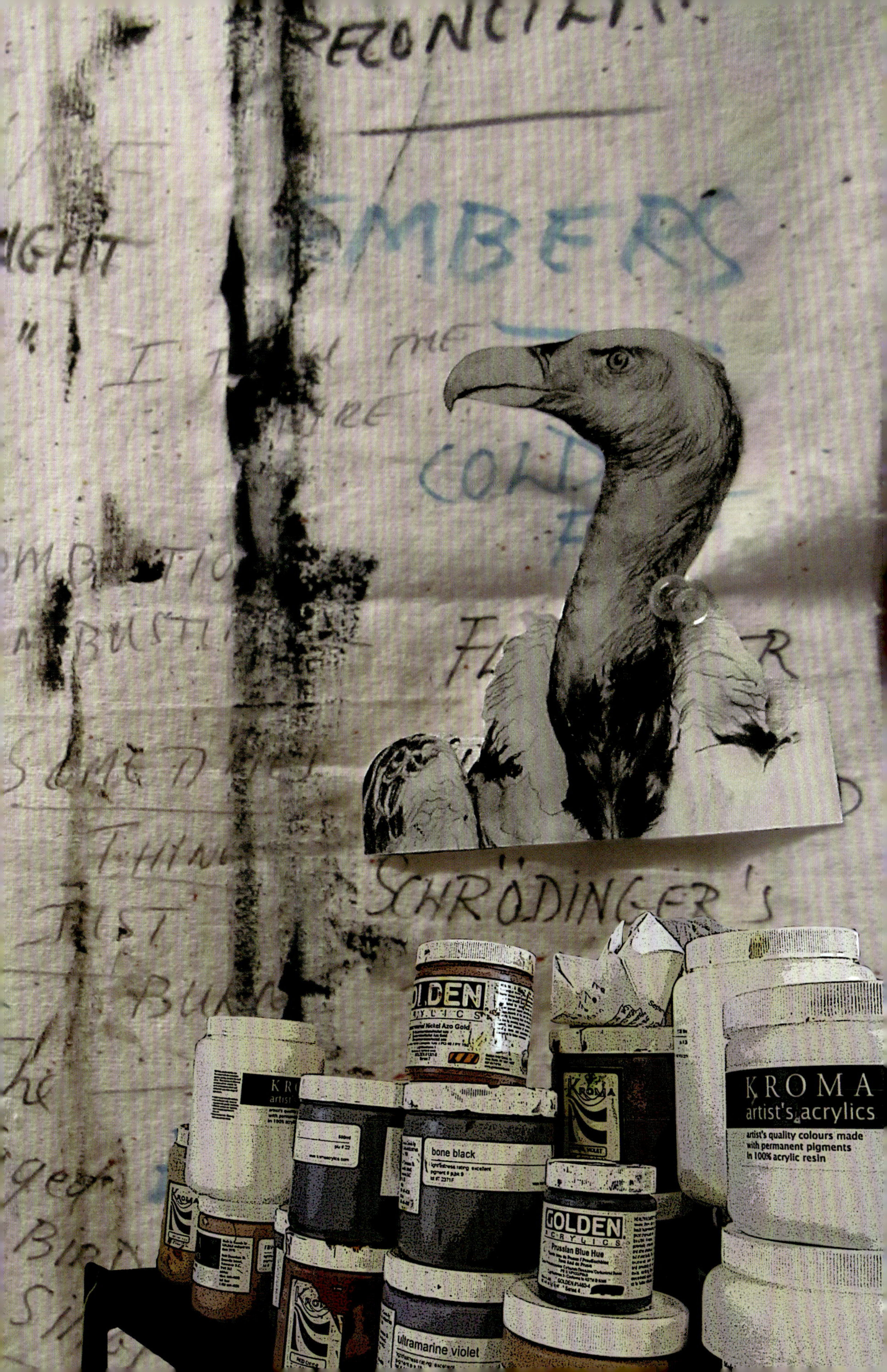
EMBERS
SCHRÖDINGER'S
GOLDEN
KROMA
artist's acrylics
artist's quality colours made
with permanent pigments
in 100% acrylic resin
bone black
GOLDEN
ACRYLICS
Prussian Blue Hue
ultramarine violet

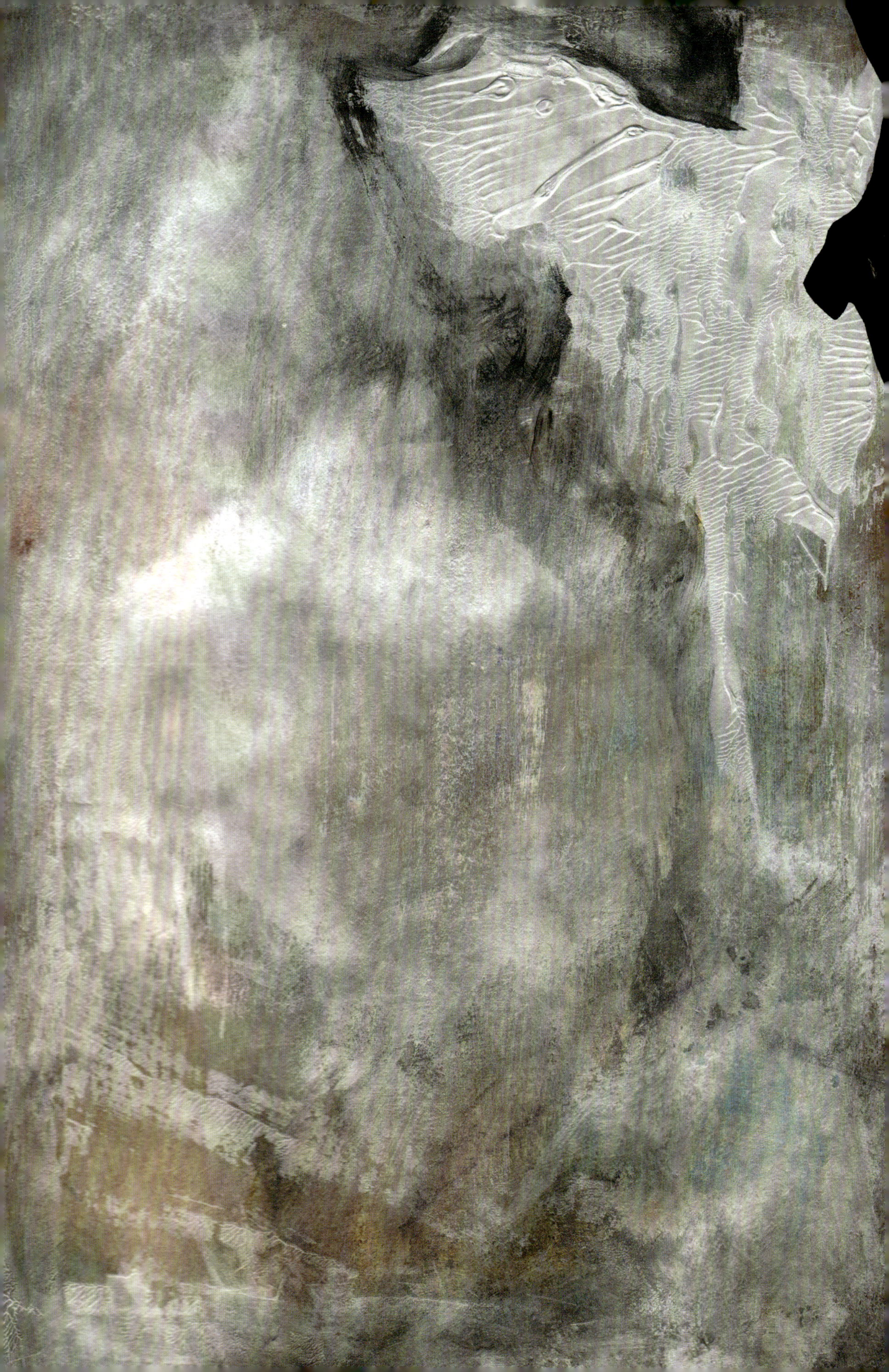

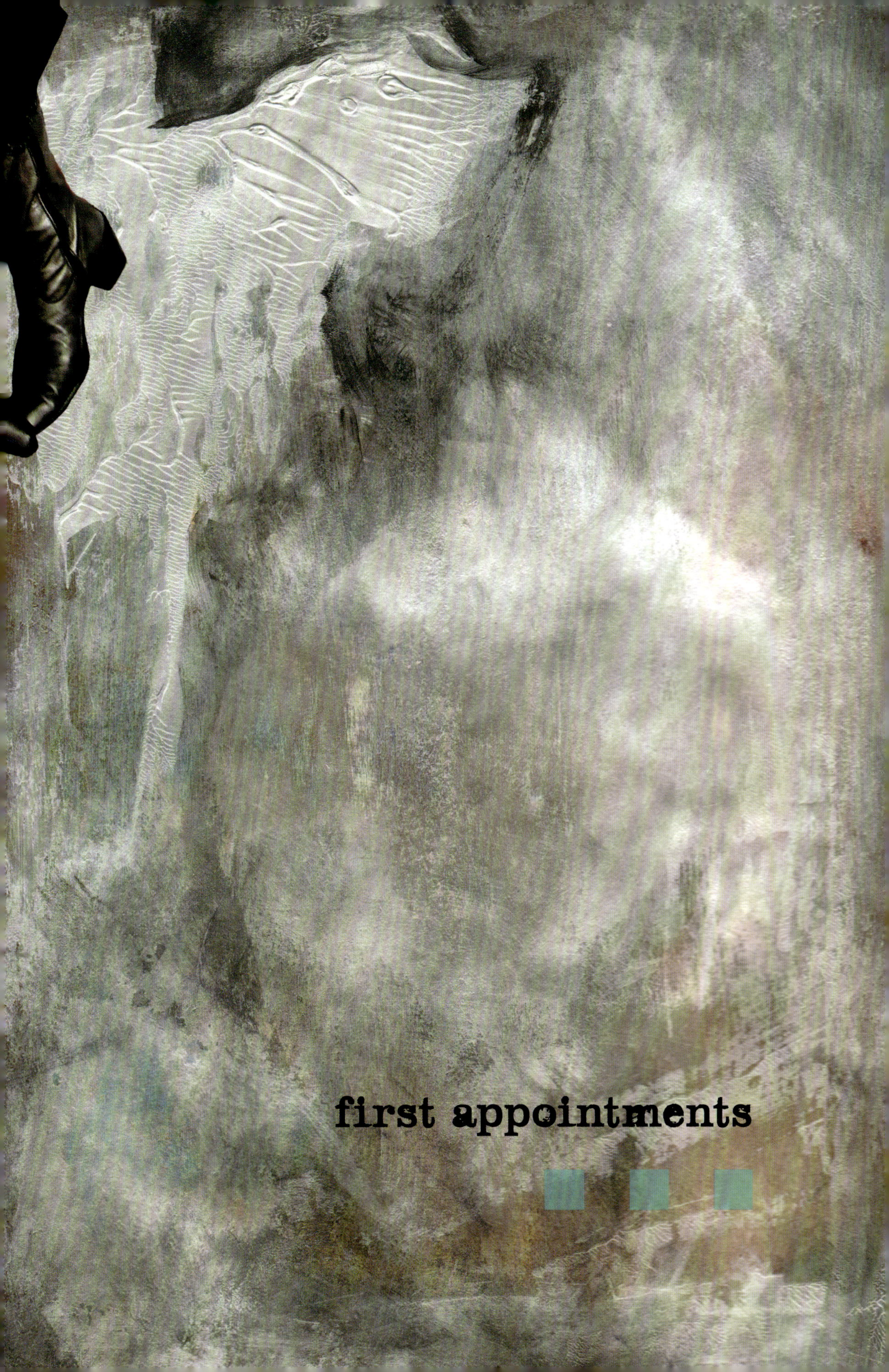

first appointments

My first appointment with the oncologist is a long and gruelling session. Because of the spread of the cancer, Dr. O is recommending everything: chemotherapy, radiation, and hormone therapy. I am impressed with his thoroughness and his kindness, if not excited by the information. He is treating me like a human being and not a widget to be processed. I am flooded with more information than I can possibly absorb in one sitting. Doug takes notes. He will continue to do so throughout every appointment.

The protocol Dr. O has decided on is six sessions, spaced three weeks apart, over three and a half months. The first three cycles of treatment will be with

Cyclophosphamide
Epirubicin
and Fluorouracil

also known as 5FU which makes me snicker in a very juvenile way. Then a switch to a drug called Docetaxel for the remaining three cycles. He also wants me to consider Tamoxifen, a common hormone therapy drug that blocks estrogen production. Although I have almost convinced myself to have chemotherapy and radiation, I am skeptical about this drug given all my research. When he tells me it would only increase my chance of survival 3% to 6%,I draw a line in the sand that for now he skirts.

He asks what I know about relative and absolute statistics and I give him the five-minute washing machine analogy that I found on cancer.org. You buy a new washing machine and have a 10% chance of needing service in the first year. If you use bleach the risk of needing service in the first year increases by 5% to 15%. The 5% increase from 10% to 15% is considered an absolute risk. The same risk increase from 10% to 15% is a 50% increase in terms of relative risk. Drug companies, doctors, and most of the medical profession deliver statistics in terms of relative risk. Dr. O doesn't. Yet one more reason to trust him. That and his laugh.

He cites a list of potential side effects: nausea, fatigue, low white blood cells ... Each side effect appears to have a drug to manage it. I suspect there is one for everything but death and who knows, maybe someone is at work on one now. Dr. O warns me there is zero chance of keeping my hair. My eyebrows and eyelashes? He shrugs.

50/50?

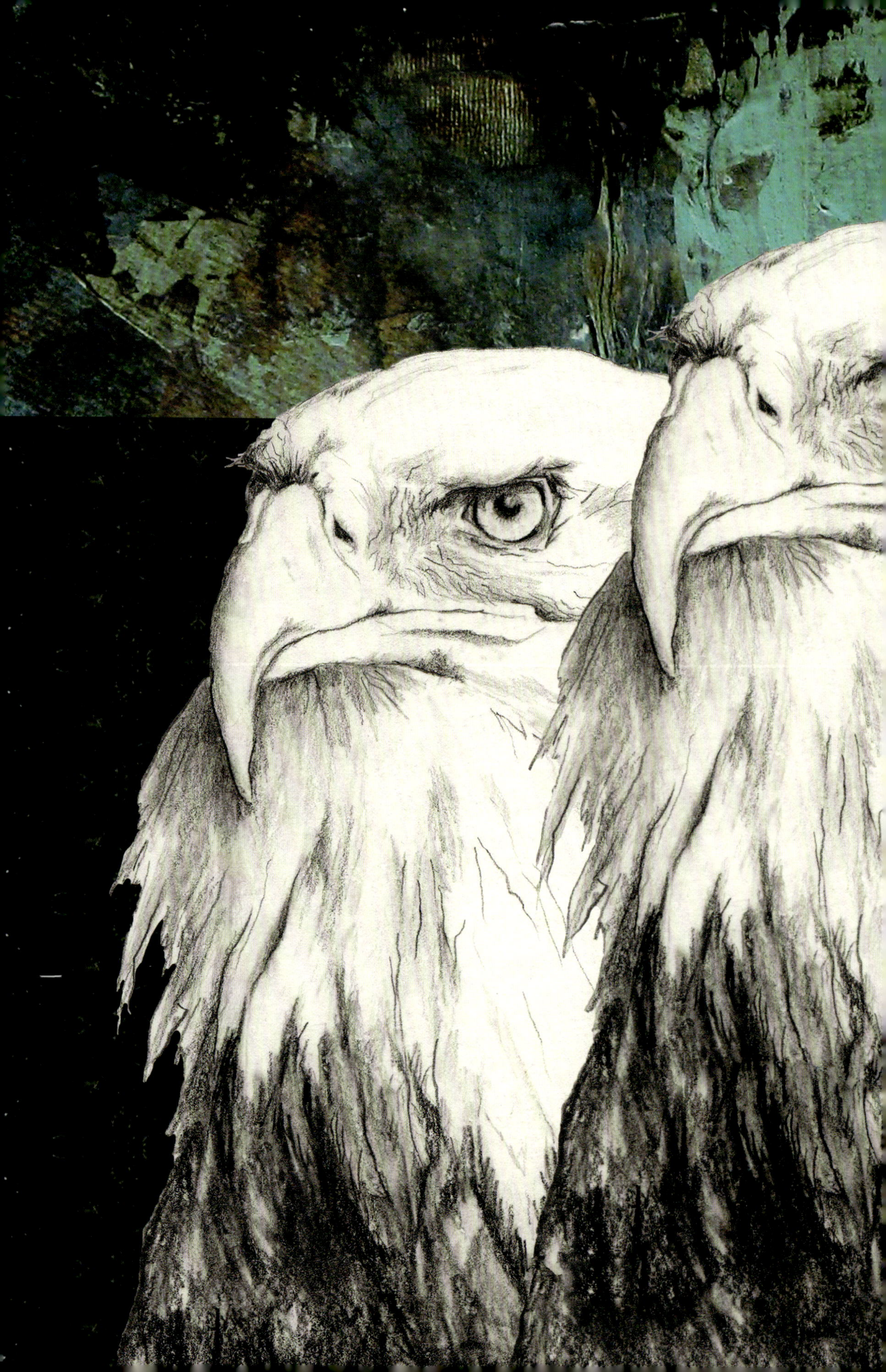

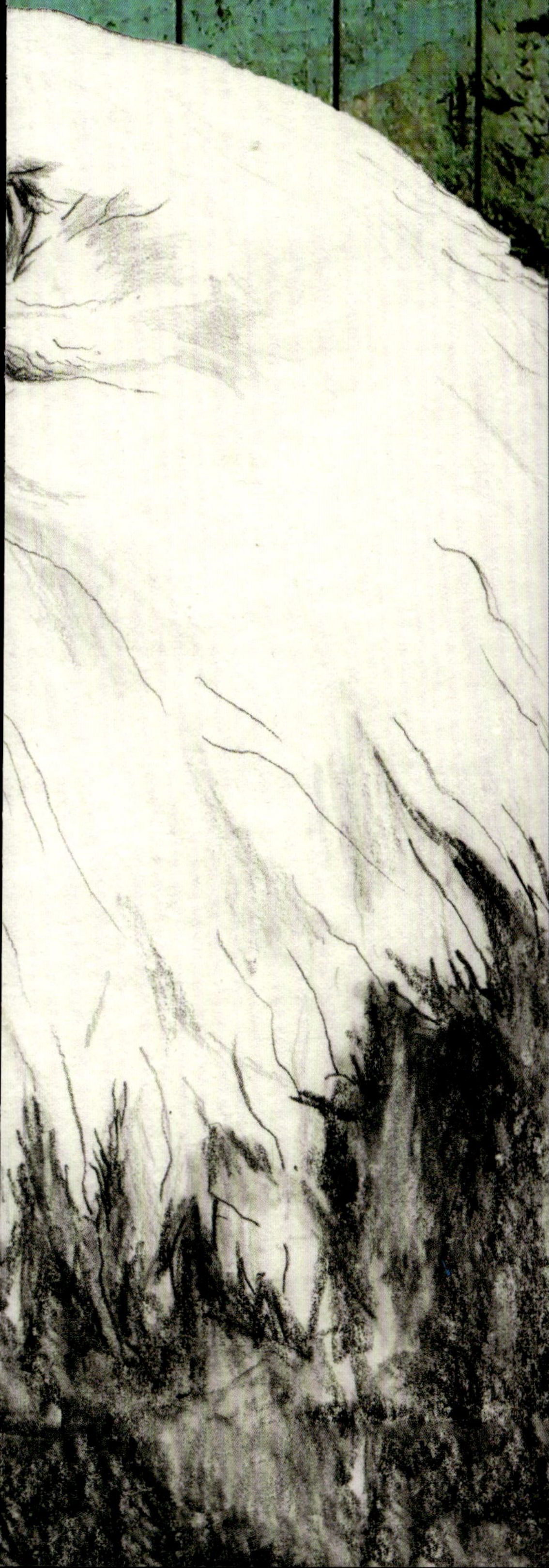

When my mother was faced with the same threat, she bought a wig and waited for her hair to fall out. After several months of chemotherapy she retained a full, impressive head of hair. When I ask if she knows anyone else who did not lose their hair she says "Yes, my friend Madeline's uncle." Really? What happened? Mom looks me in the eye and quips, "He died." We are practically rolling on the floor with laughter. Just as we did the time we went to pick up quilting to stuff her bra until she could get a prosthesis. We could only find a massive half-metre-long-bag. Although my mother is far better endowed than I, this amount was still excessive. At the counter the clerk asked us what we were making. Neither of us could choke out an answer.

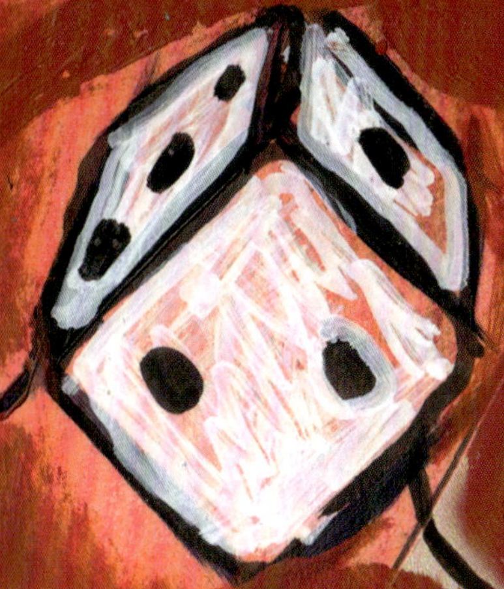

I tell Dr. O I plan to seek alternative care in addition to the traditional treatment he recommends. He is not particularly pleased but we come to an agreement. I will level with him about what the homeopath is doing and if he can honestly, without prejudice, tell me it is dangerous to my health, I will stop. Otherwise, we agree to disagree. I am booked to start my treatments mid-December.

There is a test called the Oncotype DX that determines the probable success of the chemotherapy regime for your particular genetic type based on your tumour's tissue sample, with a 99% accuracy. Depending on where your numbers fall you can make up your mind whether to put yourself through the rigours of chemo. Unfortunately, there is only one lab in California that carries out the testing. While insurance companies in some provinces routinely pay for the test, I will have to pay myself. I make the decision not to. A decision I will come to regret.

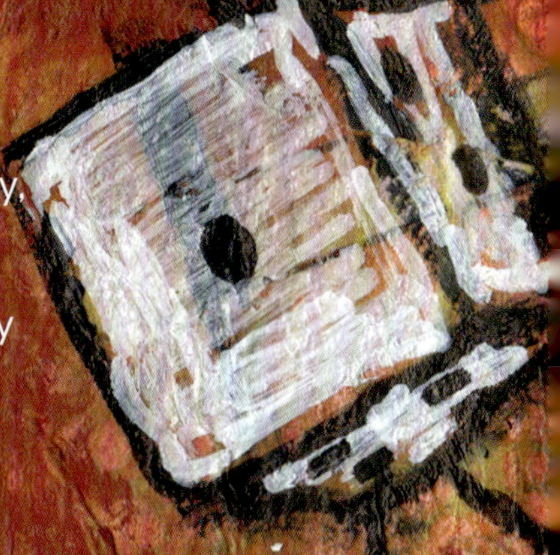

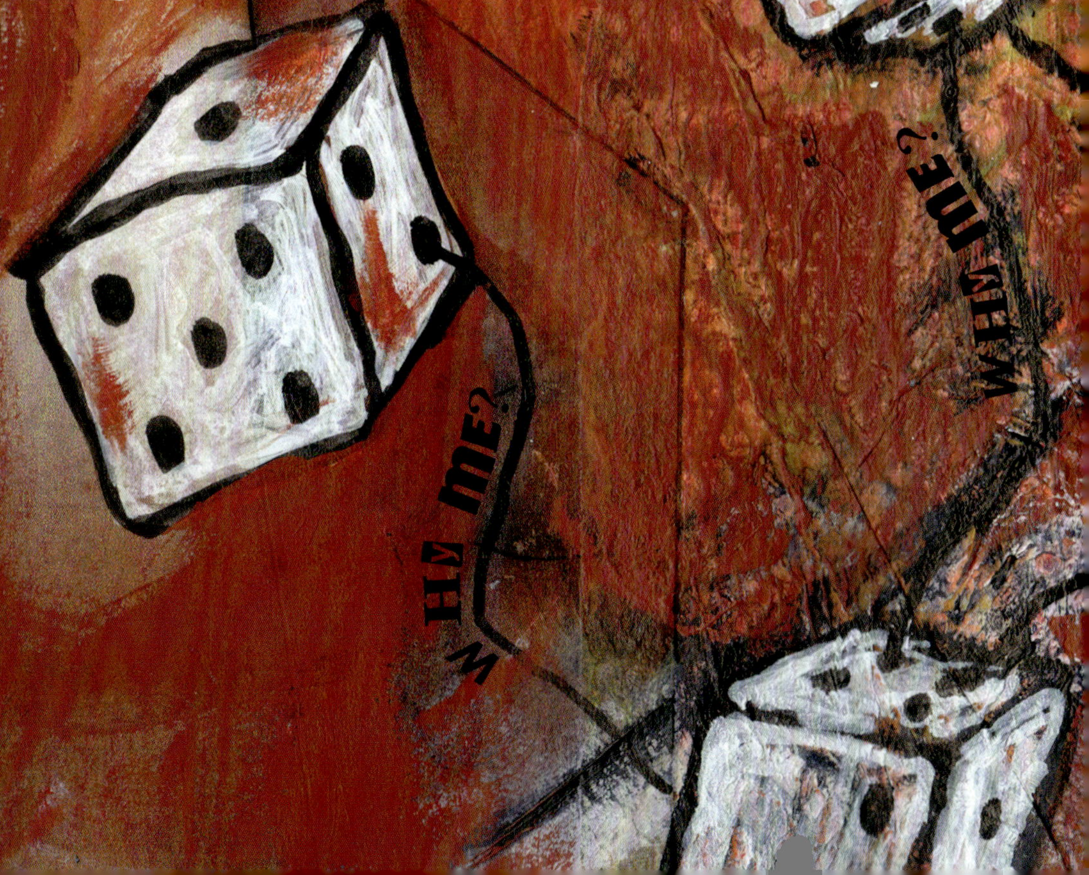

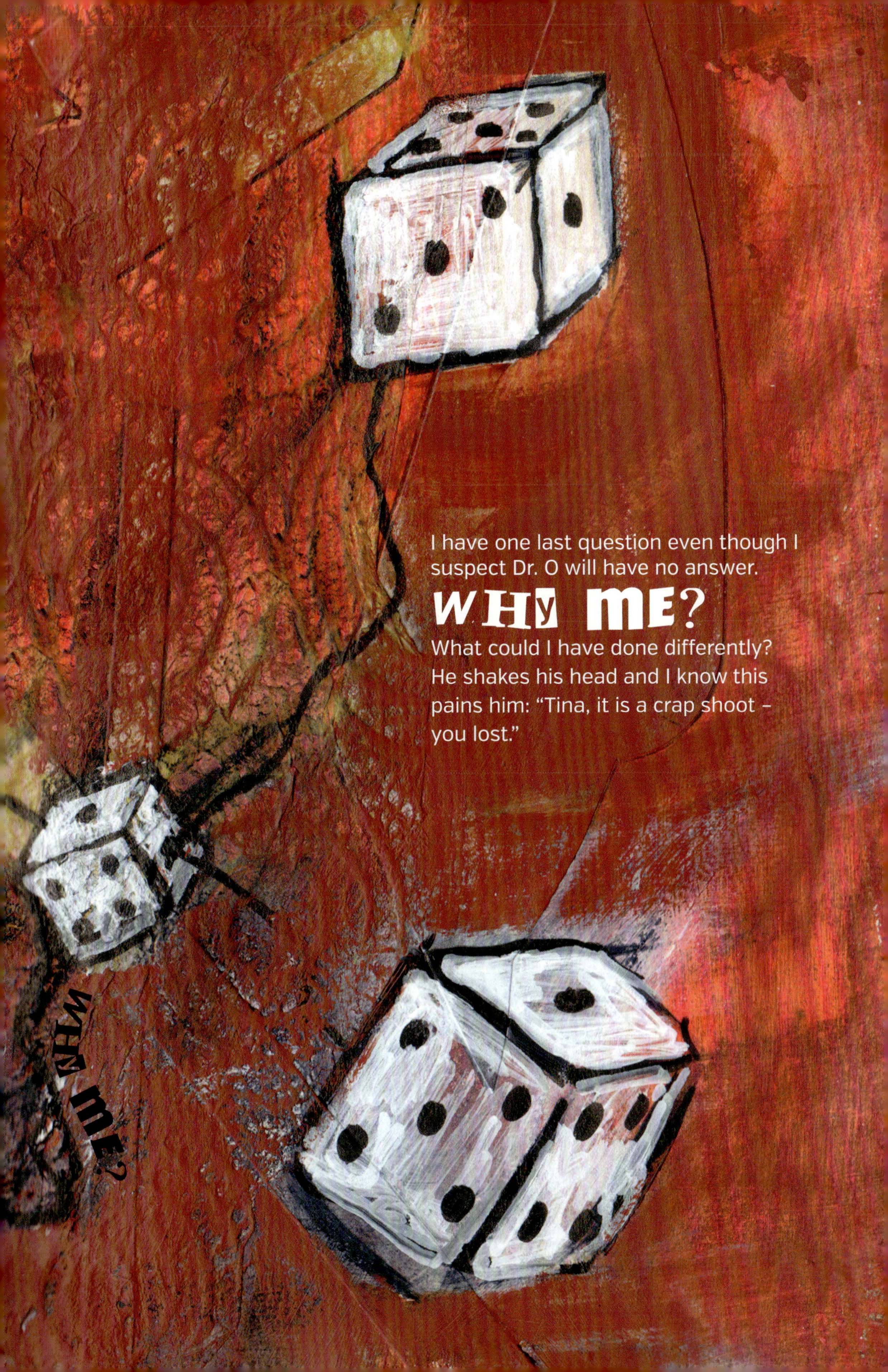

I have one last question even though I suspect Dr. O will have no answer.

WHY ME?

What could I have done differently? He shakes his head and I know this pains him: "Tina, it is a crap shoot – you lost."

My radiation oncologist, Dr. R, is also kind, listens well, understands my fears. She is thorough and inundates me with yet more information. But since radiation is several months away, I revert to my earlier strategy of one thing at a time and decide to focus on the chemotherapy. Dr. R is marginally less skeptical regarding alternative treatment.

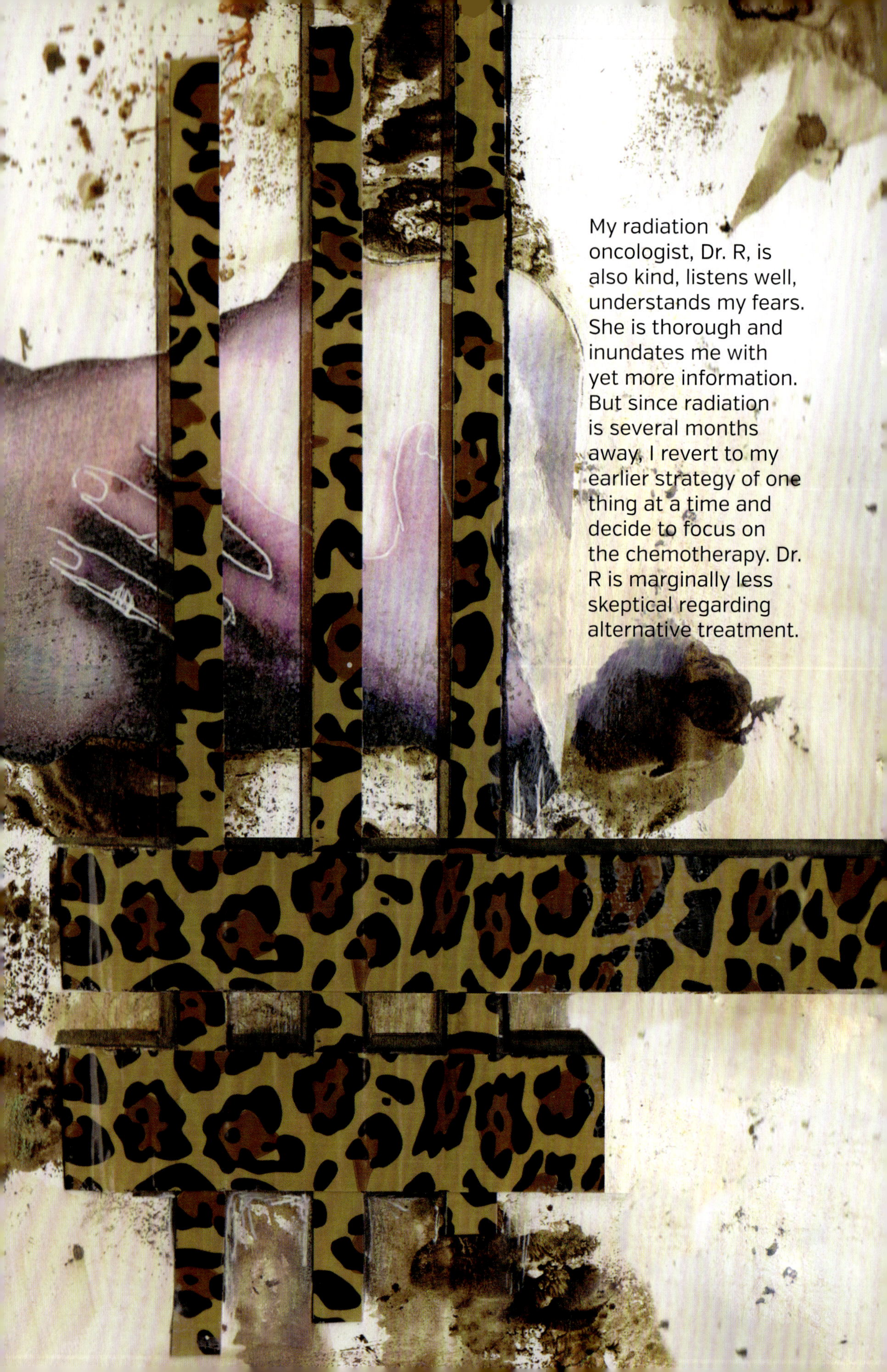

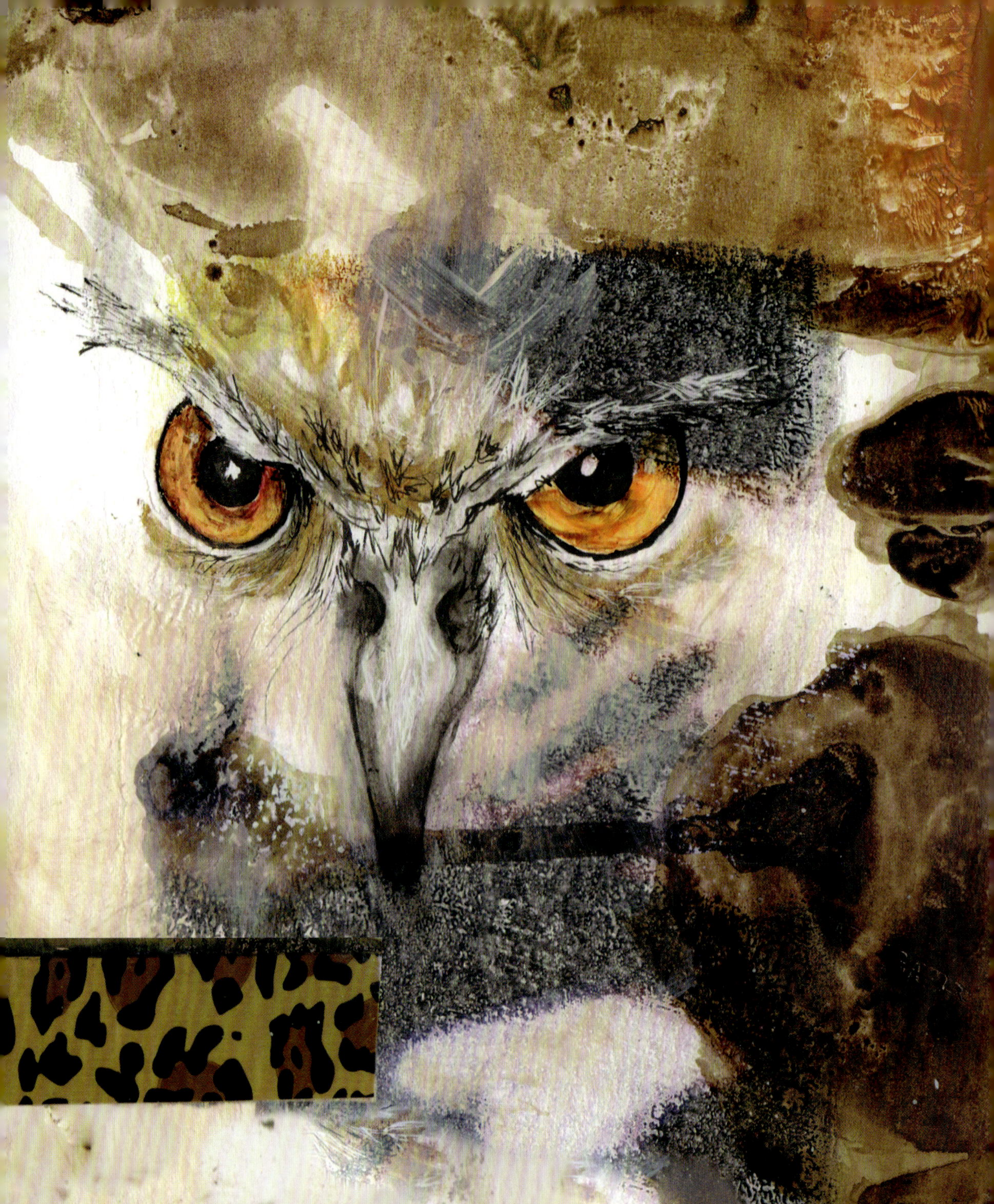

I have one more appointment during this long and arduous week, with a homeopathic doctor. Dr. H recommends a combination of infusions, vitamins, supplements and acupuncture spaced around my treatments. I am batting three for three as I am impressed with her as well. She is the only one who does not disapprove of my raw food diet. She convinces me to give up coffee ... at least for now. I can replace it with green tea. Is that even a real drink?

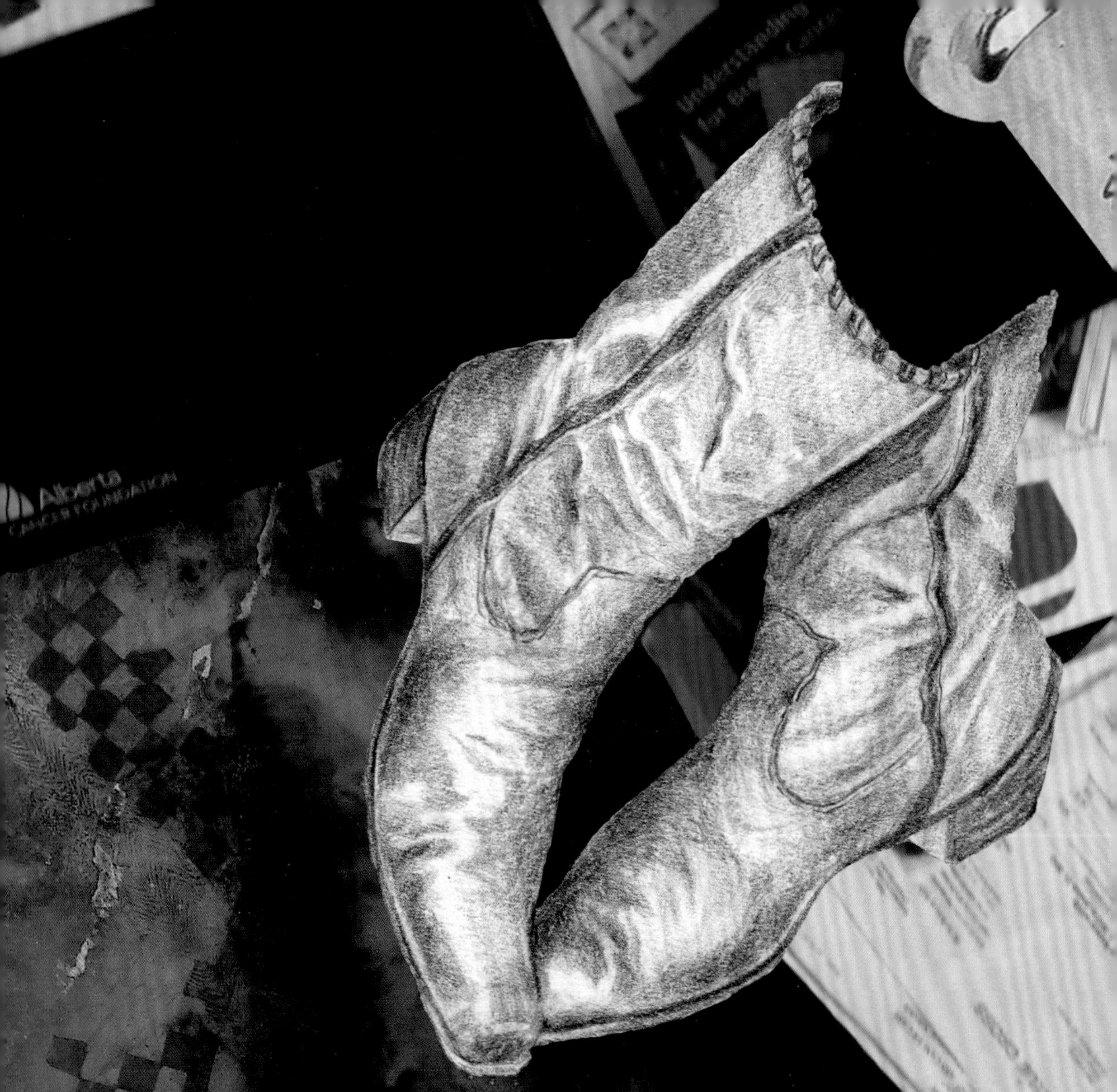

In my spare time, I catch up on the mountains of reading material that have been given to me. I find in one of the very first medical reports a recommendation for a biopsy on a lump in my left breast. Left, not right. The biopsy was never performed, and though I could feel the lump, I assumed that it was not a problem. The discovery sends me into a tailspin and I call my surgeon, Dr. S, who has agreed to act as my family doctor while I am waiting to find another. He has not seen this particular report and apologizes for its slipping through the cracks. Over the weekend he consults with a colleague and in a subsequent phone call sounds less worried.

On the following Monday he examines the offending lump. It is a cyst. When he brings out a very large

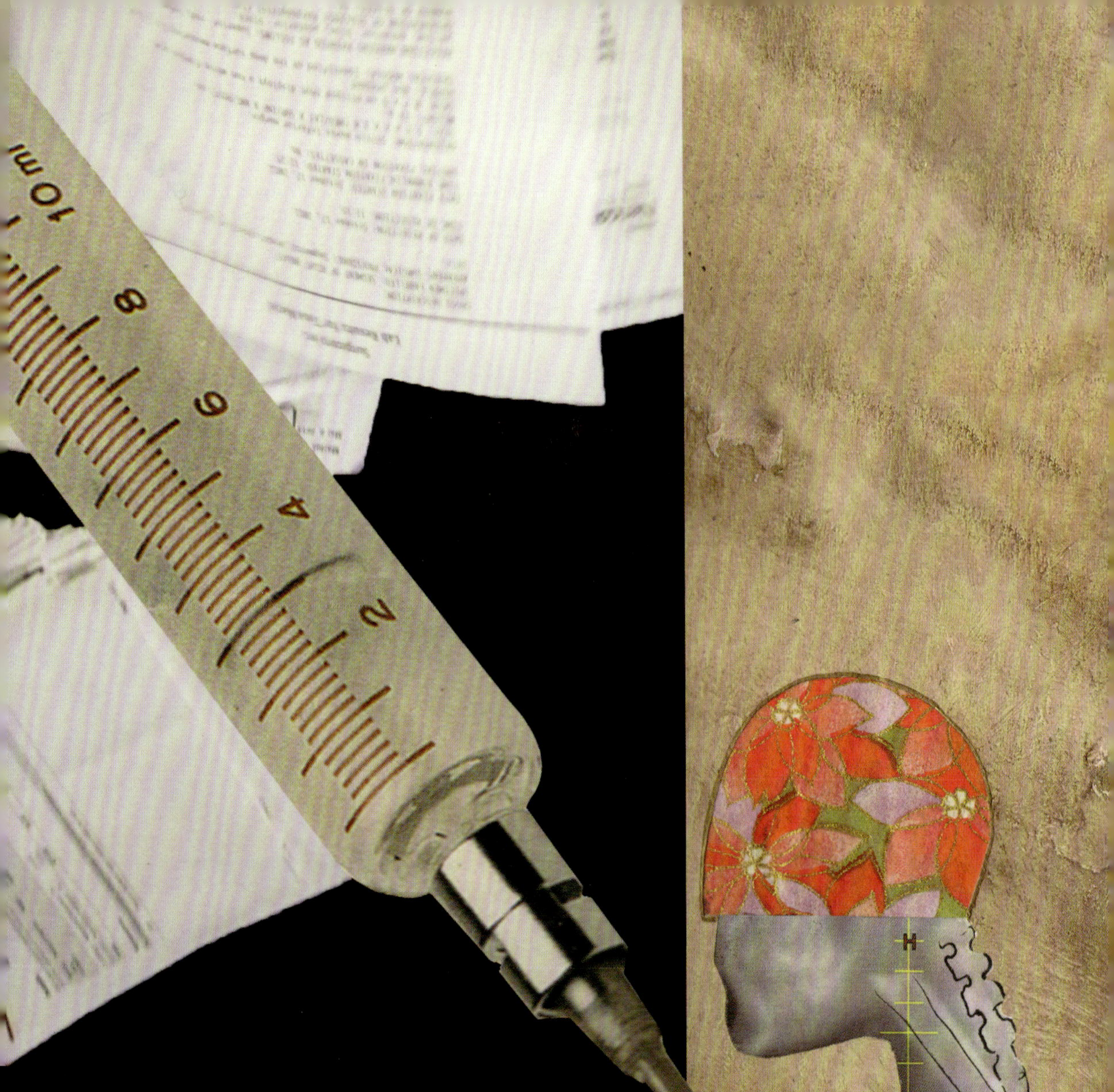

syringe I politely inquire about freezing. Apparently my choice is one painful poke or two. One please. Fascinated, I watch as he fills two vials with a straw coloured liquid. I can't believe either that one small lump could hold that much fluid or that I just watched him stick several millimetres of needle into my breast and barely flinched. He doesn't suspect anything serious.

This incident has both scared the crap out of me and has dissipated many of my reservations about further treatment.

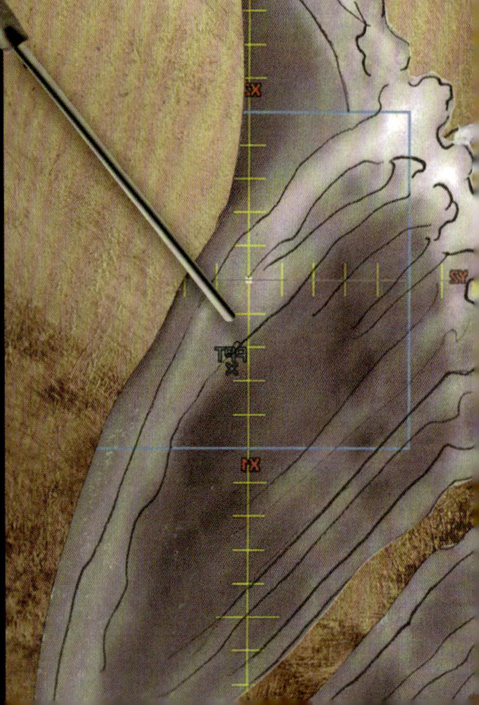

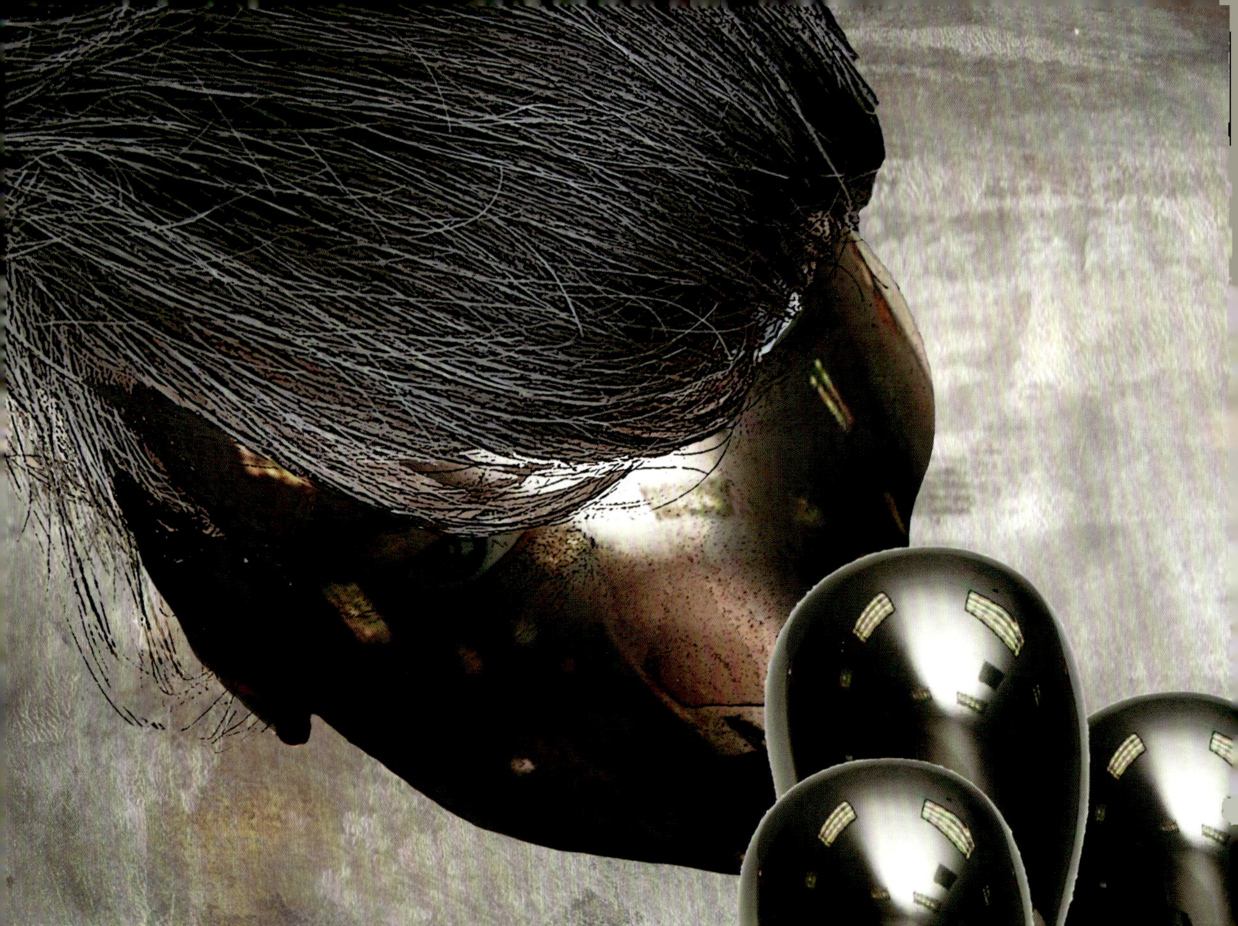

At the Canadian Cancer Society there is a roomful of wigs in a wide range of colours, floor to ceiling. I stopped dyeing my hair several years ago so in trying to find a wig close to my short cropped silvery grey I try on a white one first. Looking back at me in the mirror is my grandmother.

I try a red one with bangs, shoulder length, and see my niece staring back at me, only with a few more wrinkles. Something shorter, streaks, suburban. My sister takes up residence in the mirror.

At one point I am positive I look like my father in drag. Doug is laughing so hard he can barely manage to snap the pictures he is taking in case I want to make my mind up later. In the midst of the merriment I become very quiet. I don't want to be here. I don't want a wig. Somehow I don't remember being asked. It's just one of those things you do when you get cancer. I take the red wig out of sympathy for the woman who has been helping me. She doesn't understand my reluctance. As per usual, I'm being uncooperative.

Petulant. Problematic.

At home the wig hangs on the corner of the mirror, the abandoned mop in a commercial. On the days I want to be someone else I try it on. It never leaves the house.

I believe it is a fine choice for people who aren't me. My mother is a little shocked and discreetly suggests if it is a question of money she would be happy to buy me a wig. It is not about the cost. It is about trying to find my place in all of this. About trying to stay me.

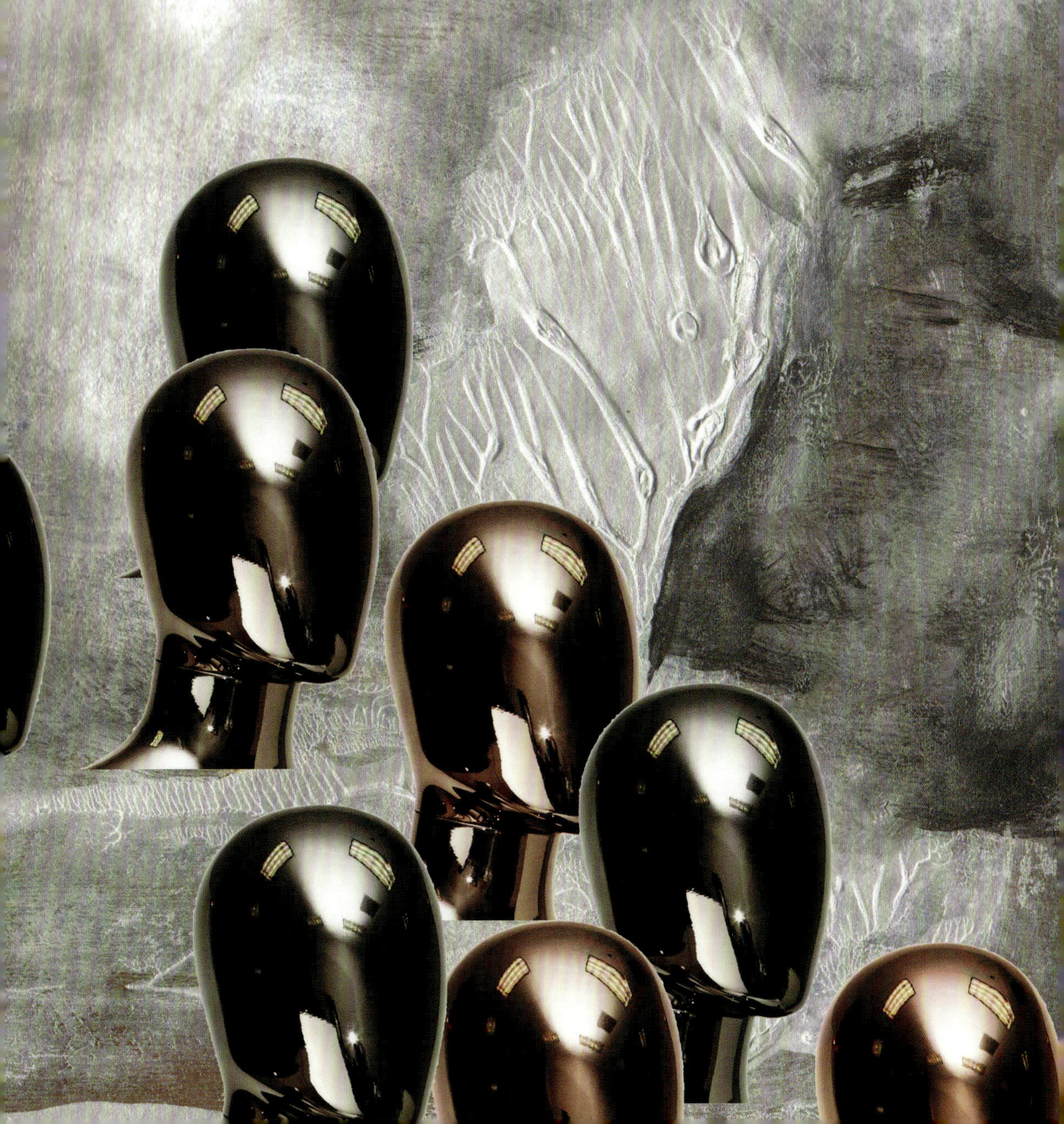

I need an ECG to determine if there is a risk of my heart stopping during chemotherapy. Doug drops me off in front of the building before parking the car. I am walking up the steps travel mug in hand when I miss the second step and go down like a felled tree. Flashing thorough my head is the thought that I have spent thousands on my dental work and I am about to smash my face into a concrete block. I manage to pull my arm under my body to absorb some of the impact but not enough to save my chin. I lie there in the cold. Unmoving. This is the first time in days I have been still. I hear people around me. Are you OK? Can you move? Why does the earth never open up and swallow you when you need it to? I retain my hold on my mug and haven't spilled a drop.

I struggle to my feet just as Doug appears. He is incredulous. He left me alone for five minutes. My chin and knee are bleeding and swelling rapidly. I limp into the clinic. The receptionist directs Doug to the family practitioner down the hall for an ice pack and bandages. I sit in a chair in the waiting room feeling foolish and conspicuous. This is all my fault for not paying attention. I am not living in the moment.

Can you blame me?

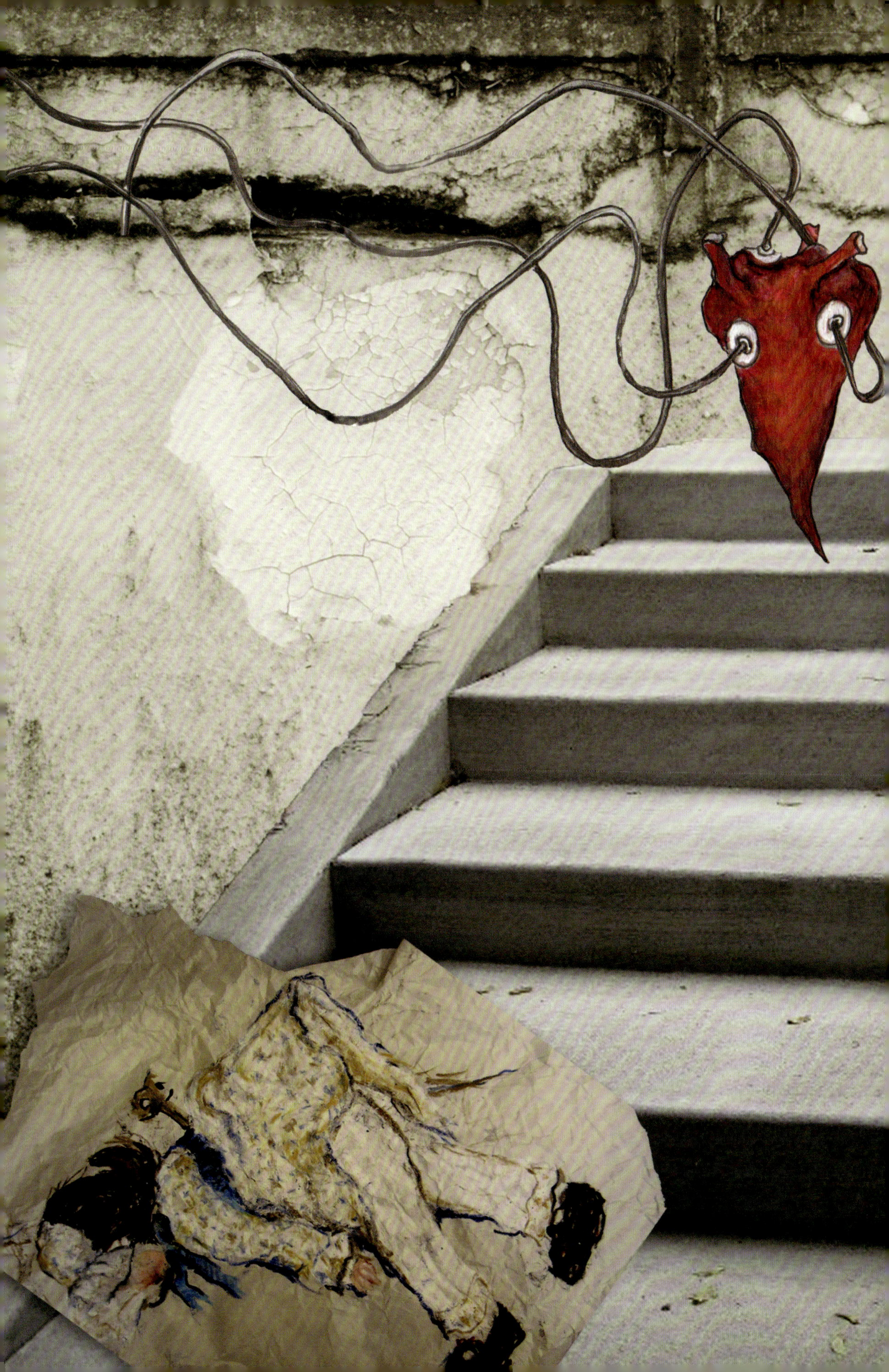

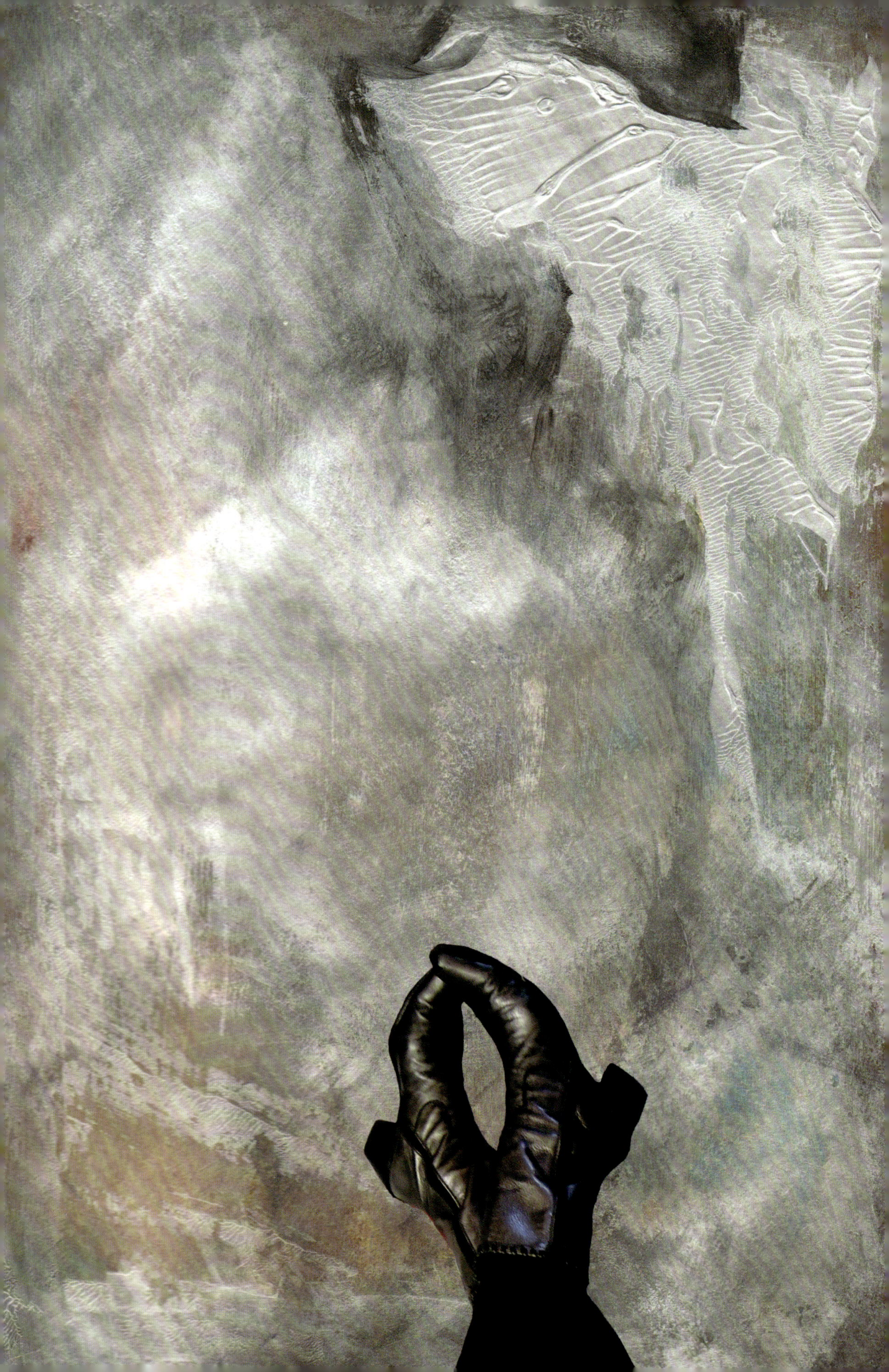

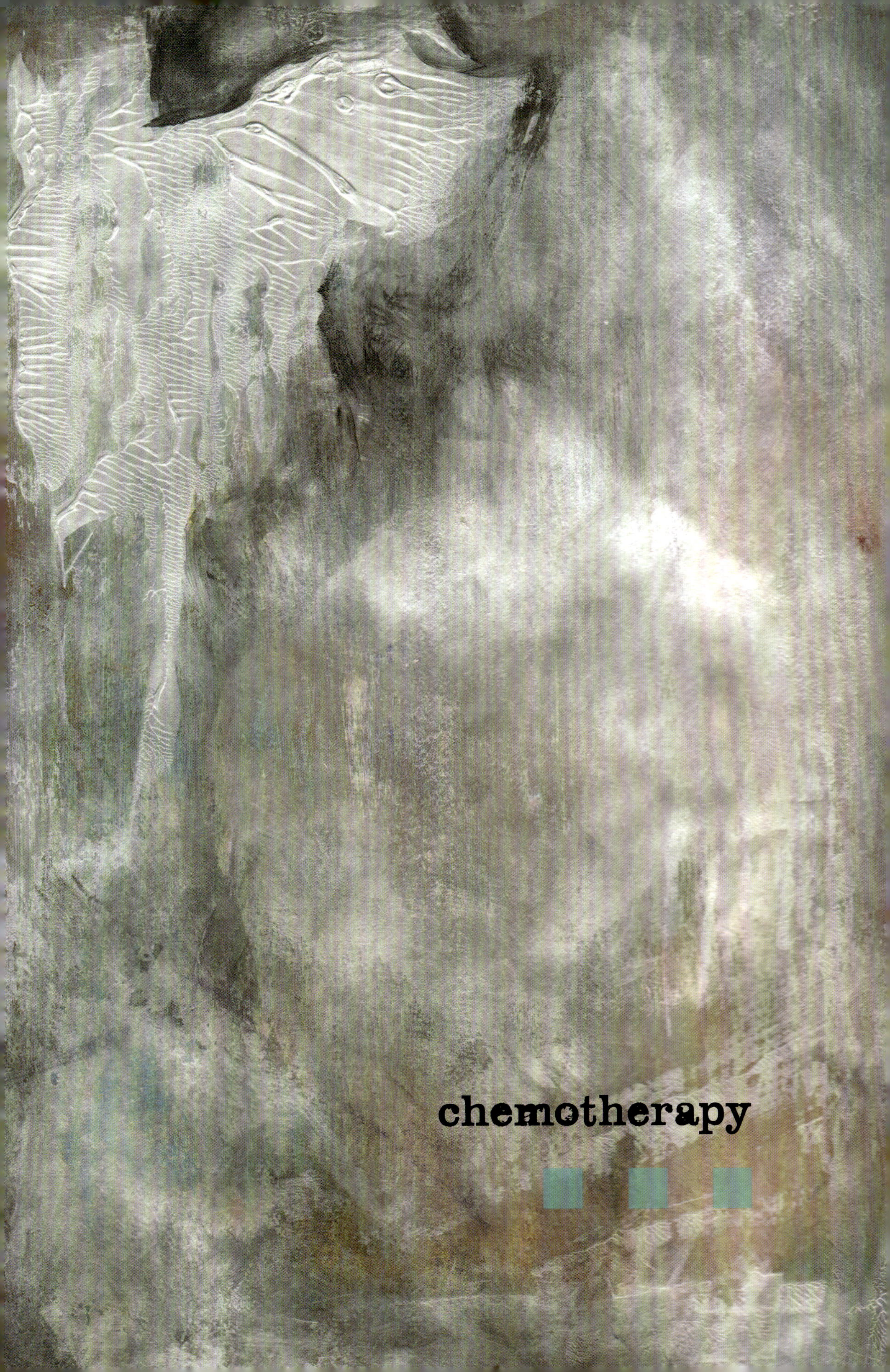
chemotherapy

The day before my chemotherapy starts, I have blood tests at the hospital, then another appointment with my oncologist. At the lab you take a number like at the butchers. The room is very cold. At least my veins cooperate. In Dr. O's waiting room I fill out yet another form: contact information, health problems, current medications, herbal supplements, even vacation plans over the next several weeks. There is a lengthy list of symptoms that I am supposed to check off if I am experiencing any of them. One is anxiety. In a moment of rebellion I refuse to check that box.

Fuck'em.

Dr. O shakes his head when he sees my battered face. People have been staring at Doug with thinly veiled hostility and I want to wear a sign proclaiming “It’s not his fault. I am a klutz.” Or maybe put it on the other side of the “I have Cancer” t-shirt.

My ECG has revealed a heart murmur. A murmur? More like a scream. Not enough to put me in a risk category. Just another grain of rice on the wet tissue that is my life.

Before treatment I also have my first acupuncture session. Apparently poking holes in you helps you to relax - though I could have lived without the one between the eyes. Afterwards, I have an IV drip with Vitamin C. I am in such unfamiliar territory. Every step requires a huge amount of trust. Am I doing the right things???

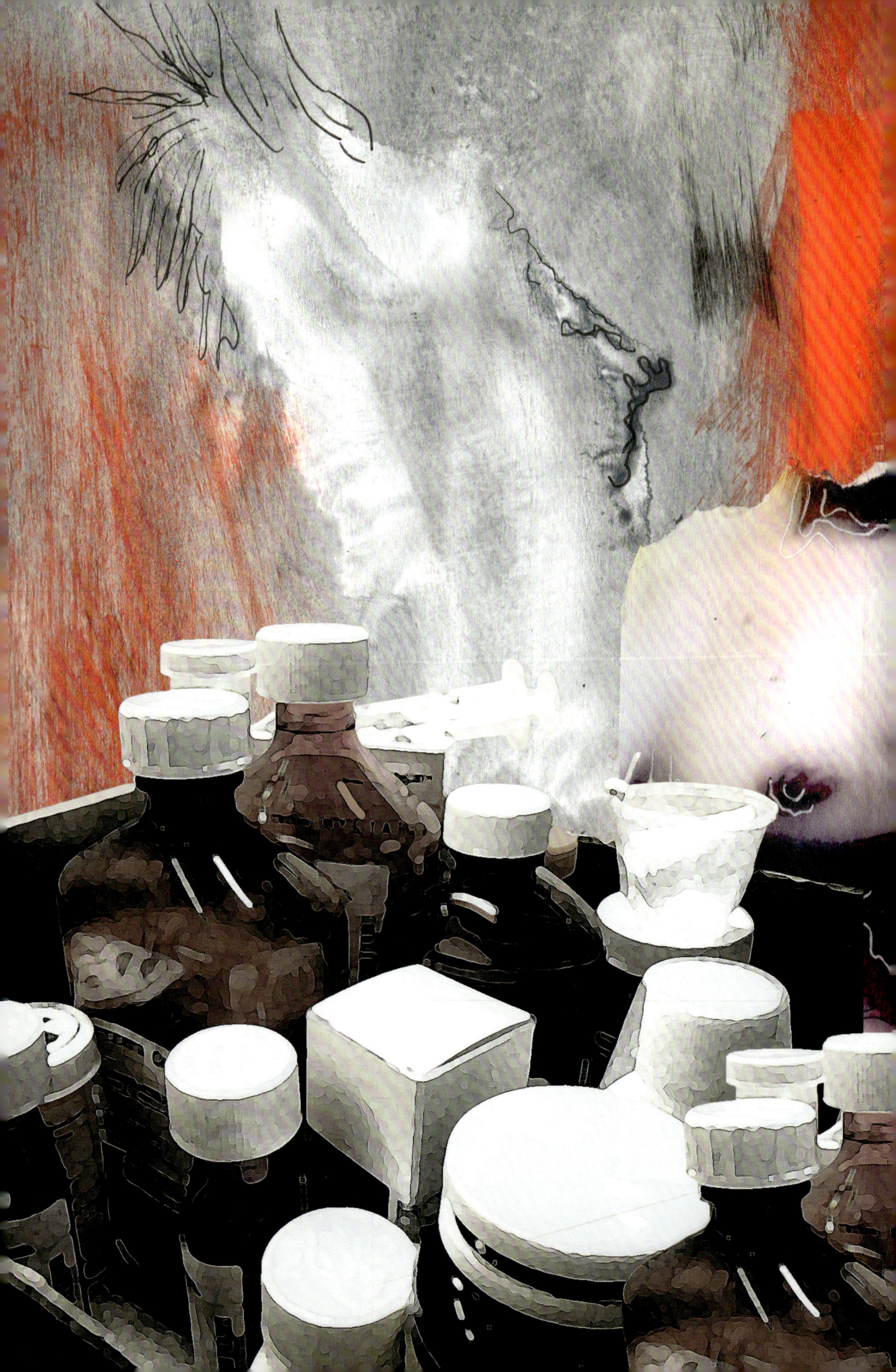

I stop at the pharmacist's
to fill my prescriptions:

an **anti-nausea drug**
steroid pills
antihistamine

Because I frequently choke when I attempt to swallow pills the pharmacist concocts a liquid mixture. Even the act of filling prescriptions is foreign to me. I can count on one hand the number of times I have taken any medications. Now the bottom shelf in the bedroom is full.

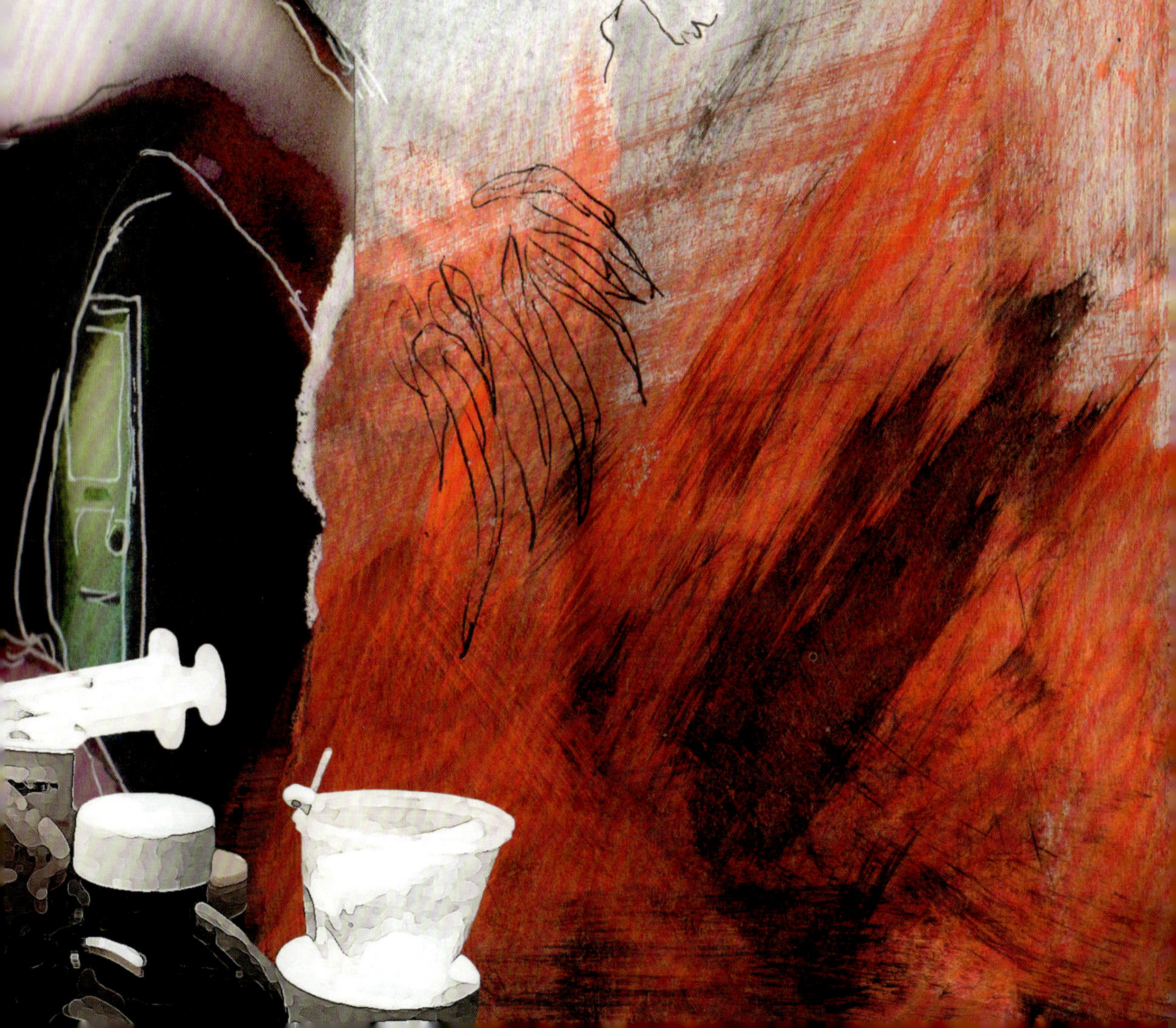

Today is the first day of my chemotherapy treatment. I produce my red cancer card I.D. with all my information on it. I am asked the now familiar questions. Name? Can you spell it? Birthday? Over and over. Apparently the surgery ward isn't the only place that people are attempting to sneak into.

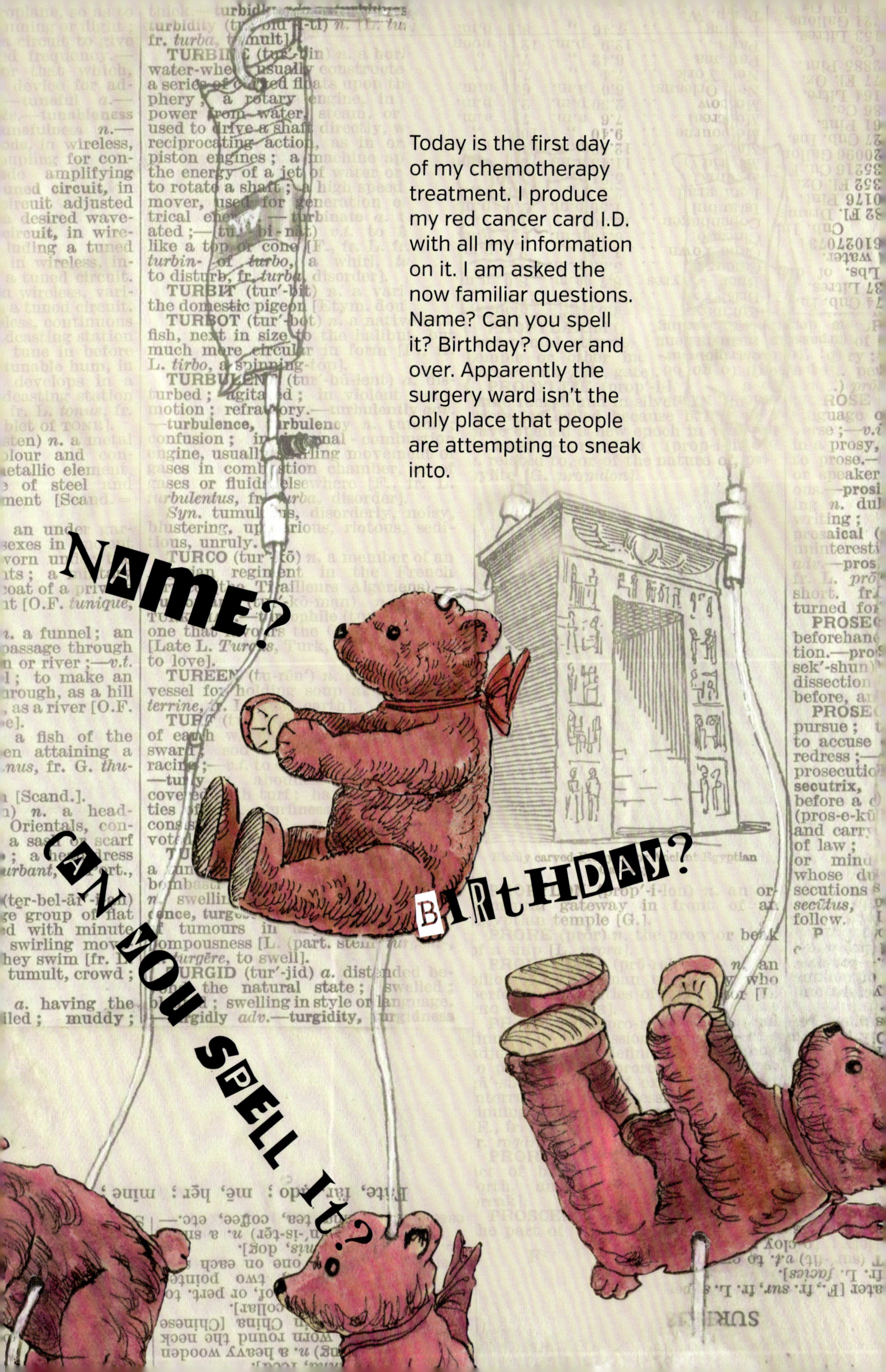

The ward is full of traumatized looking people. A look I am sure is reflected on my face. Many of them are women ... young women. The nurse informs me my blood pressure is low, my heart rate high. I tell her I have always had extremely low blood pressure. When I check it at the local pharmacy I can hear the machine chortling at me.

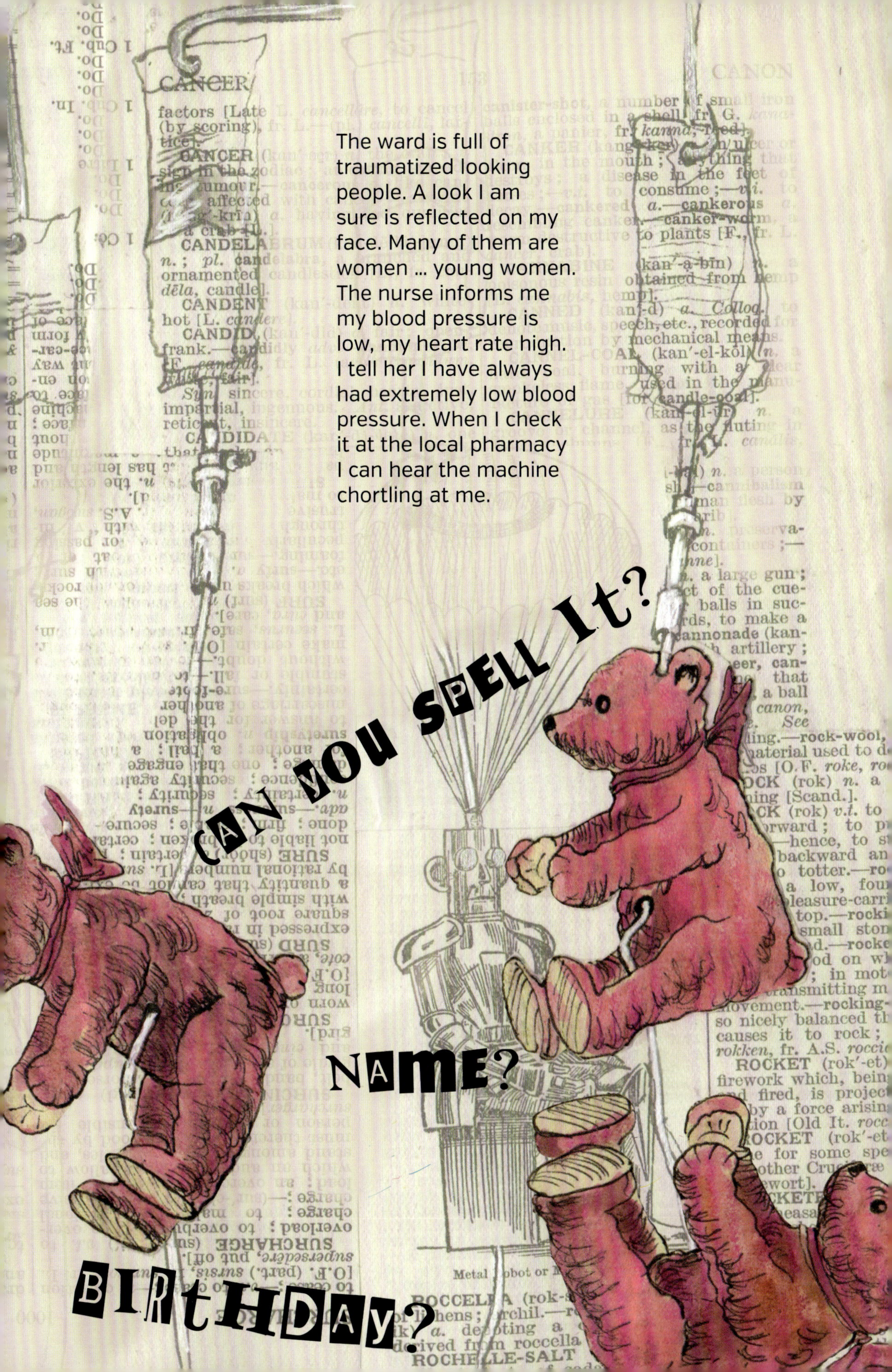

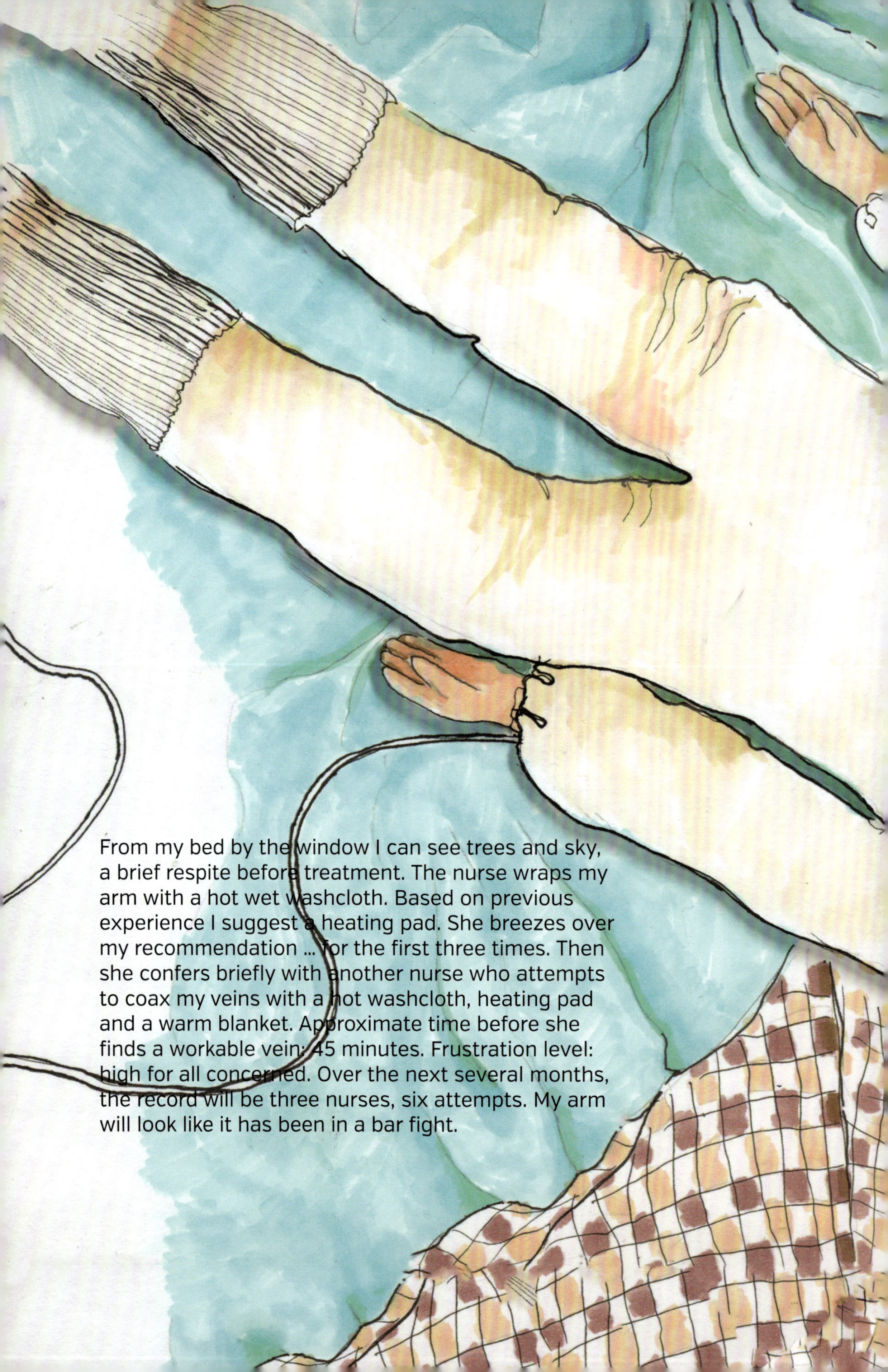

From my bed by the window I can see trees and sky, a brief respite before treatment. The nurse wraps my arm with a hot wet washcloth. Based on previous experience I suggest a heating pad. She breezes over my recommendation ... for the first three times. Then she confers briefly with another nurse who attempts to coax my veins with a hot washcloth, heating pad and a warm blanket. Approximate time before she finds a workable vein: 45 minutes. Frustration level: high for all concerned. Over the next several months, the record will be three nurses, six attempts. My arm will look like it has been in a bar fight.

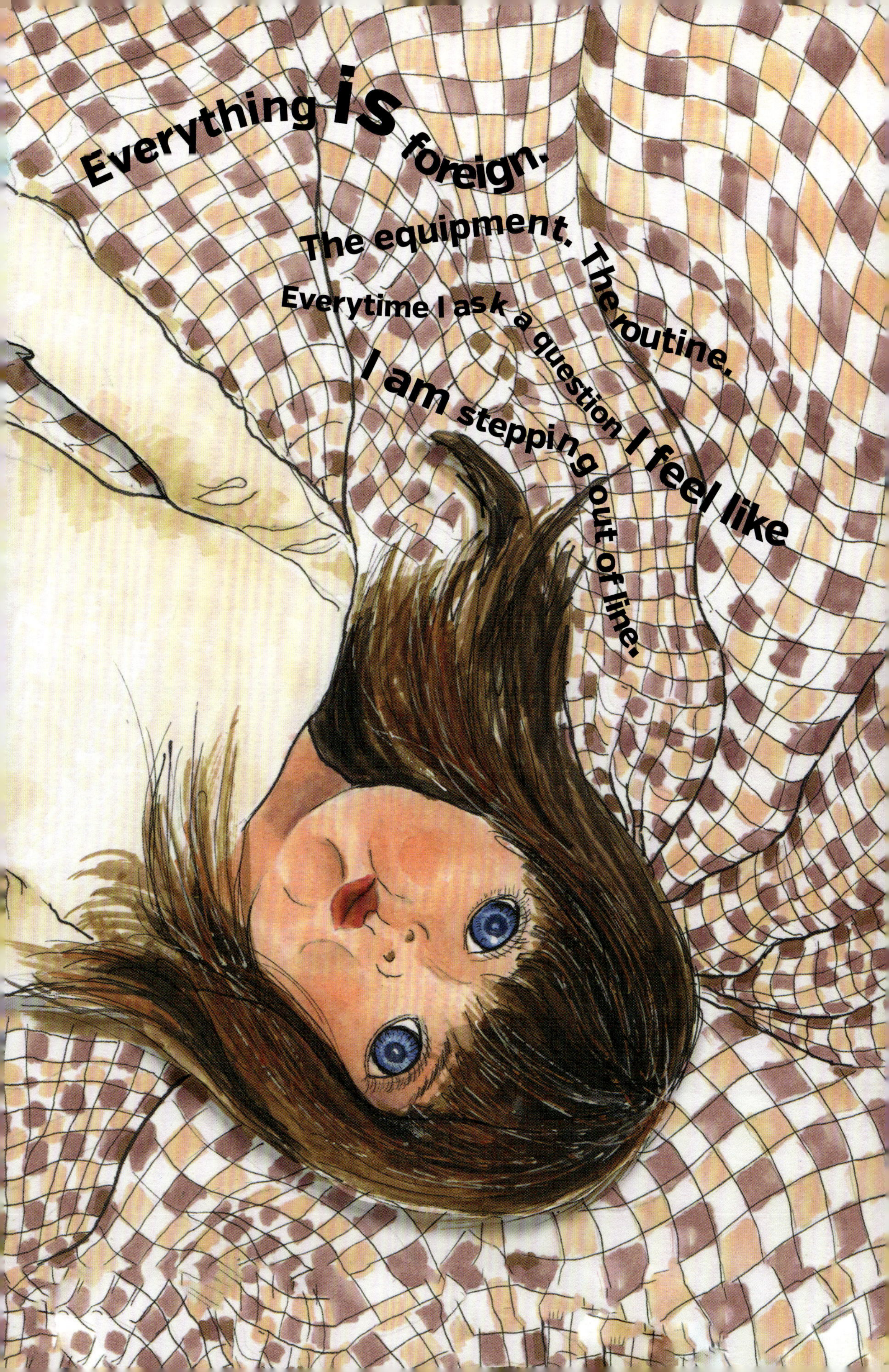
Everything is foreign.
The equipment. The routine.
Everytime I ask a question I feel like
I am stepping out of line.

I am given a combination of steroids and anti-histamine by IV. But the Epirubicin has to be injected into my veins by hand. In preparation the nurse dons goggles, a heavy apron and gloves, then picks up a vial of liquid that is a noxious fluorescent red colour. Do I have this straight? You have all this protective gear in the event YOU are accidentally splashed but you shoot this into my body?

I flash to my refusal to check the "anxiety box" on the form. I am almost crippled by my non-existent anxiety.

At the slightest burning sensation or pain, I am supposed to let them know. Three vials are pumped into my arm. I judge it successful.

My arm isn't smoking.

Now my veins are flushed with saline and I am hooked to a bag with the second batch of drugs: Cyclophosphamide and Fluorouracil. It drips slowly over the next 45 minutes. At one point my bladder which is about the size of a pea, is full. I unplug from the power source and drag all the gear along with me into the bathroom. We make quite a parade. It is a feat to unzip my jeans with one hand. I make a mental note in the future to wear a skirt. I am more than a little high from the drugs. The woman in the mirror washing her hands has a massive bruise on her chin, dark circles under her eyes. I don't know who this woman is. But I know one of us has to be strong. I just don't know why it has to be me.

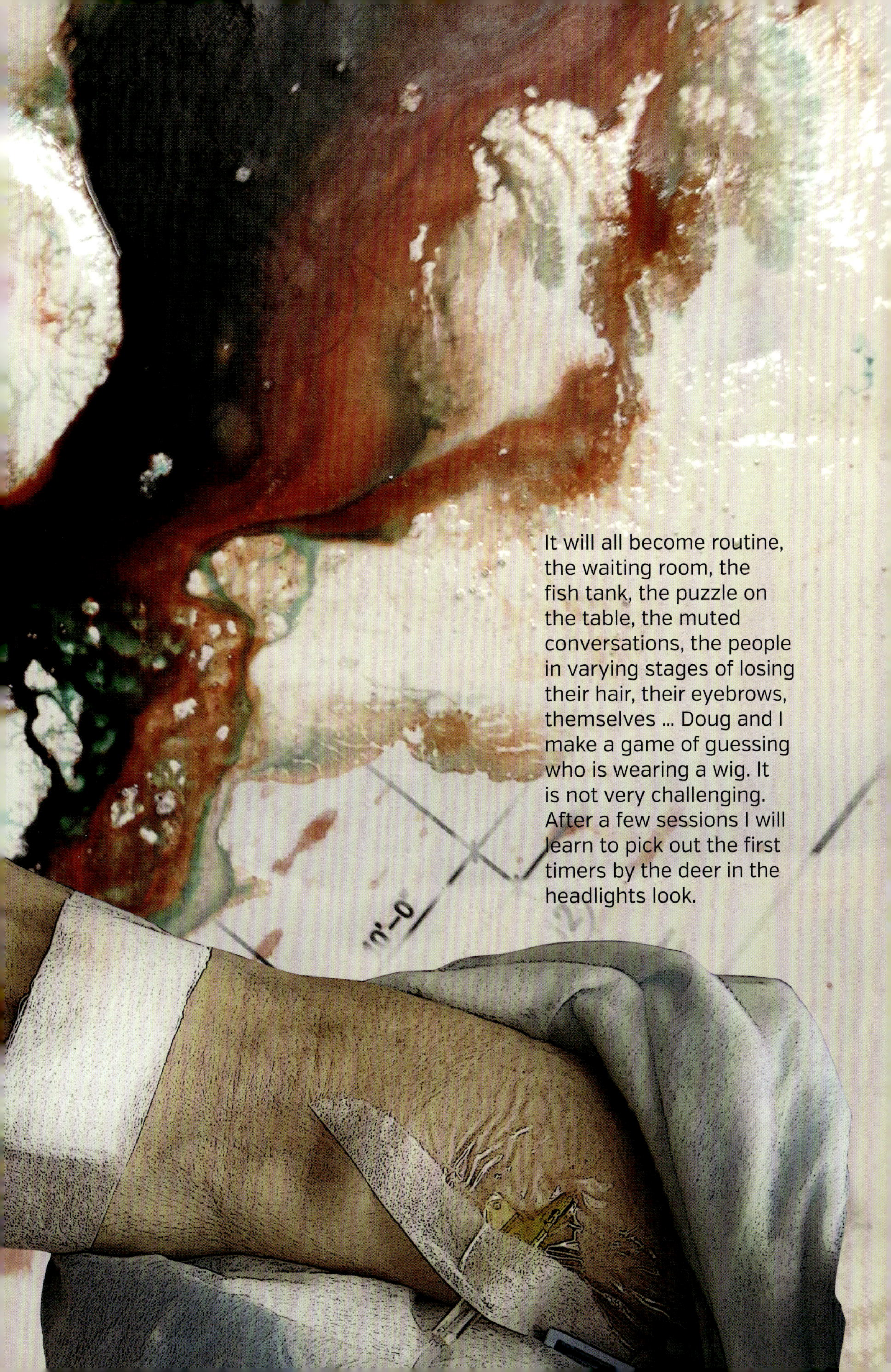

It will all become routine, the waiting room, the fish tank, the puzzle on the table, the muted conversations, the people in varying stages of losing their hair, their eyebrows, themselves ... Doug and I make a game of guessing who is wearing a wig. It is not very challenging. After a few sessions I will learn to pick out the first timers by the deer in the headlights look.

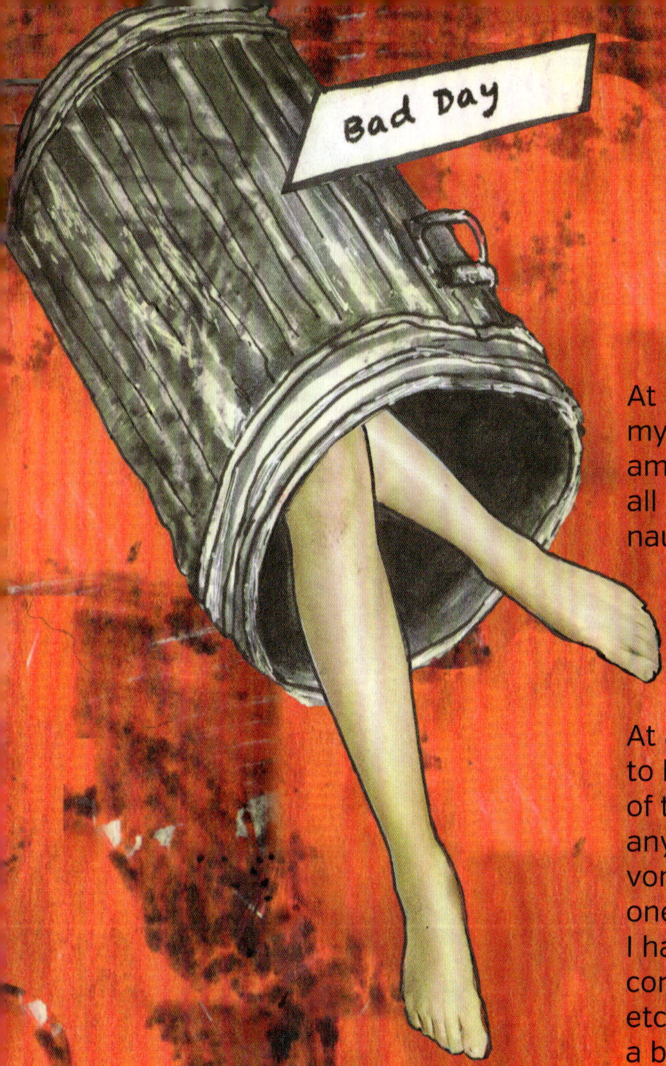

At home I take a few calls from my family and friends. I tell them I am taking all of this in stride. After all I am extremely healthy. No, no nausea yet.

At about 11:00 p.m. I start to heave. I have a horror of throwing up. I would do anything in my power to not vomit but it appears this is one more thing over which I have no control. Doug, his concern and helplessness etched on his face, places a bucket beside the couch. The nausea comes in waves. By morning the worst has subsided to a constant queasiness. The anti-nausea drugs don't help.

I have a permanent metallic taste in my mouth. Food is iffy right now. I accept that my raw food diet is not going to work. I need to consume all the calories I can keep down. This will make my mother very happy as we are all coming home for Christmas and now she will be able to make her traditional cabbage rolls and turkey.

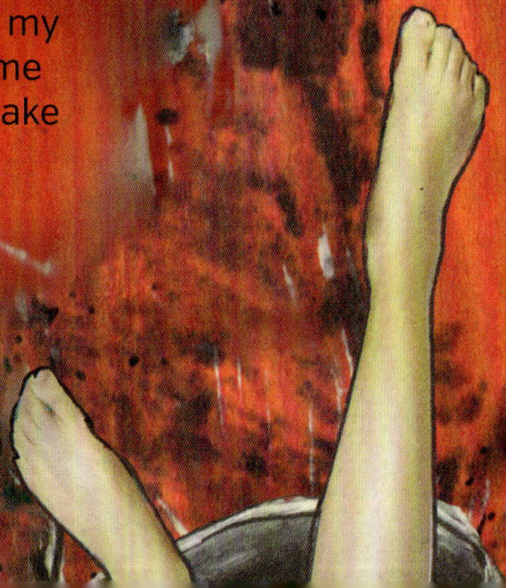

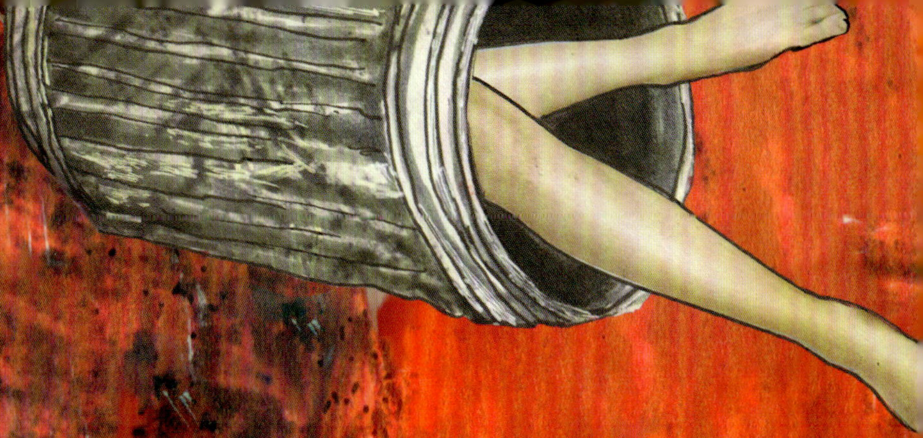

I stop taking the steroid drugs on Sunday morning out of fear I may be overcome by uncontrollable fury. I am mildly bitchy. What if it's a sign of impending roid rage?

I find myself praying, a prayer remarkably similar to the one I recited for most of my teenage years.

Dear God. It's me. Please get me out of this one and I will never do this again.

No. Really.

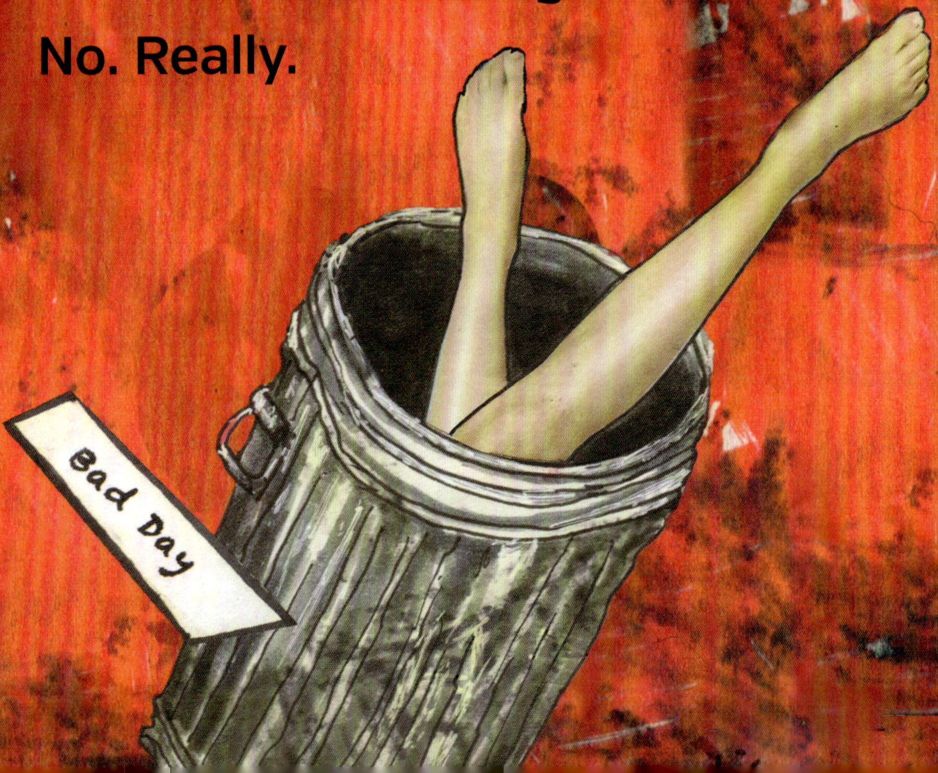

Four days later my friend Alan's sister Nadine, who has had breast cancer, calls to ask how my first treatment went. When I tell her, she briskly informs me, "Get your ass back into the oncologist's office and let him know that anti-nausea drug was useless."

Apparently there are hundreds.

You start at the top of the list and work your way down. Vaguely I recall Dr. O's claim that there is a drug for almost everything. I had assumed he meant only one per condition. Another important lesson, for which I am grateful.

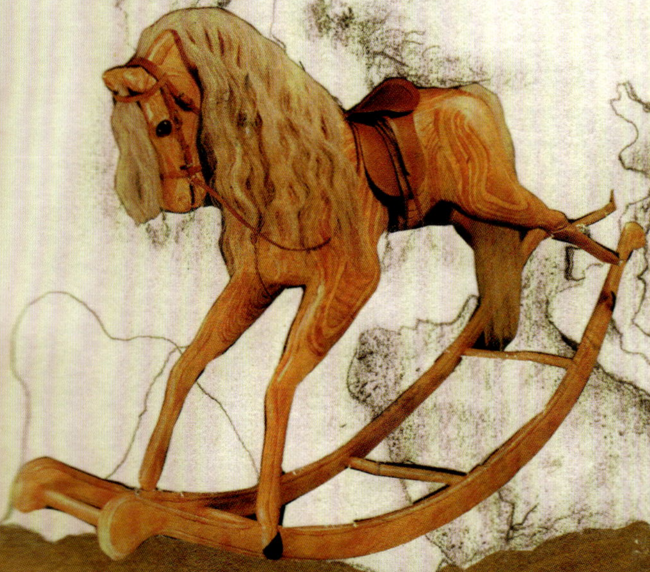

Christmas at my mother's is a quiet and peaceful respite. I have time to reflect and rest, interspersed with visits from people I know. We play cards and pretend everything is fine.

I have been told that my hair could start to fall out in as little as two weeks. When my Mom was going through chemo 20 years ago there'd been some evidence that cooling your head before chemo could prevent hair loss. On one of our first trips into Saskatoon for her treatment I pulled into a service station and picked up a 2.5 kilo bag of ice from the outside fridge.

Mom wrapped the bag in a towel and balanced it precariously on her head.

We laughed so hard it was all I could do to drive.

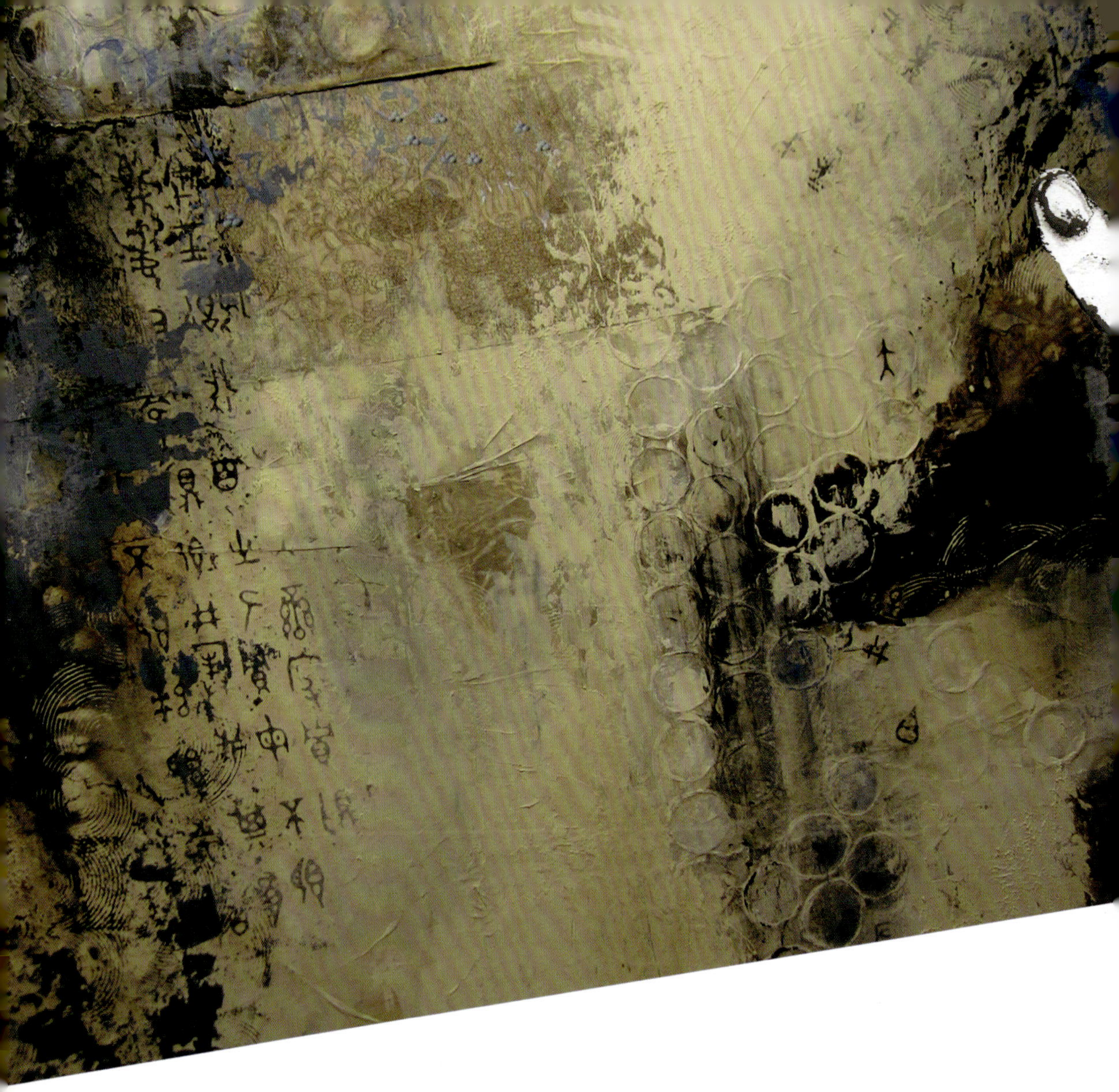

Sure enough between Christmas and New Years I start shedding in handfuls. My hair is everywhere: in my food, on my pillow, sticking to my clothes. This at least is one thing I can control.

I decide it is coming off.

By this time I am staying with my friend Marcelle. Her kitchen has a stunning vista of the river valley. It is sunny and cold with the kind of light that only a perfect prairie winter day provides. Nice day to shave your head. I have decided to do it in the kitchen rather than the bathroom with it's large mirror. Somehow the diminutive size of a hand mirror makes the procedure easier to face.

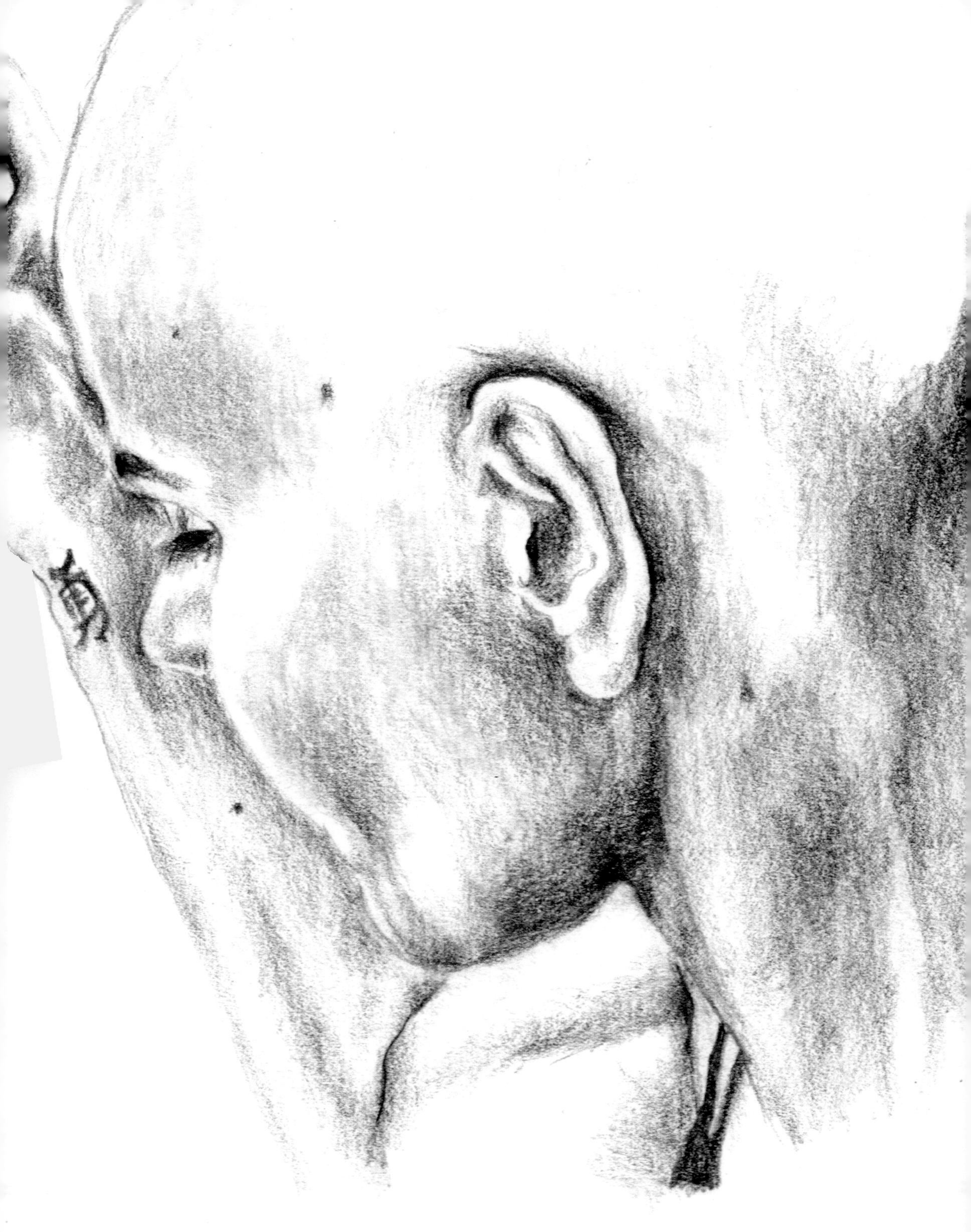

I have purchased a head shaver appropriately called “Balder.” Marcelle shaves. Doug shoots a video with my camera while she and I talk about all the things we did when we were growing up. We have been friends since we were 12 and have seen each other through bad marriages, career changes, family problems and countless life traumas. I think we can count this as another.

My scalp is smooth, strange, unfamiliar. Images of Ripley in ***Alien*** flash through my mind. Maybe I should buy camouflage pants and sleeveless white T-shirts. Wear combat boots. Build up my triceps. Kicking this thing's ass requires me to act the part. Doug objects to my buying a flamethrower but as I point out he can't watch me all the time. I don't cry. I am struck by the ritualistic nature of what we are doing: in some cultures head-shaving is a preparation for a major rite of passage.

All the hair on my body falls out except my eyelashes and eyebrows.

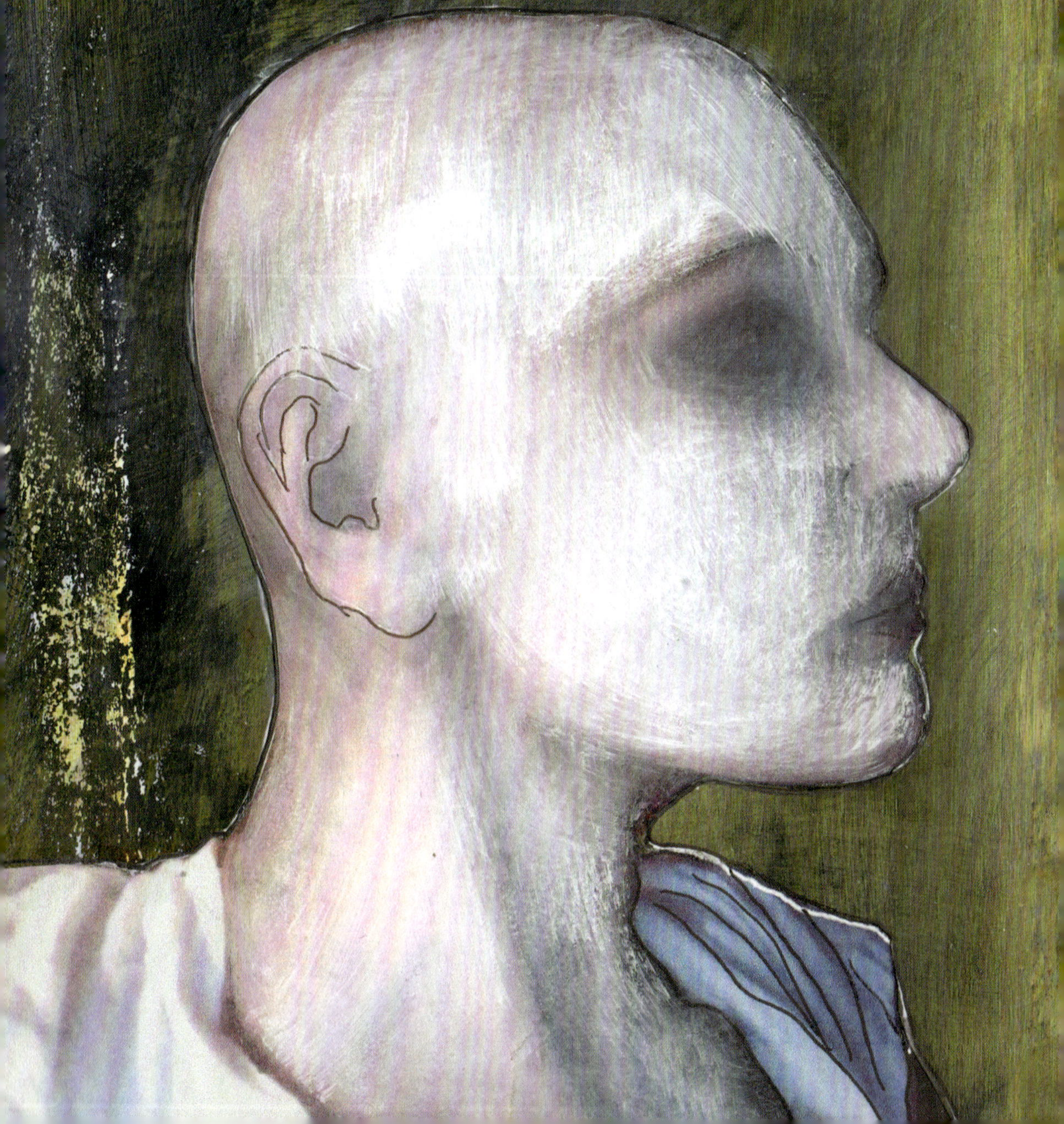

ROR

There are advantages. Having eliminated shampooing and conditioning my hair along with shaving my legs and underarms I can now with complete honesty say, give me five minutes to shower. In fact, after three minutes I'm pretty much in there doing the mambo. Not having to blow-dry or style saves me another ten minutes. I find myself with time on my hands – perhaps I can use it to find the enlightenment this experience is supposed to bring me.

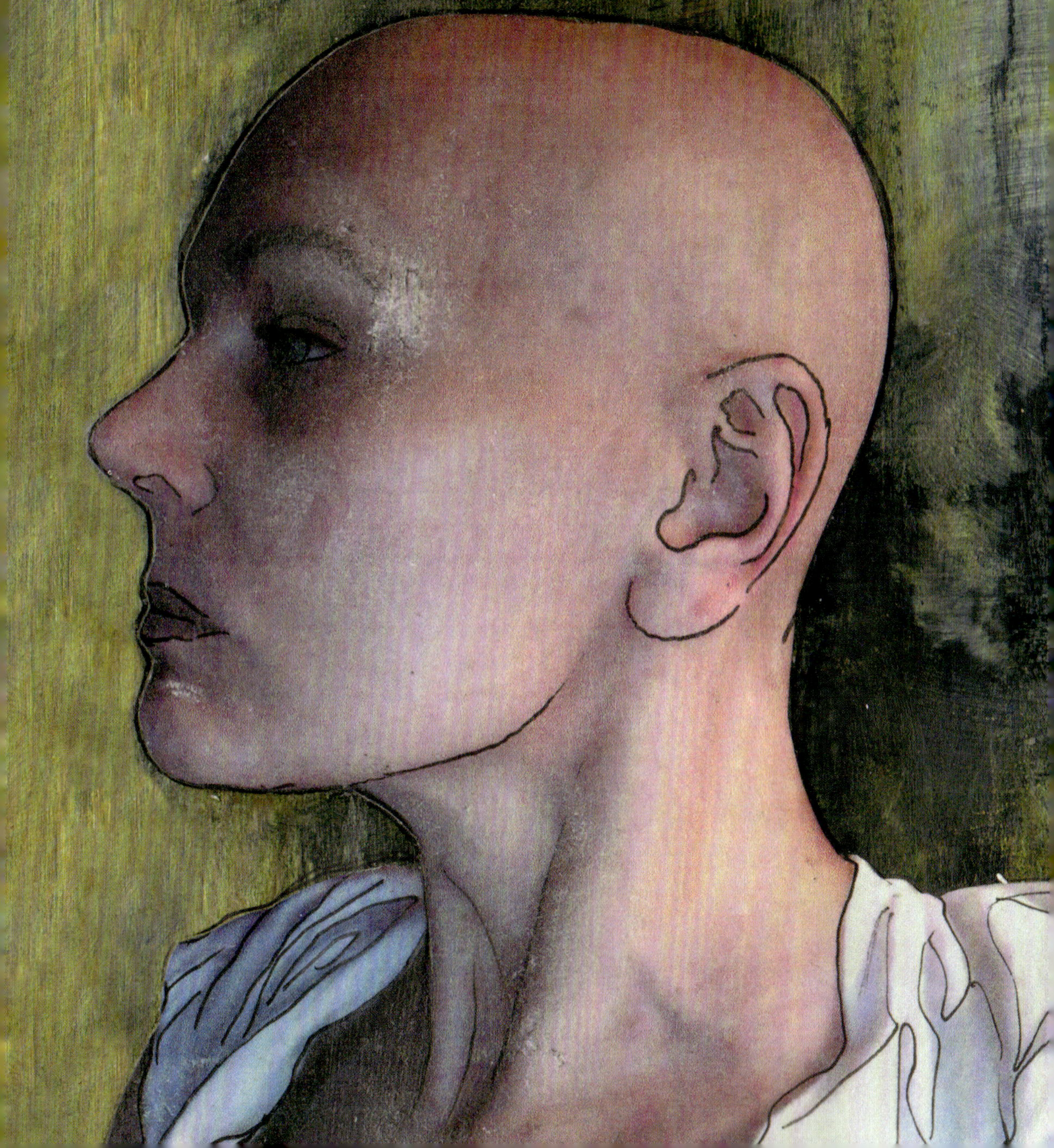

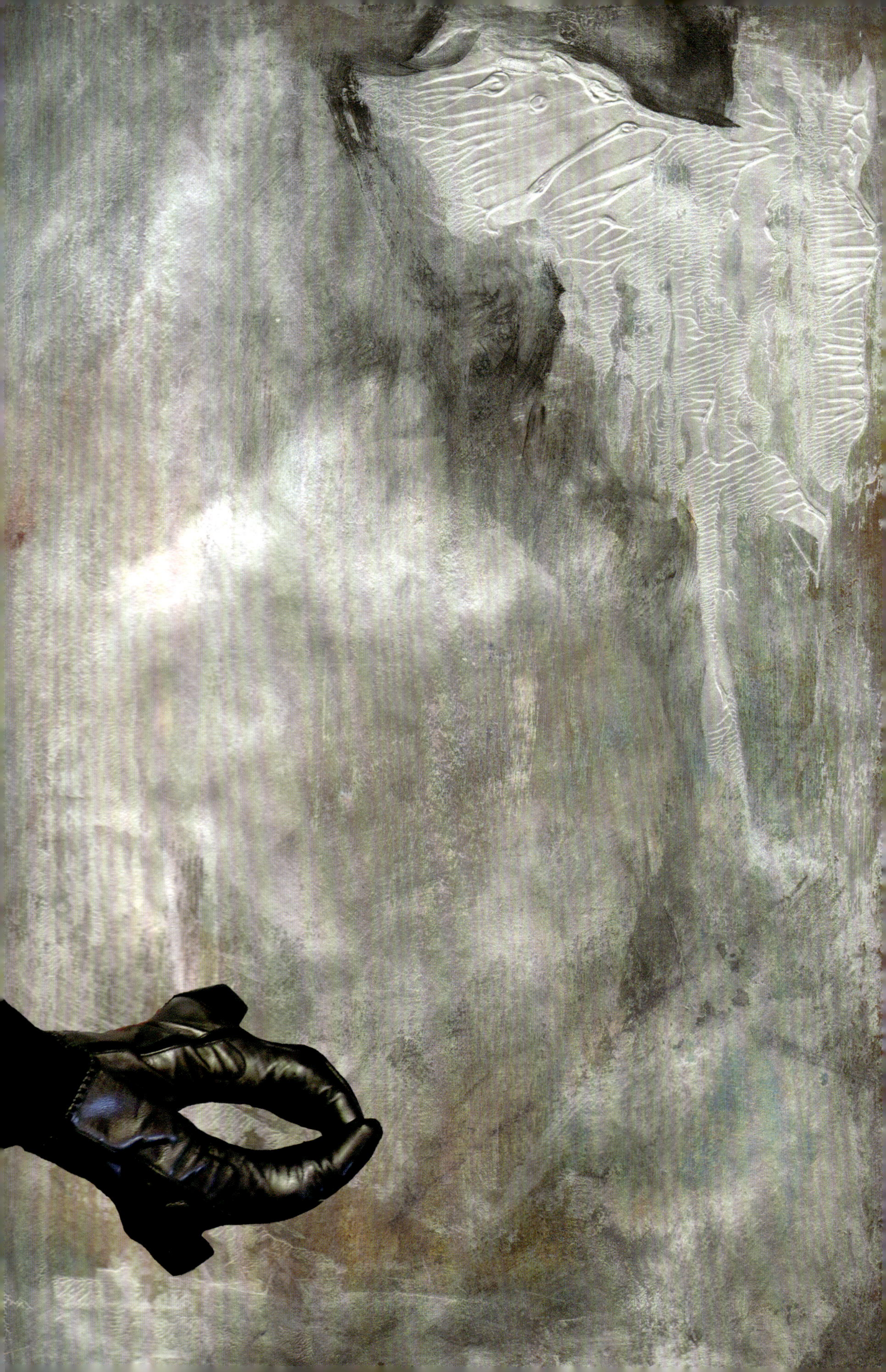

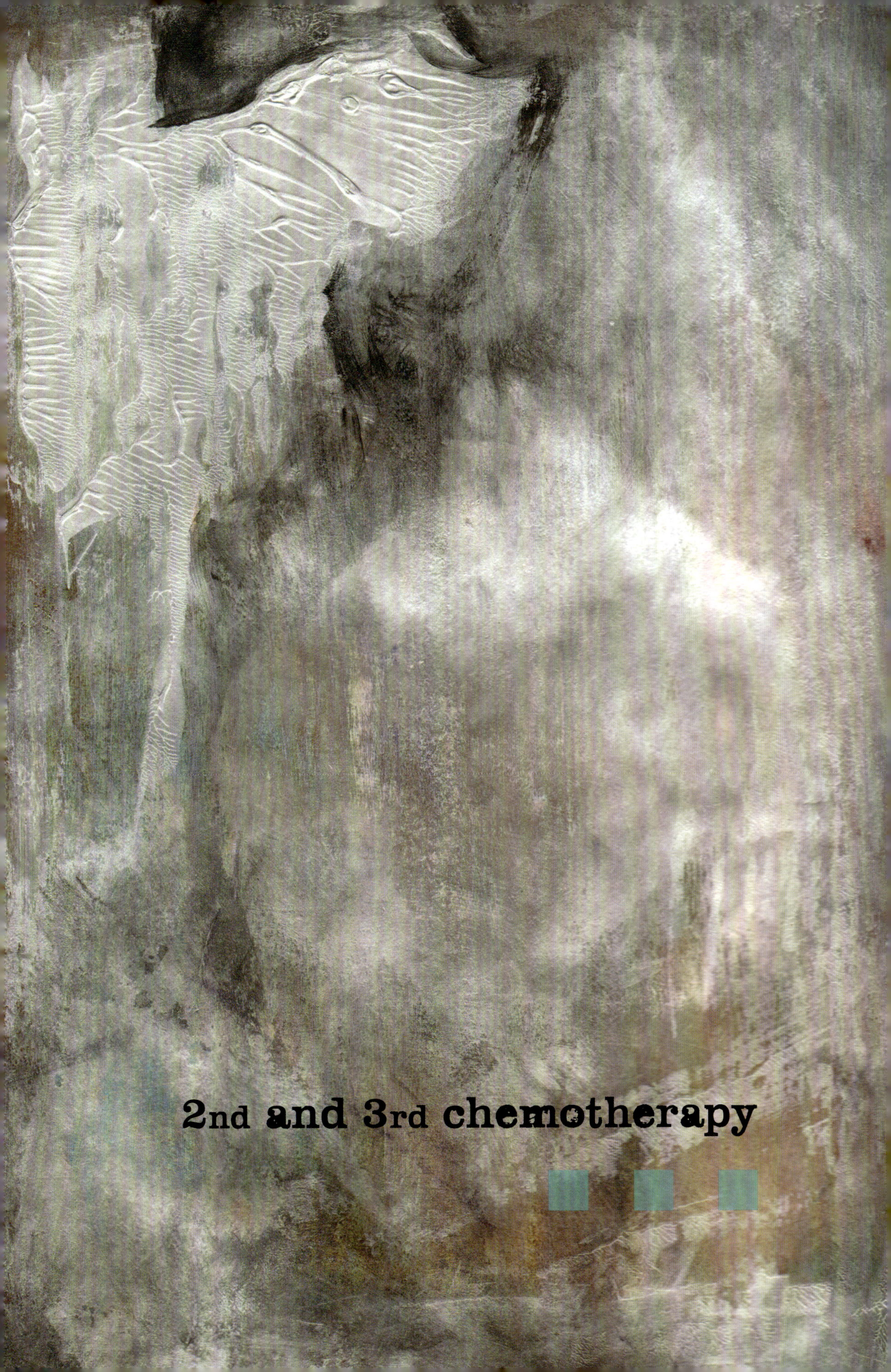

2nd and 3rd chemotherapy

A new year.

I begin my second chemotherapy treatment on January 6th.

Most of the nursing staff are very caring and genuine. It has to be difficult for them. All that fear. I am stunned at the number of people having treatment who are alone. Doug packs my snacks, makes tea, fetches ice, distracts me, tries to keep me calm. As they stick needles into me, he grips my hand. On the bad days he bears the marks of my nails.

Today I have a male nurse who actually gets a needle into my vein on the first try. He is the second person to attempt it but it's still an improvement. He asks me what I do for a living.

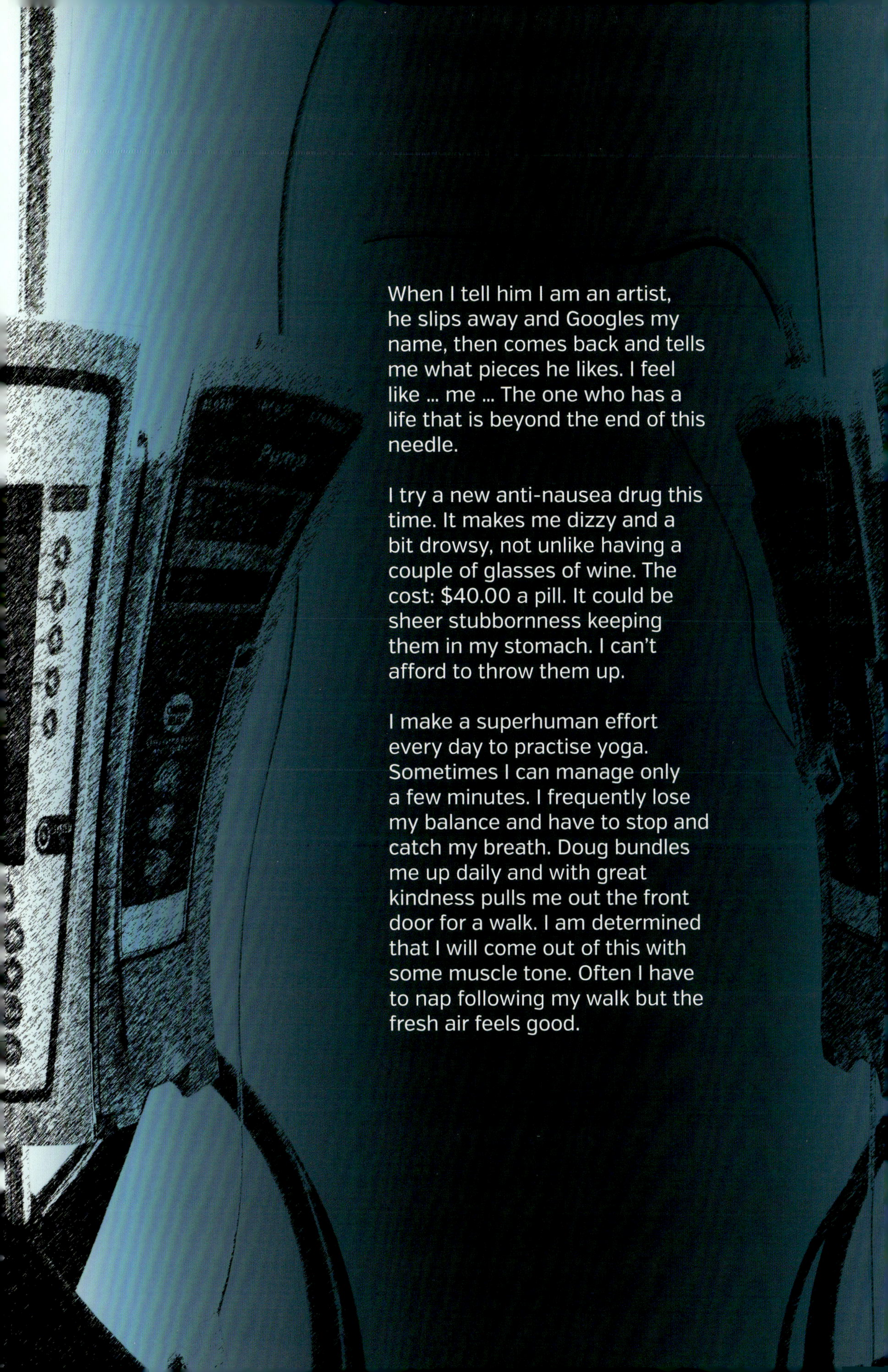

When I tell him I am an artist, he slips away and Googles my name, then comes back and tells me what pieces he likes. I feel like ... me ... The one who has a life that is beyond the end of this needle.

I try a new anti-nausea drug this time. It makes me dizzy and a bit drowsy, not unlike having a couple of glasses of wine. The cost: $40.00 a pill. It could be sheer stubbornness keeping them in my stomach. I can't afford to throw them up.

I make a superhuman effort every day to practise yoga. Sometimes I can manage only a few minutes. I frequently lose my balance and have to stop and catch my breath. Doug bundles me up daily and with great kindness pulls me out the front door for a walk. I am determined that I will come out of this with some muscle tone. Often I have to nap following my walk but the fresh air feels good.

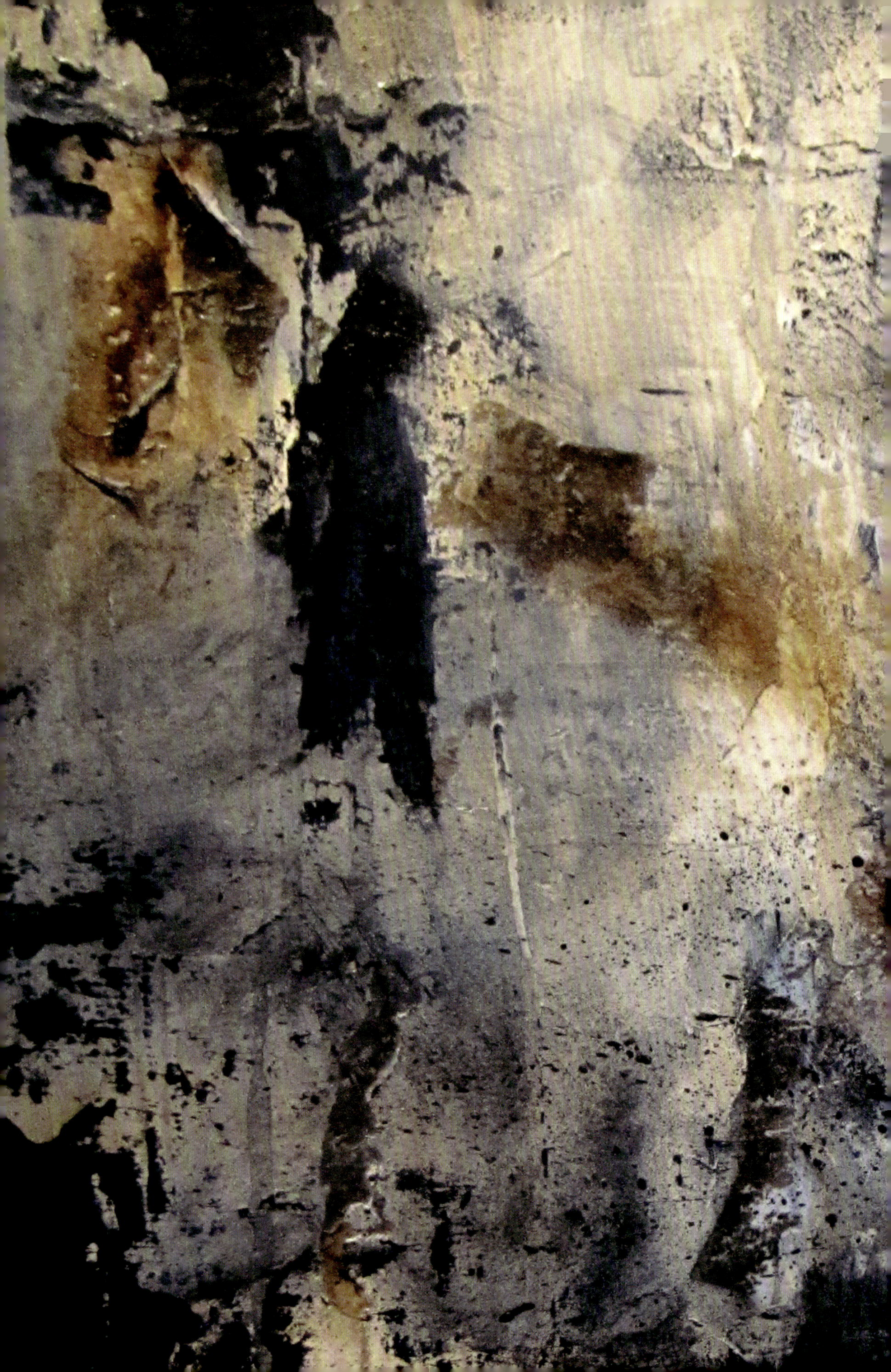

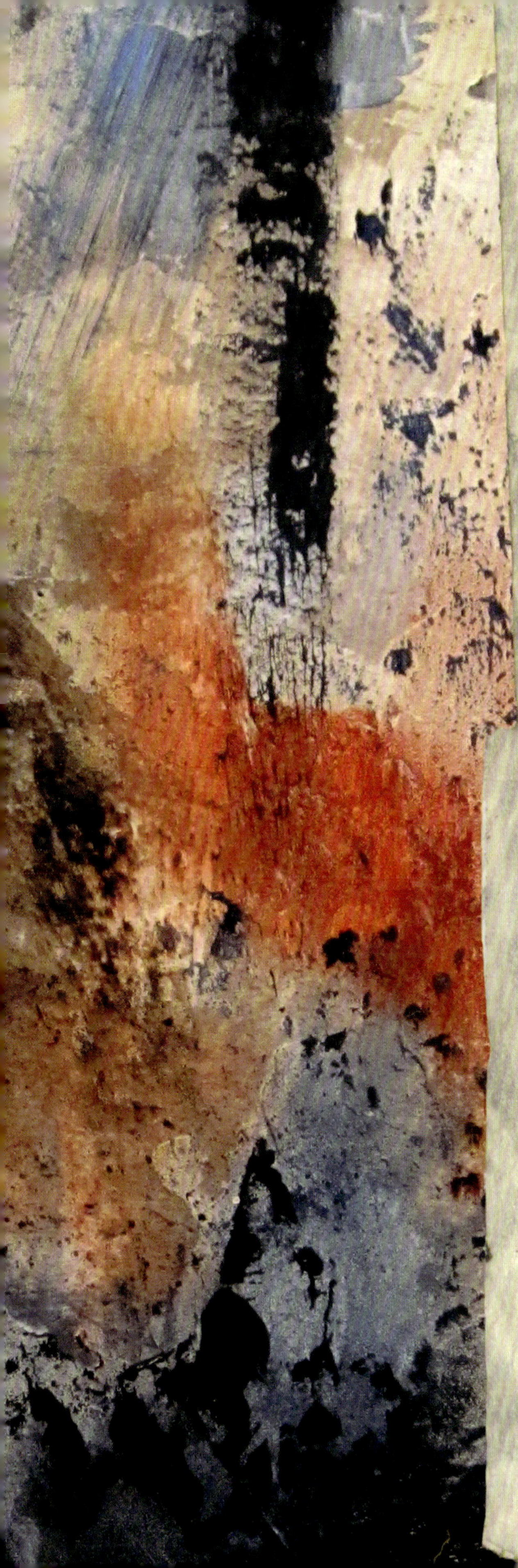

When I thought about chemo before starting treatment it was like a montage: I am breezing into appointments dressed chicly in black, trying on hats with my friends, curling up on the couch reading Dostoevsky. Standing on a cliff like ***The French Lieutenant's Woman*** while the wind buffets my overly slim body and solitary tears occasionally drip over my pale but still lovely face. Months slip by and seasons change, but the entire ordeal only lasts five minutes, as any good montage should. Then the music swells and the screen fades to black.

Instead of the montage I have **side effects.**

Chronic nasal drip. My nose is raw and starting to scab.

Hemorrhoids. The first time I see all that blood in the toilet bowl I almost pass out. Surely, this can't be normal.

Thrush. Mouth sores. The inside of my mouth has what feels like threads buried under the skin. Not painful, just alien.

Nausea. Comes and goes. The taste of food is horrific, the texture worse. Doug patiently cooks dinner only to be told I can't eat that. My go-to's are fruit and vegetable smoothies with homeopathic supplements blended in or homemade chicken soup.

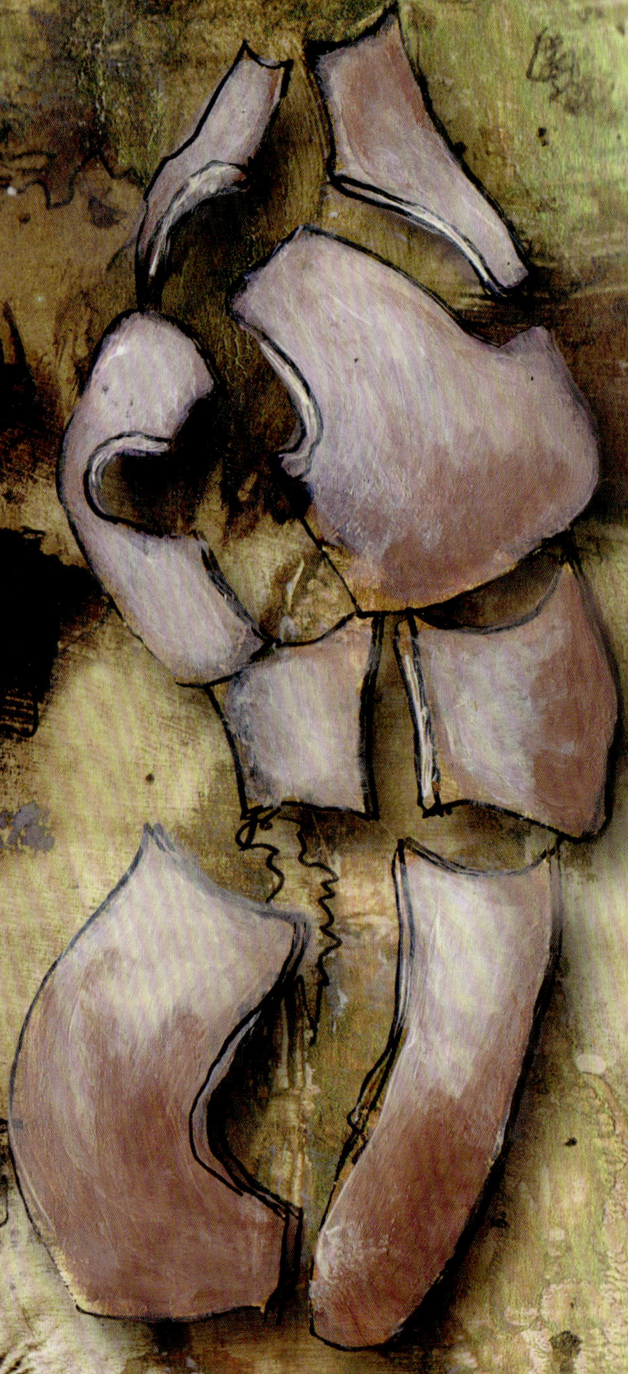

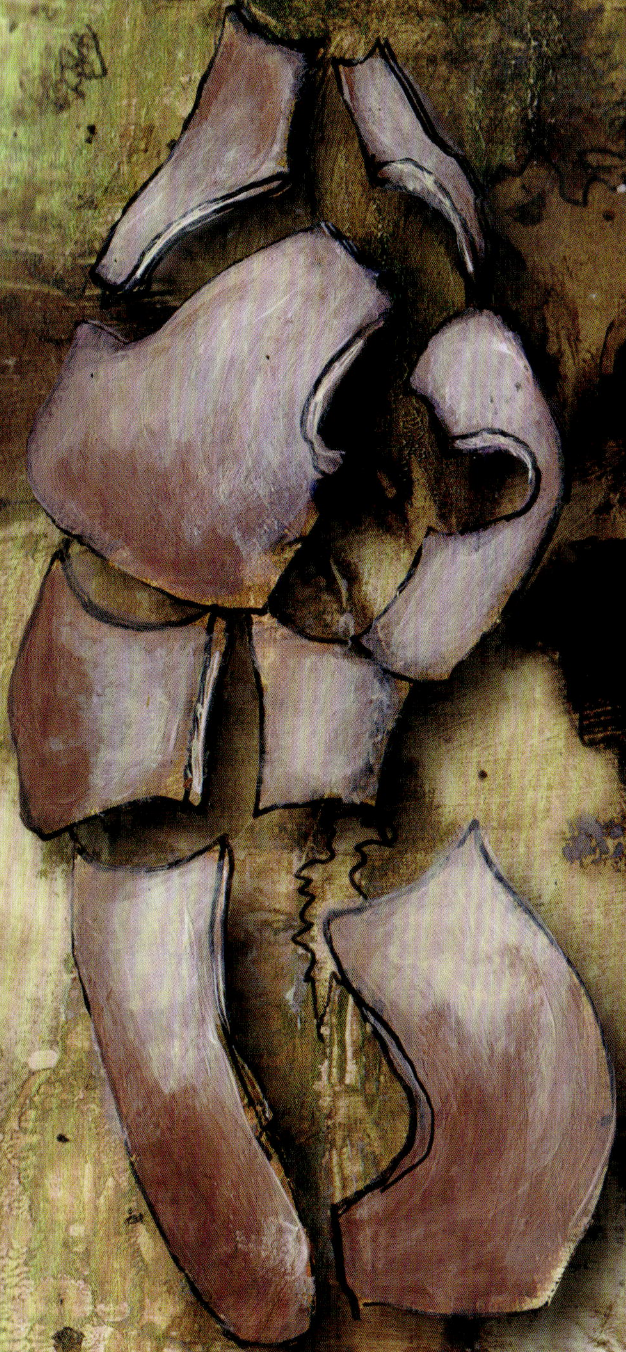

On a good day, I can have eggs. The sharp edges of crackers are painful. Cheese is slimy and intolerable.

My intolerance of food lasts at least 18 days of the 21-day cycle of chemo drugs. Three days of feeling human and eating, then I begin again.

Fatigue. My constant companion. It can't be powered through or solved with napping or diet. I am on the mat. Pinned. A more apt metaphor: an anvil on my chest.

My nipple leaks blue radioactive dye for several weeks, a disconcerting residue from surgery that chooses to show up now along with everything else.

scaring small children

In January I attend a cancer workshop for women. The idea is to leave us feeling we have taken back some of the control wrested from us during our various treatments. The first half concentrates on make up and skin care and sets what I think will be the tone for an empowering afternoon. It is surprising and moving to see how many companies are donating to women struggling with drastic appearance changes.

The second half of the workshop is presented by a woman whose specialty is hair loss. She has brought hats, scarves and wigs, and a number of edicts: "You have to be covered up when you leave the house: hat, wig, scarf … you don't want people to know there is anything wrong with you." "Every day with hair is a good day." "Don't shave your head completely." "You don't want to be running around bald and scaring small children."

you don't want people to know

you have to be covered up

you don't want to be running around bald

I am one of several women attending who has already lost her hair. Admittedly I am the only one who does not have my head covered. Still I am shocked at her comments and the subtext. It is not acceptable to look sick. Neither in the workshop nor on the organization's website is there any mention of baldness as an option let alone how to do it well.

you have to be covered up

That night I write a letter expressing my concerns and ask them to seriously take another look at the message they are sending. It is not empowering to be told that you must hide your cancer in order to be accepted. It is not empowering to made to feel uncomfortable about your appearance, your diagnosis. I do receive an immediate answer and an apology.

don't shave your head

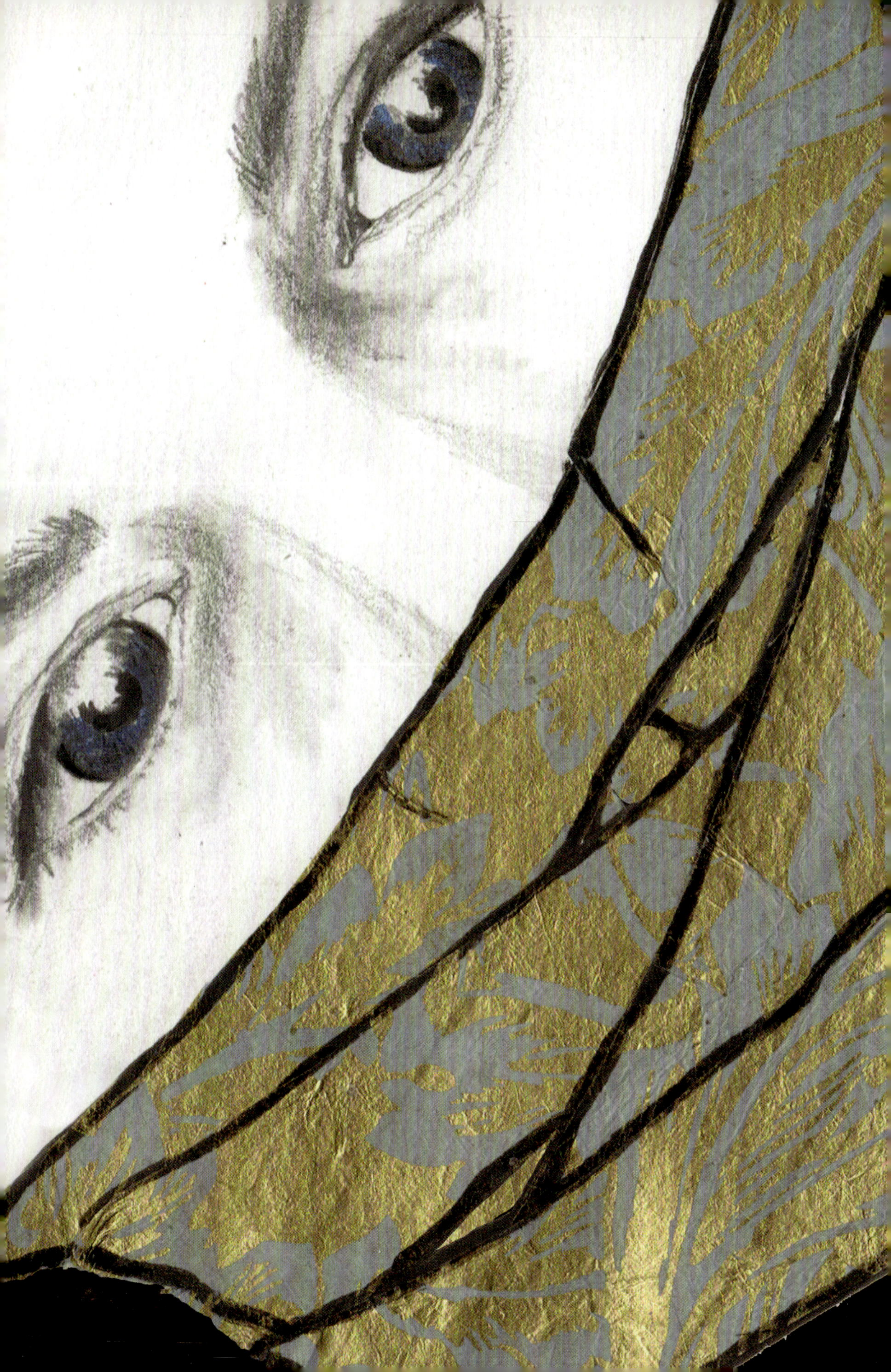

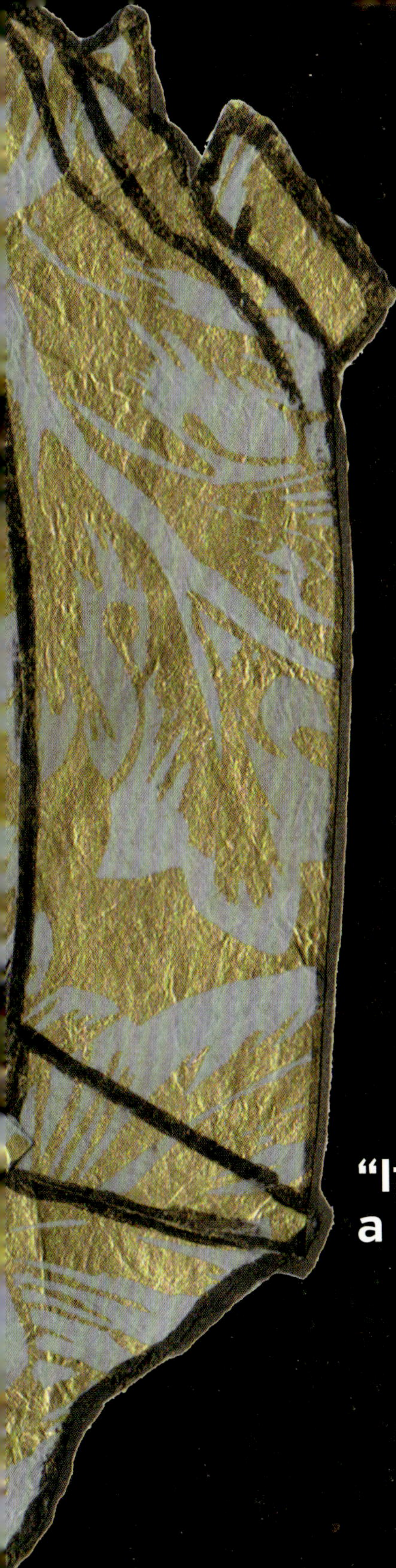

Not for the first time I suspect that in voicing my displeasure with the system, with this disease, I have broken one more unwritten law. The law of the stiff upper lip. I am suffering from erectile dysfunction of the lip. I am causing discomfort to people. The good patients. The ones who do what they are told no questions asked. My loose lips are flapping in the breeze like Fido's ears when he hangs his head out the window on a car ride.

In my naivety, I thought that I was in a reasonably sophisticated urban environment. I live in Alberta, home of the oil rigger and the cowboy. But symphonies, galleries, theatre, festivals are also a big part of the culture. I spend a morning at an art school I attended years ago, and the reactions to my baldness surprise me. Admittedly I have a take-no-prisoners attitude about whipping off my hat. But I anticipated less shock here where shock value is a main currency. What is it about bald women that is so jarring? Doug's opinion:

"It is different for men. We have a pattern named after us."

Our friend, Frank, is kind enough to tell me I look "hot" and that is what the students are staring at. I am not sold on the theory. The looks waver between "that poor woman, is she sick?" and "OMG what on earth is she thinking!" I am quite obviously not a punk rocker - not at my age. The temporary tattoos on the back of my skull probably don't help.

Not long afterward at the mall I fall in love with and buy a dinner plate size pair of Prada sunglasses. Although I still hope that my eyelashes and eyebrows won't fall out, if they do, these babies will cover everything. I feel incredibly chic and slightly broke. There is no problem so large it cannot be solved by Prada. Later when we meet up with our friends, Marjan and Colin, I am wearing a retro 60s coat in a vibrant turquoise colour and my new sunglasses. I feel unstoppable. Marjan tells me that every head turned as I sail through the door.

People's reactions continue to surprise me, for good and ill. I am sitting alone in a coffee shop, when a young man walks over to my table. He looks a little awkward. "I don't know why you made the choice you did but, you look fantastic." He walks away.

At the clinic, during my routine blood work, a young woman yells from across the room "Hey! You look beautiful bald."

A small child in the street asks her mother "Is that a man or a lady?" Her mother is uncomfortable, unable to meet my eyes.

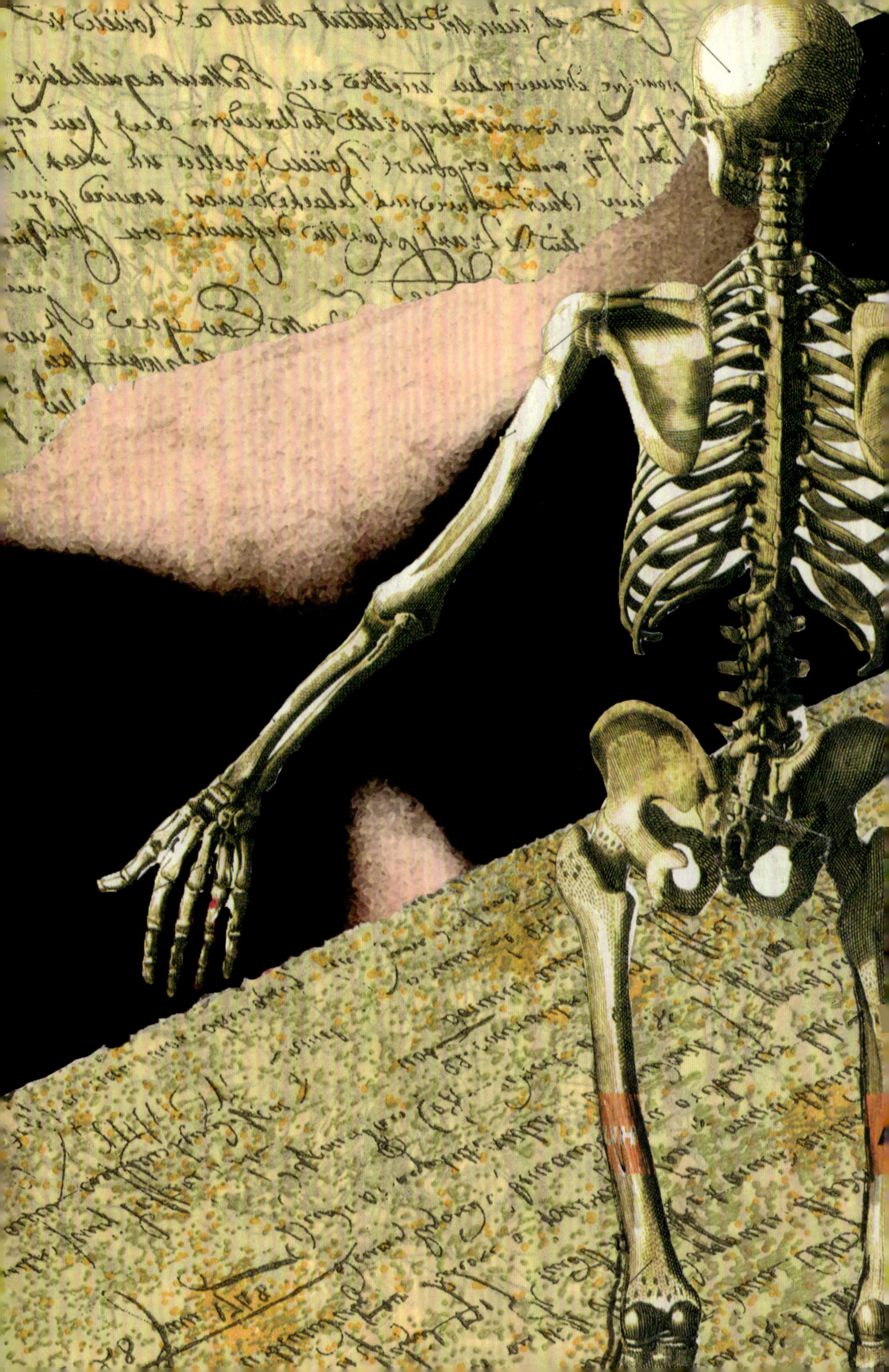

For my next appointment, I have Dr. O's substitute. She is cold, clinical and humourless. Just the facts ma'am. Just the facts. I make the mistake of asking about my upcoming switch to the drug Docetaxel. I have been reading about it and am worried. I seek reassurance. I have asked the wrong person.

She details the potential side effects. I might notice changes in my nails and skin. I might experience neuropathy. An extreme drop in white blood cells might compromise my immune system. I might stop breathing while the drugs are being administered. I take it all pretty much in stride until she mentions severe swelling in the legs and feet. What can I do about it? Keep your legs up.

Wear compression stockings. With these?

I say, pointing to my stiletto leopard print boots. You have got to be fucking kidding me! She looks shocked. Doug is snickering behind his hand. He knows my lifelong love affair with footwear.

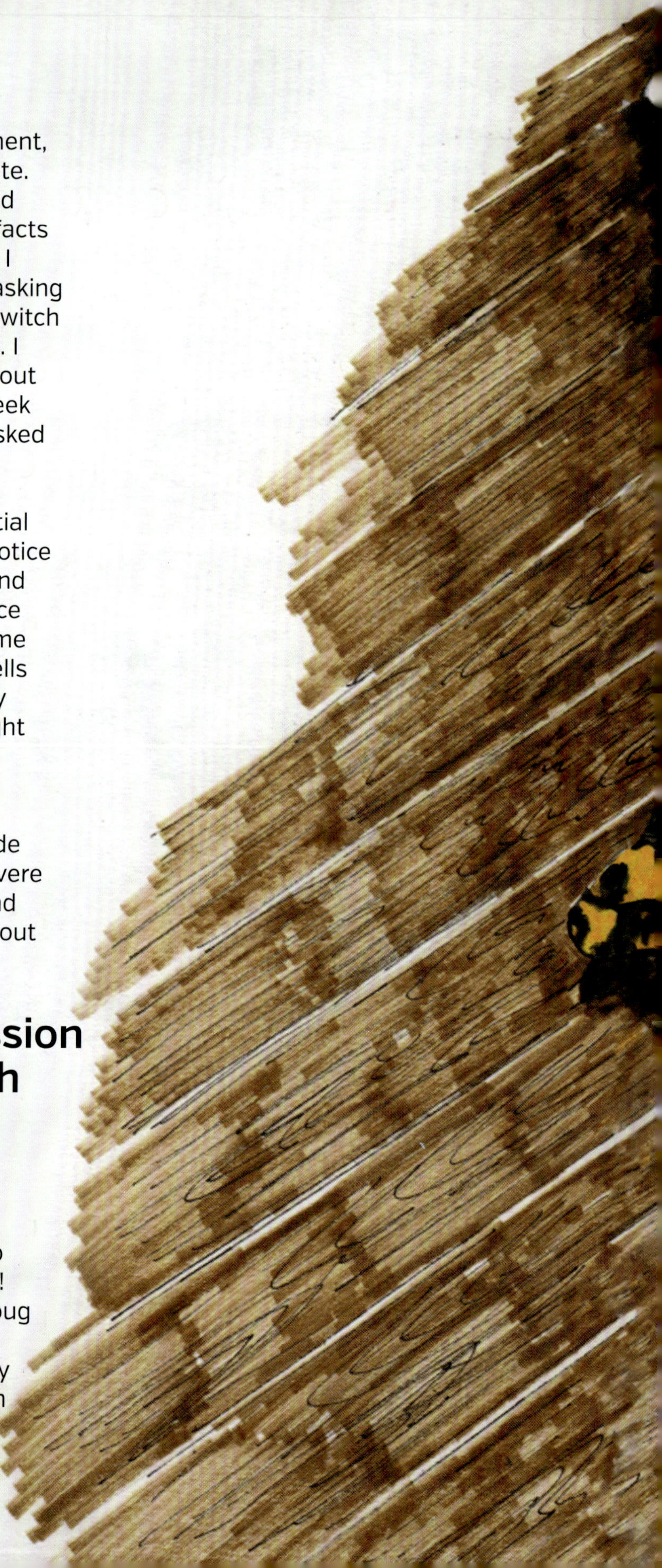

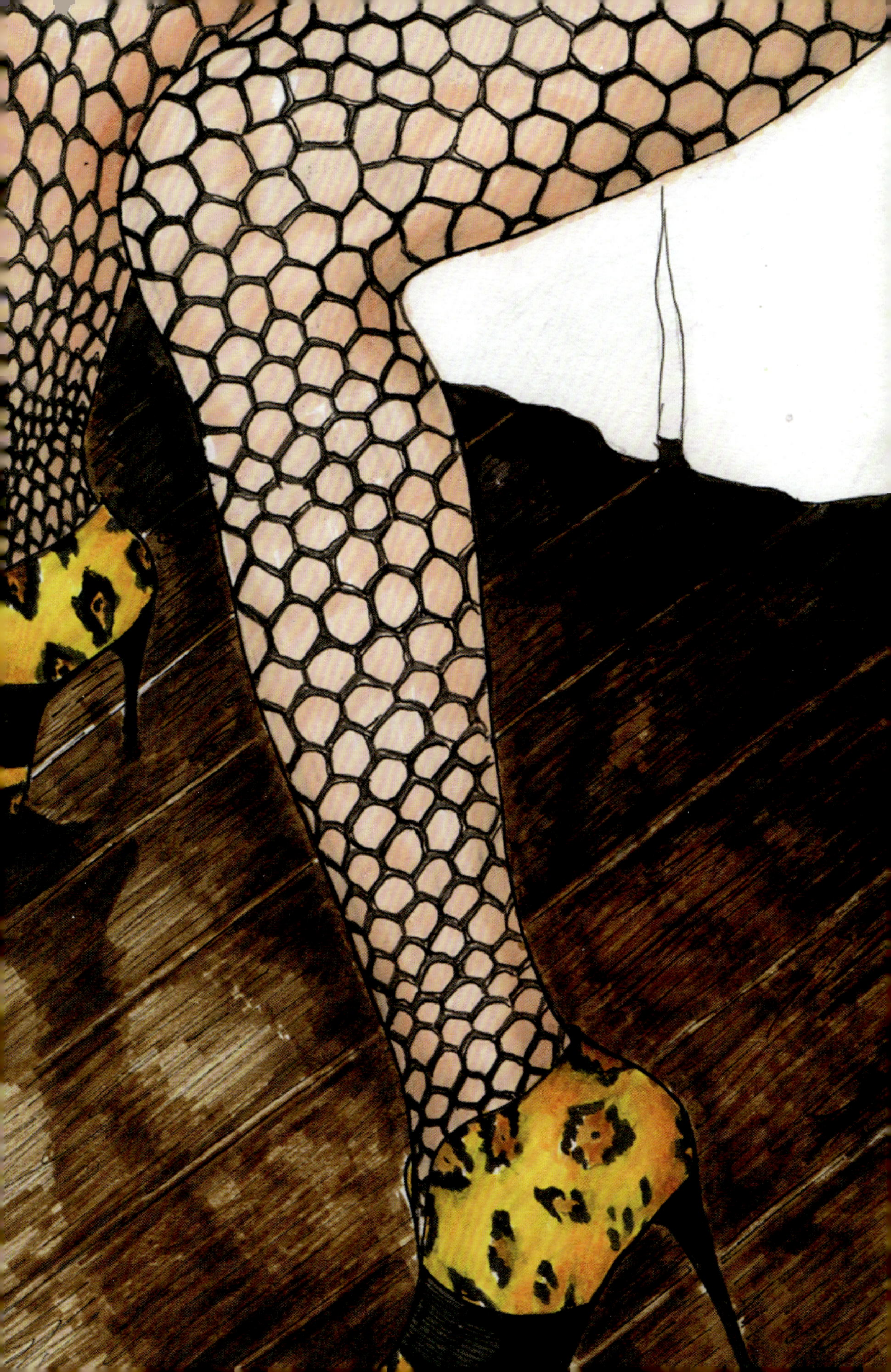

Because treatment has been going well, I decide to visit my mother again. After all, what can happen? Doug is dropping me off; my brother Jeff is picking me up.

The flight is a gong show. Welcome to chemo fog brain. I end up in the wrong seat and have to move. When I collect my luggage I put my handbag down and walk away and don't realize until I am halfway across the airport that it is sitting by the carousel, abandoned. Already exhausted, I make the trek back to fetch it. Outside, I let go of the luggage cart for just a moment and it runs off the curb hurtling into the path of an oncoming vehicle. Luckily it is my brother and he slams on the brakes. As he puts my luggage into the car he asks me where Mom is. How should I know? I thought she was with you. She came in to meet me at the gate and I was the first person off the aircraft. Somehow I failed to recognize my own mother. Though to be fair, she didn't see me either. When I go back, she is deep in conversation with someone she has just met.

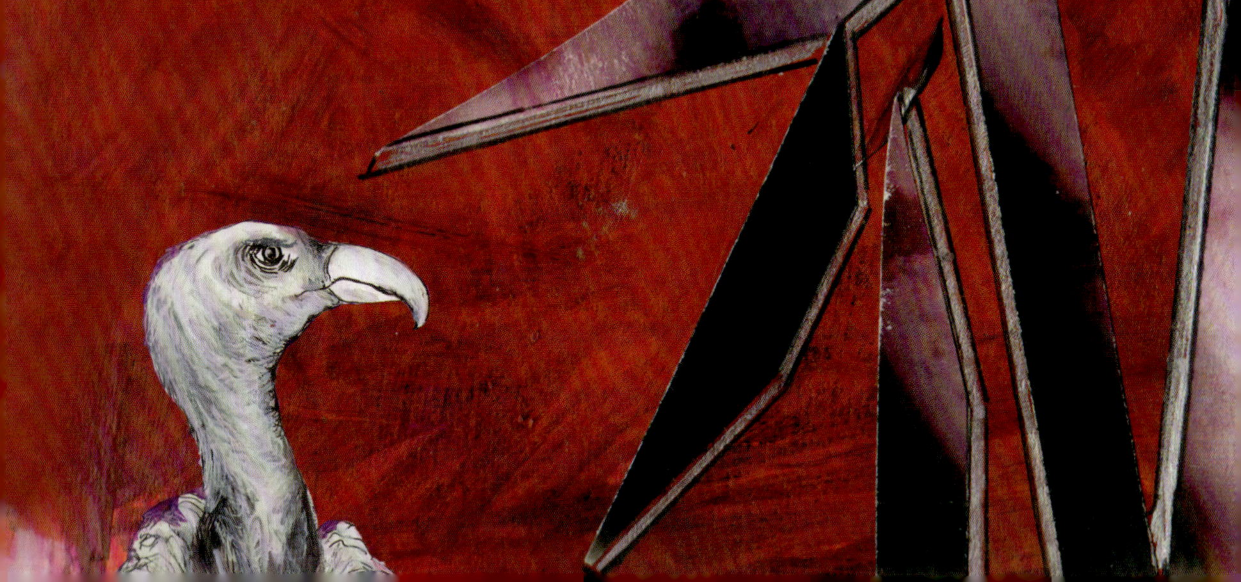

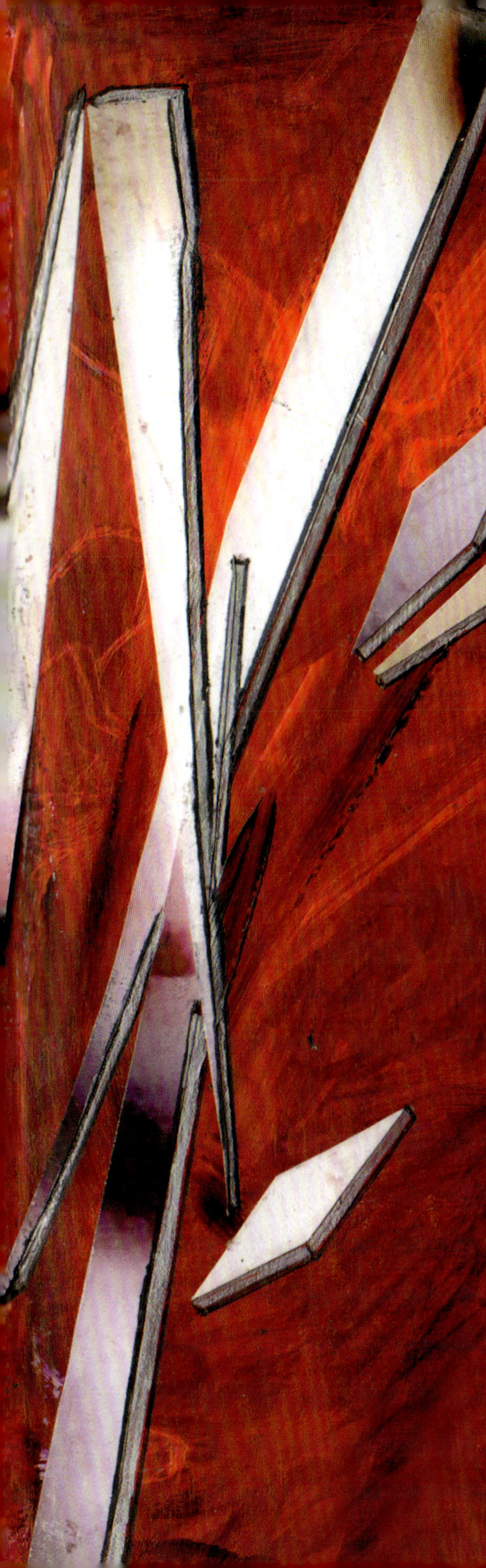

I sleep heavily for the first few days I am home. It is good for me to be with my Mom and she realizes I am doing alright. On Friday night she and I attend a banquet given in honour of an old friend, Harry Michael. I wear a hat as I am unsure what reception my bald head will get. At a party later that evening I bravely whip it off. There are murmurs of "you look great", sidelong glances, and an amazing number of people who want to touch my head. Most people ask. Not my friends ... it appears my head is now community property. I've heard pregnant women complain about their bellies becoming a site for public interaction but this is the first time I've experienced anything like it. Incidentally, I doubt rubbing it will bring you good luck.

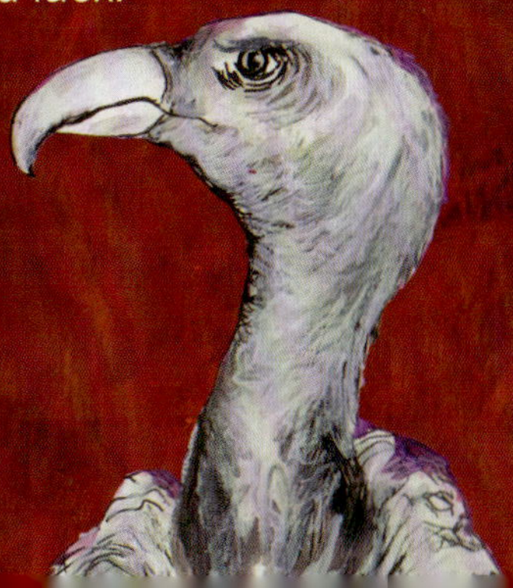

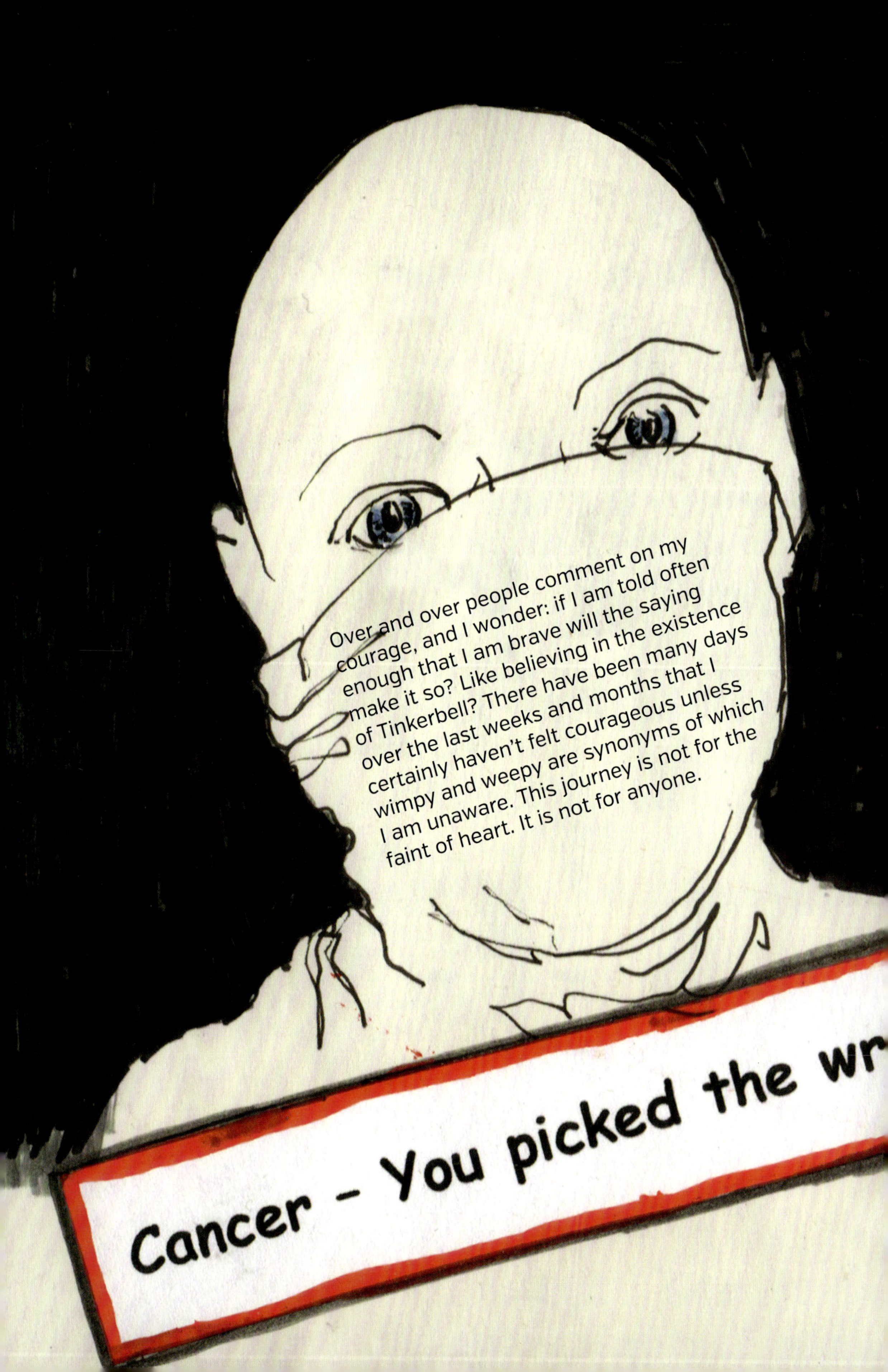
Over and over people comment on my courage, and I wonder: if I am told often enough that I am brave will the saying make it so? Like believing in the existence of Tinkerbell? There have been many days over the last weeks and months that I certainly haven't felt courageous unless wimpy and weepy are synonyms of which I am unaware. This journey is not for the faint of heart. It is not for anyone.
Cancer - You picked the wr

On the way home the airport security guard wants me to remove my hat. Apparently there's a possibility I am hiding something underneath it. When I show him I am hiding nothing, not even hair, he has the decency to look embarrassed and passes me through. On the plane I sit beside a gentleman who exchanges pleasantries with me until the hat comes off. All conversation ceases. Perhaps he thinks I am infectious.

I arrive home late. Tired. In my diminished state this trip rates as a huge accomplishment. I feel fortified for the next stage. I have no idea I will look back at the first treatments and think how easy they were.

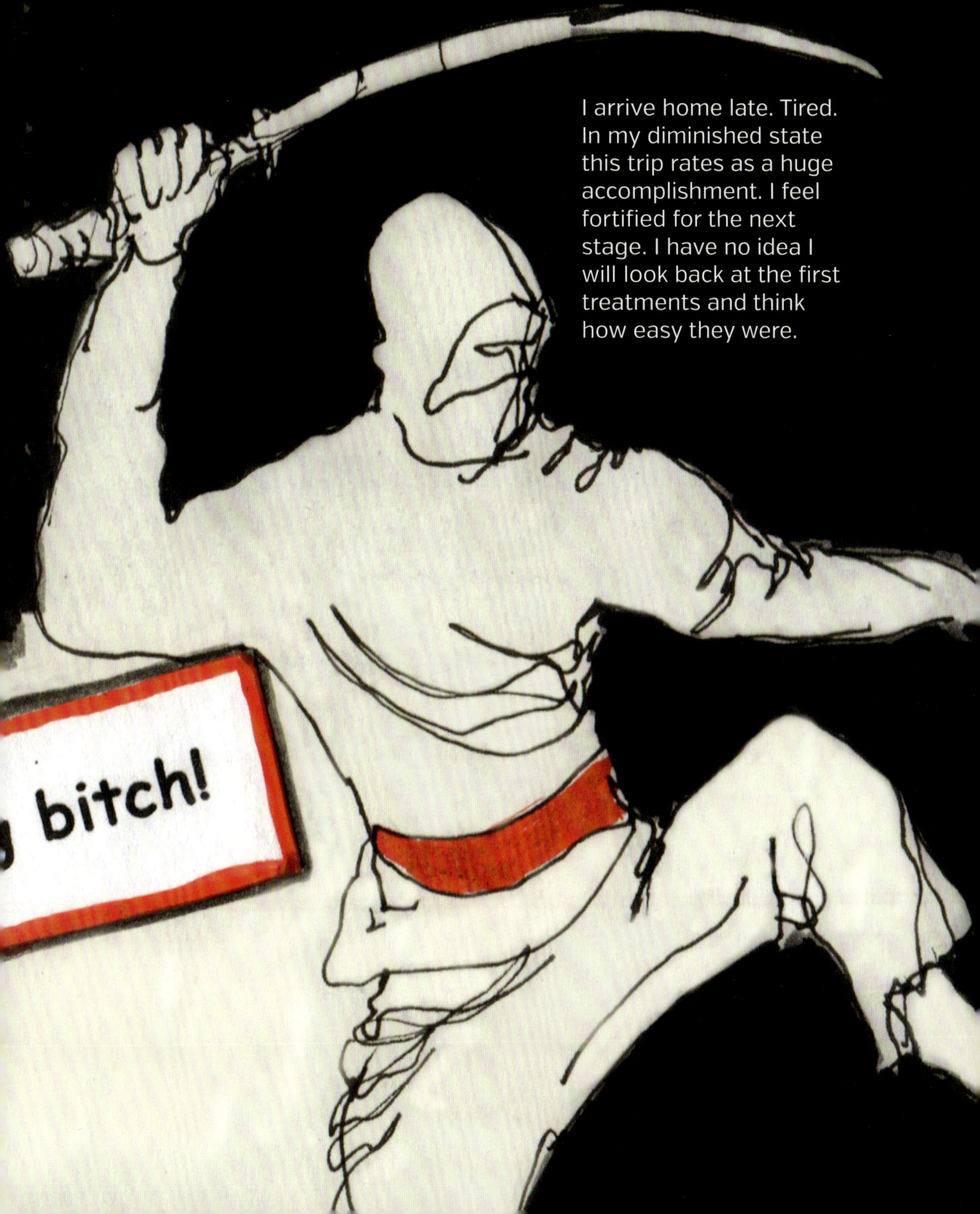

My sense of triumph is overshadowed by the loss of my eyebrows and eyelashes. It happens gradually over a few weeks. One eye retains a couple of lashes, one eyebrow has two hairs. They are valiant in the face of adversity so I refuse to pull them out. I didn't really believe this was going to happen. Not to me. I draw pictures in my sketchbook of things I look like: lizards, turtles, a tennis ball, a couple of Harry Potter characters. There's a whole series of them, none of them very flattering.

The eyebrows I ordered months ago prove to be almost impossible to glue on straight and I appear either sardonic or confused. They don't move with your skin. The eyebrow tattoos are the same. Unless I'm planning on having Botox injections to freeze my forehead I can't envision this working. I purchase several kinds of eyebrow pencils and powder.

What kind of art instructor am I if I can't draw on a couple of eyebrows?

Over the next several months, I am asked repeatedly where I got my highly realistic eyebrows.

I also give up attempting to attach false eyelashes to a naked lid, after losing one in the middle of a lunch and finding it clinging spider-like to my cheekbone. I use eyeliner but have to be careful not to poke myself in the eye as there is nothing to stop the brush from slipping off.

I change my mind about people who shave their heads for fundraising or to show solidarity with people who are undergoing cancer treatment. Their hearts may be in the right place but a bald head is only half the way there. I find myself thinking, if you really want to go all the way try plucking out your eyebrows and eyelashes. Only then can you know what I look at in the morning when I wake up.

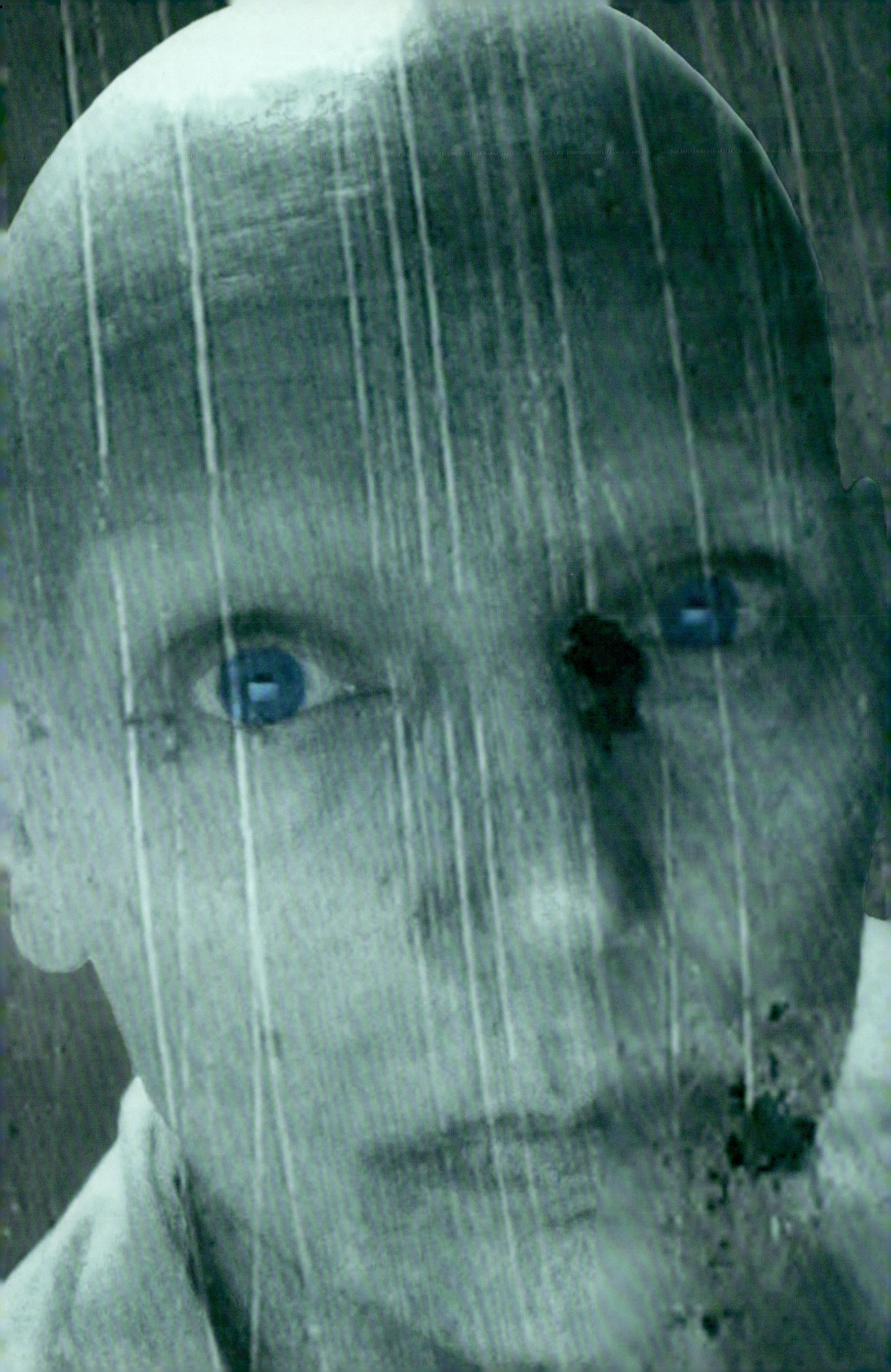

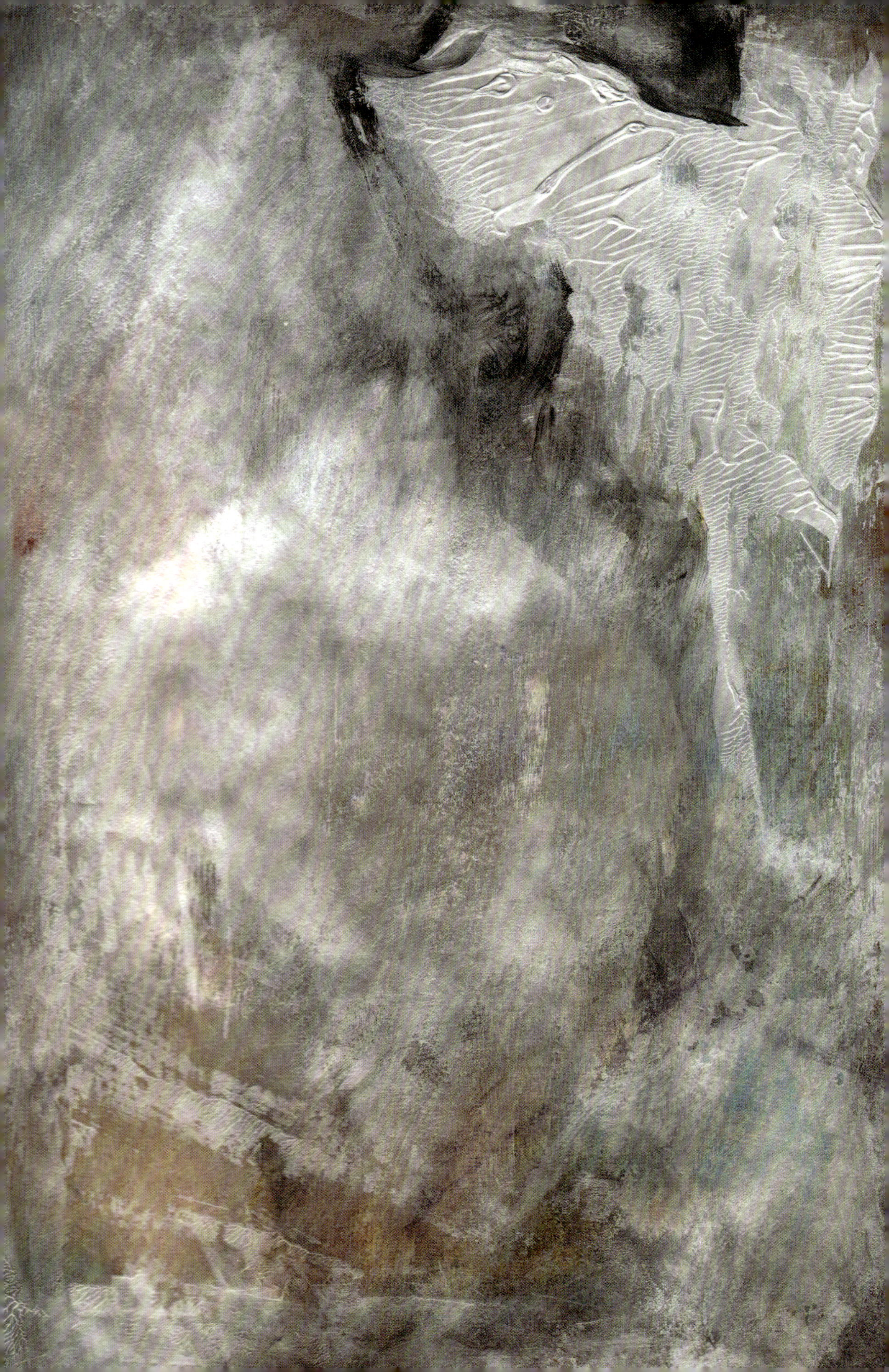

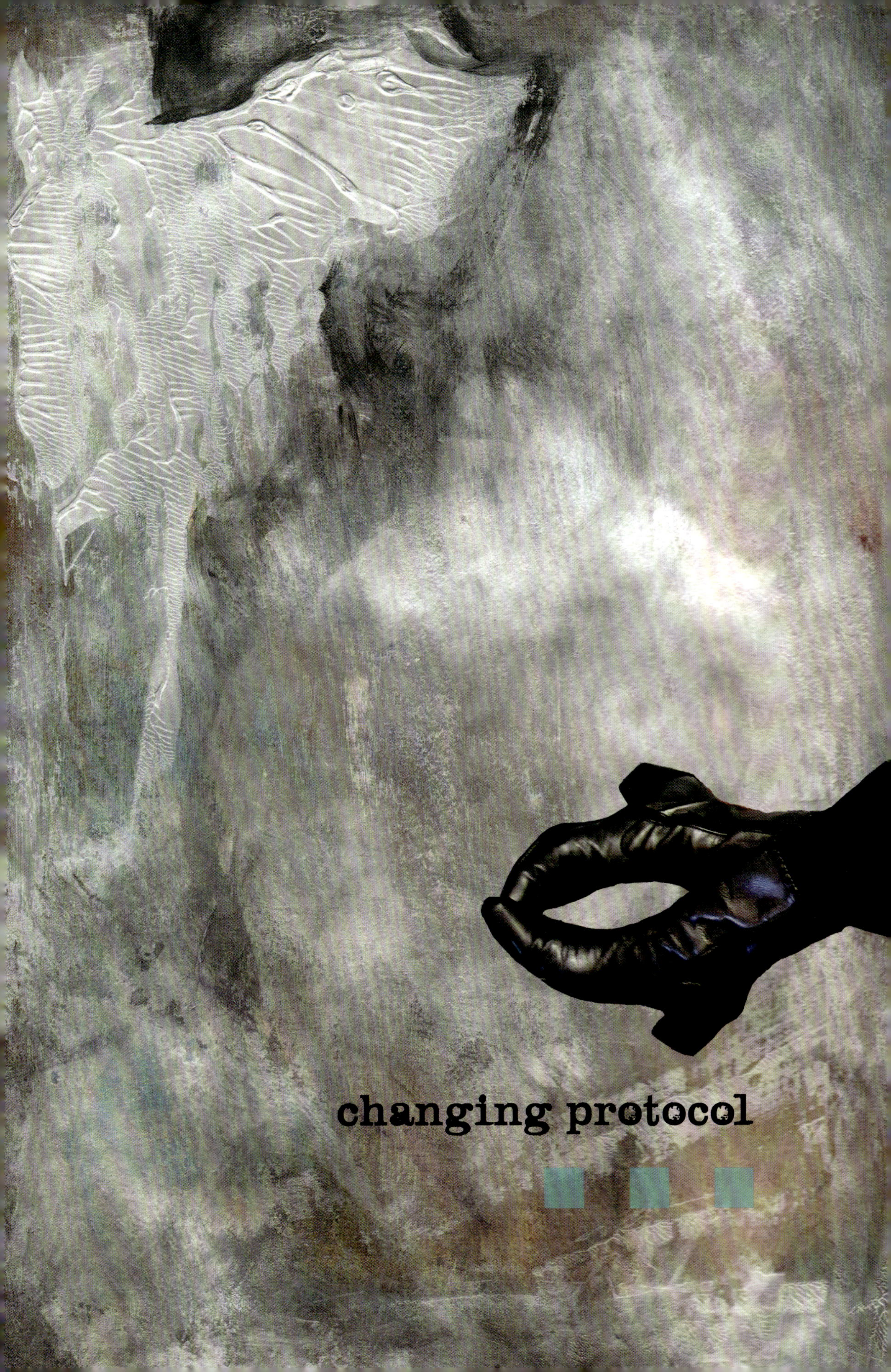

changing protocol

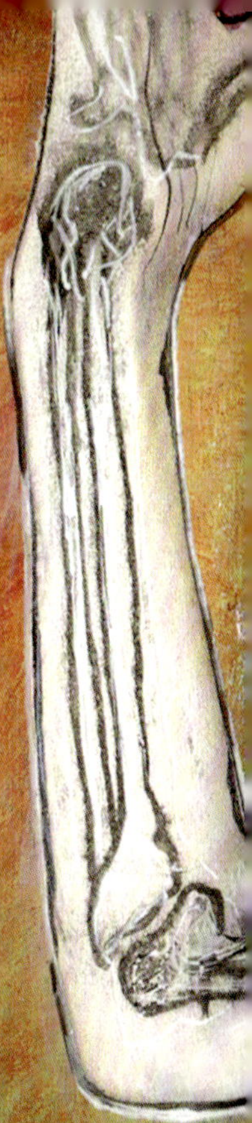

My protocol is changing for the last three sessions. Dr. O prescribes Neulasta to counteract the neutropenia (a severe drop in the white blood cells) that the new chemo drug causes. Unfortunately, its side effect is intense bone pain. He casually mentions it is expensive, and, thinking he means in the range of the anti-nausea drugs which were $40 a pill, I don't ask further. Later I discover it is $2600 per dose.

I am directed to an agency to help sort out the $7800 I will have to pay for the drug. My insurance company tells me they will refund it after I spend the money. But I explain to the agency woman that the first big insurance claim I sent in for my prescriptions was lost. The company maintained I never provided the receipts. I had the photocopies but they refused to pay without the originals. Their representative was worse than unhelpful. They did not lose things. It was out of her control. Not her problem. She hung up. In an act of desperation I called the pharmacist, who assured me it was a common occurrence and she could re-issue "originals." It took almost two months to be reimbursed. I am not optimistic about being paid quickly for this new batch of drugs.

The woman at the agency arranges for the drug company to cover the first batch of Neulasta; another agency agrees to advance the money to pay for the second one. How do people with no money, no insurance, or will to fight manage? Do they simply go without?

You have to administer the drug yourself. Doug receives a lesson from the oncologist's nurse, who fills a syringe and shows him how to inject it. They practice by stabbing the bed in the examining room. "Jam it in," she says. "Don't try to be kind." After several attempts he finally masters it. I am wary as my skin is a lot thinner than Naugahyde. And the bed is less jumpy and less prone to complaining.

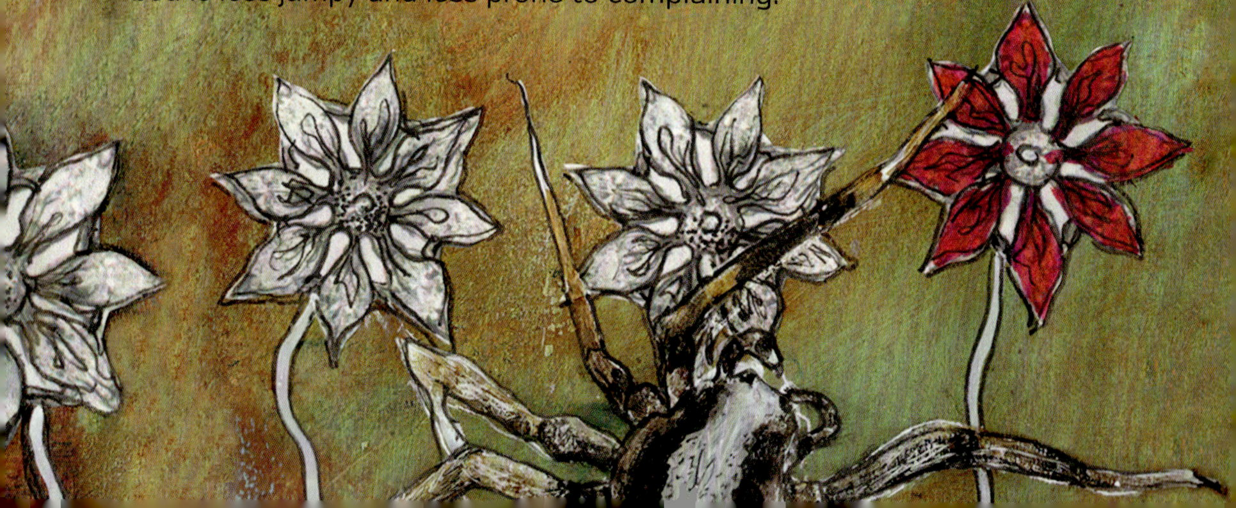

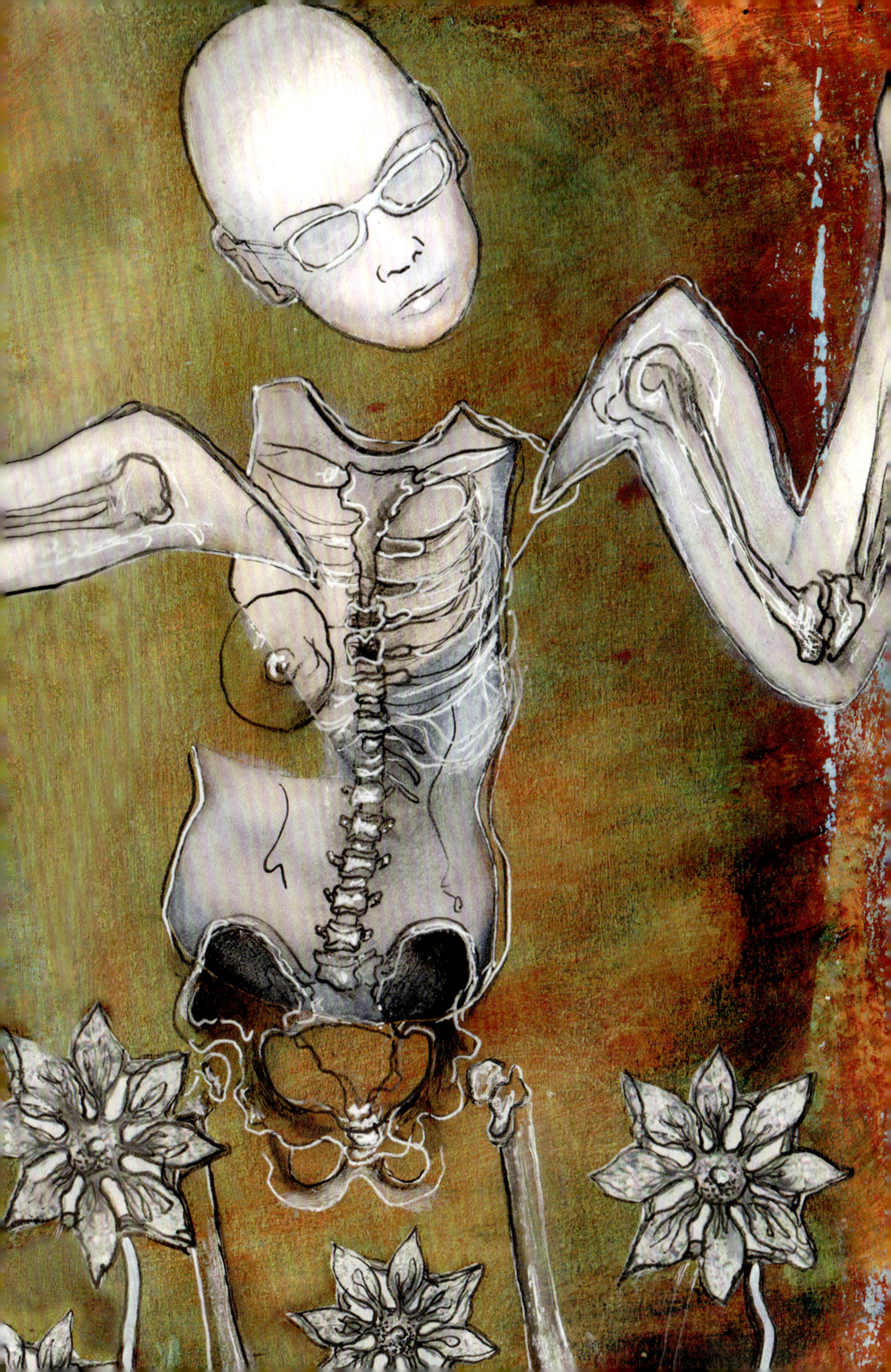

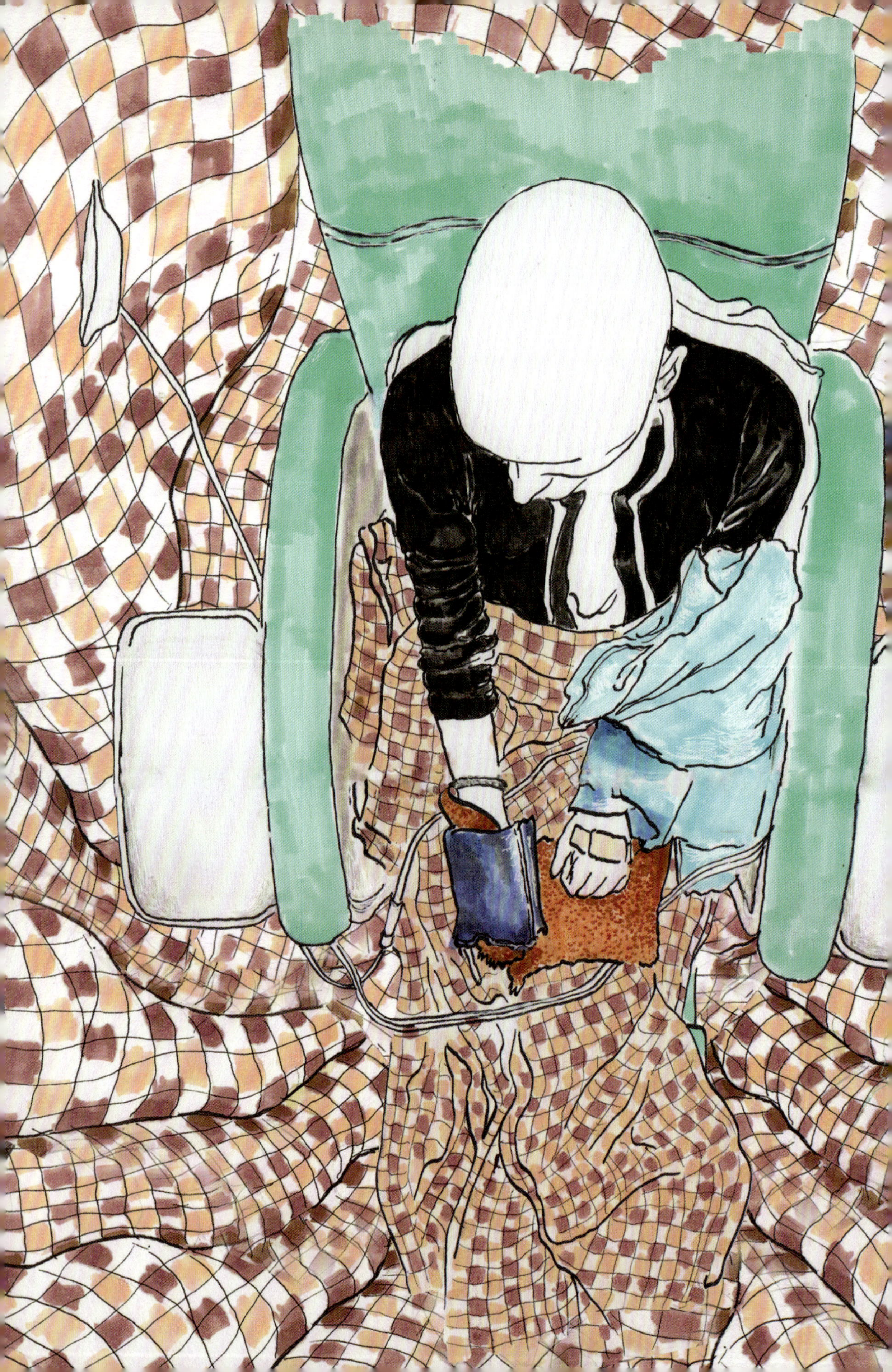

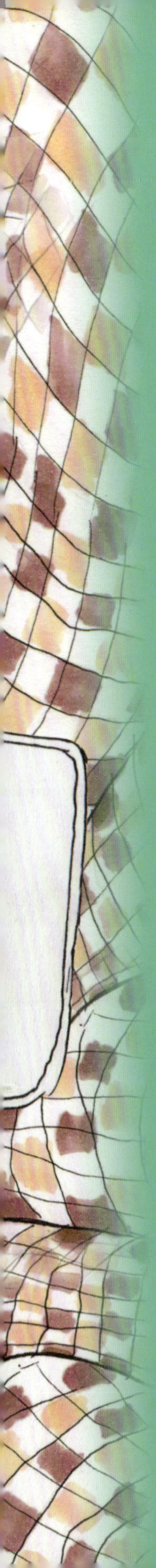

The next morning the chemotherapy with the new drug goes without incident. I am closely monitored by the nursing staff as a small percentage of people react immediately to the drug. I don't appear to be one of them so they put band-aids on the injection sites and send me home. This is what happens:

Friday February 17 evening: I have the usual loopiness on the Benadryl and steroids.

Saturday February 18: I remain loopy. That afternoon I lie on my stomach on the bed while Doug tries to give me the Neulasta. He simply cannot *not* be kind. At the first prick I jump. He jumps. The needle flies through the air and lands, thankfully, on the bed not the floor. All I can think of is the cost. On the second attempt, I tell him, Jab! He does. We both look startled.

Sunday February 19: the pain in my hips starts. Like electric currents or flashing lights. If light were painful. I start on a painkiller, Naproxin.

I wake up. The clock says three in the morning. I feel a little funny. I pull myself out of bed and stumble into the bathroom. When I turn on the light, I barely recognize my reflection. My face is swollen, my eyes are mere slits and both the inside and outside of my lips are visible. My tongue fills my entire mouth and it briefly crosses my mind that if it gets much worse I won't be able to breathe. I do the only sensible thing and decide to go back to bed. I have had enough. I will either wake up in the morning or I won't. Surprisingly I fall asleep.

Monday February 20: Doug panics at the sight of my face and wants to rush me to the hospital. To my surprise, I look marginally improved from last night. He can't believe I didn't wake him. After much begging from me, he agrees to wait and during the day my face resembles a face again. I have no appetite.

Tuesday February 21: The pain continues in my hips and moves down into my legs. I have three or four mouth sores, a thick mucous nasal drip, and some neuropathy – pain and tingling in the thumbs and fingers of both hands.

Wednesday February 22: The bone pain is the same. More mouth sores, my tongue has remained swollen making it difficult to talk or swallow. I develop a rash across my chest. I have elephant skin: thick, swollen and bumpy, extremely itchy.

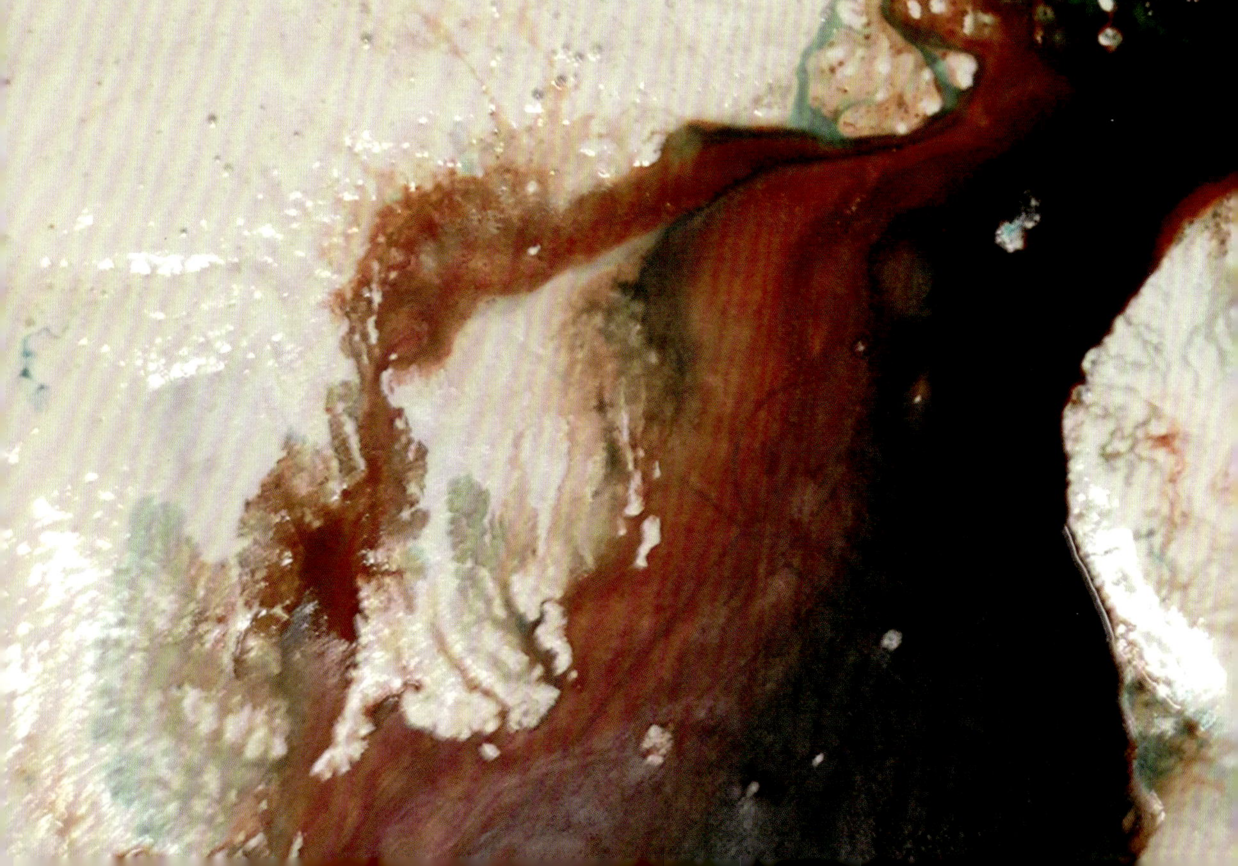

Thursday

February 23: The rash across my chest has spread up my neck. My swollen tongue and lack of appetite are making it difficult to get enough nutrition. At my last appointment the homeopath suggested adding whey protein to my smoothies when eating becomes really difficult, but I can only manage small amounts at a time.

I have reached new depths of fatigue. Today I manage in Bambi-like fashion to struggle to my feet and keep my legs under me. I can hear Thumper in the background saying “he don't walk so good – do he?” I make it from the bed to the couch.

Today is my birthday.

Friday

February 24: The rash is improving with an over-the-counter hydro-cortisone.

Saturday

February 25: My tongue is almost normal.

Sunday February 26: My left hand is developing what resembles chemical burns: a half circle on the base of my left thumb is spreading to the fingers, which are starting to itch and swell. My left heel is also burning and uncomfortable, but I hardly notice because of the pain in my hand.

Monday February 27: My right hand and palm are affected with the same strange marks. Both hands are now swollen. The burns have spread down my left arm. I have marks where the band-aids were. Echoes of the shape. My mouth sores have almost healed. Somewhere along the line, my hips have stopped hurting but it could be that everything else is distracting me from noticing.

Tuesday February 28: My right hand is practically useless. I call the Cancer Centre and report my strange symptoms. The triage nurse says my reaction is normal and suggests I take an antihistamine and Extra Strength Tylenol.

Wednesday February 29: I am consuming large amounts of Benadryl and have resumed pain killers. My hands have been dipped in a vat of acid. I am incapable of fine motor skills: doing up buttons, zippers, picking up small objects. I am seriously starting to question on what planet this treatment could possibly have an end result that is good. We take pictures to show my oncologist.

Thursday March 1: The swelling is receding. But my right heel has started to hurt. I have some sensitivity in the big toes of both feet.

I spend a lot of time on the couch in the living room. My mother phones frequently as do my sister, my brother, my friends. When I can't talk Doug fields the calls. Sometimes I talk, sometimes I cry.

Friday March 2: My appetite is returning. I am hungry but food tastes terrible.

Monday March 5: The swelling is down.

Tuesday March 6: My skin is peeling off in big leprous strips.

Although I am no Snow White I am living with the seven chemo dwarves.

Itchy
Weepy
Weary
Drippy
Achy
Queasy
Bitchy

They bring a friend:
Wimpy

I return to see Dr. O with a list of my side effects in addition to the photographs. Most of the pain has subsided and I am slightly less exhausted. I am supposed to take two more doses of this drug. The next one is tomorrow.

Dr. O is practically speechless when he sees the photographs of my hands. He has never seen this happen before. "Why didn't you come in? Phone?" I did phone, I say. I relate the message I was given. That this was "the norm." He is even more concerned when I tell him my lips, tongue and the inside of my mouth and throat were so swollen I could only swallow liquids. I should have been hospitalized, he says. He decides to try another drug from the same family. He worries that another dose of any of the "taxanes" could stop my breathing. Something I would like to continue doing.

The next day I try the new drug, Paclitaxel, to moderately improved results. A milder version of the burns on my hands returns.

A week later Dr. O hovers in the doorway to the examination room and says to Doug:

"Did you take the knives from her?"

Doug deadpans:

"I disarmed her before we left the house."

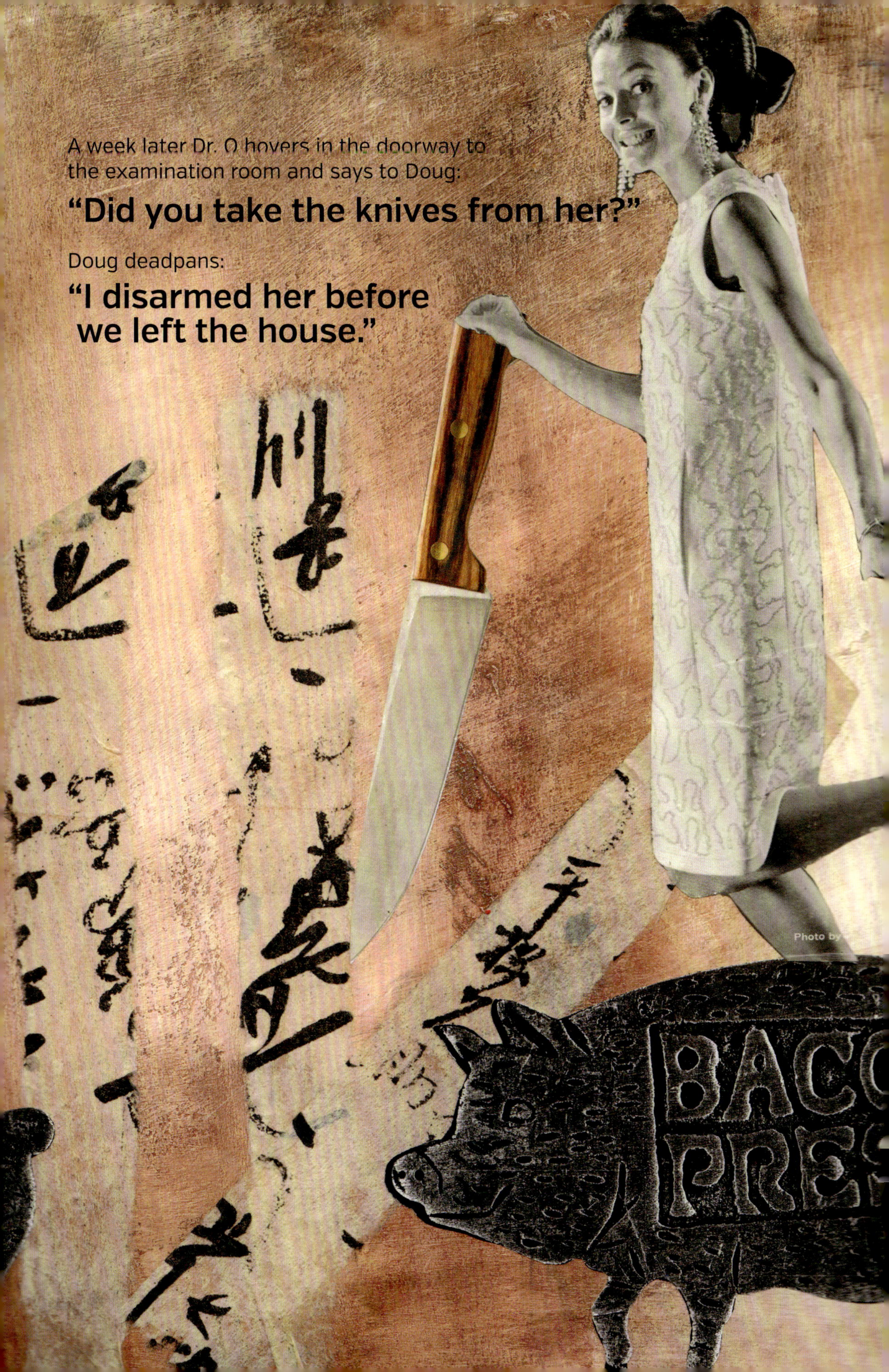

Taking into consideration my recurring symptoms and my blood work, which has plunged off the charts, Dr. O suspends my schedule. There is a strong possibility that we will have to stop completely. He tells me that approximately 20% of patients have to abandon treatment because of their inability to tolerate the drugs. I am half way between dancing in the street and worrying: What if it was not enough? He says that he honestly doesn't know exactly how much of the drug needs to be in my system to be effective. Perhaps dancing is premature. It is a challenge not to dwell on the idea that I could be "done" if not "finished." But the extra week with few, at times, no symptoms is wonderful. I can taste food. I have some energy and Doug claims I even laughed once.

Following a two-week break, Dr. O offers a lower dose, if I am willing. Any red flag symptoms, we call it a day. Instead of two treatments, 21 days apart, I will now have six weekly doses. I can't decide if I am proud of my perseverance or incredibly disappointed with myself for agreeing. I could have walked away.

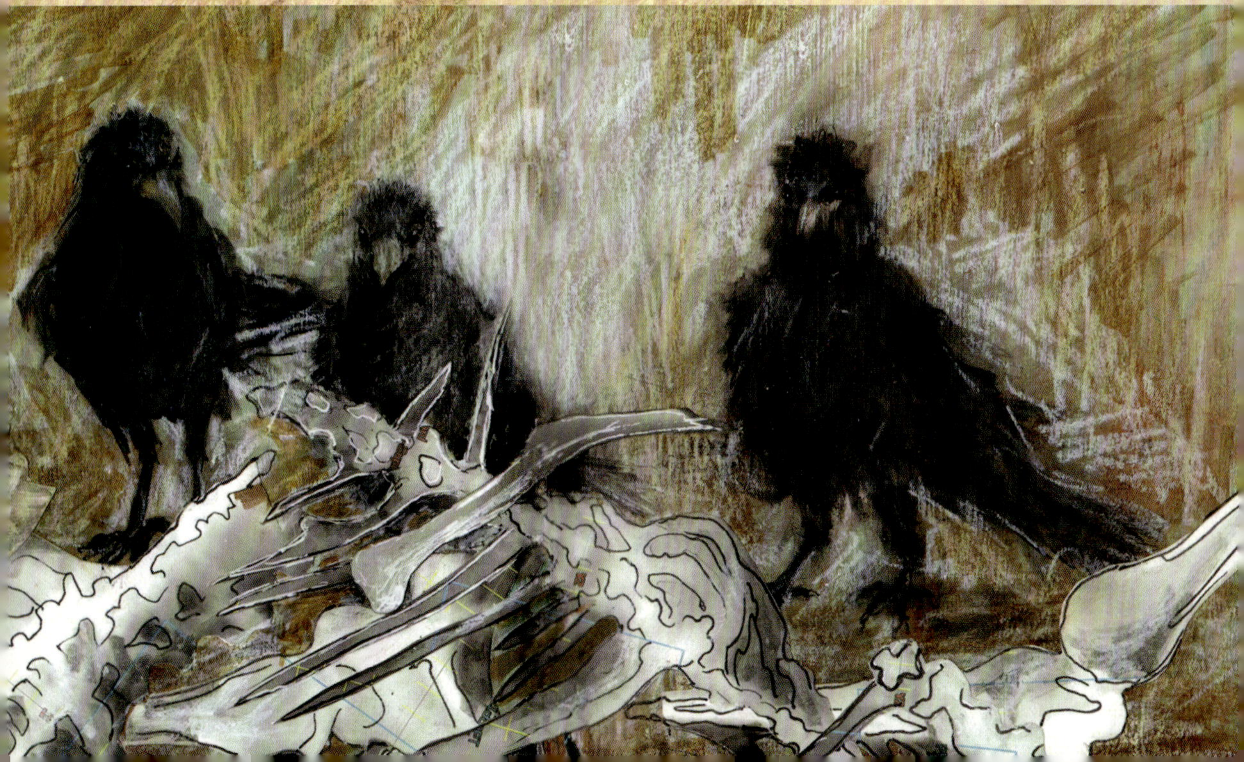

The following day I ask what dose I am being given. When the nurse shows me the written instructions I know they are wrong. She is more than a bit patronizing. Doug refers to the notes we have. I refuse to go any further until she calls Dr. O. She returns half an hour later and yes: the dosage was incorrect. We continue. I am one of the lucky ones. There are a half-dozen bad reactions to treatment happening all around me. The crash cart has to be called.

Unfortunately some of the side effects are not reversible and will simply run their course over the next several months. I will lose my fingernails, perhaps my toenails. I knew there was a possibility of nail abnormalities: ridges, lines, perhaps some discoloration. Although I believed I was becoming inured to the possible reactions ... I am floored. My oncologist shakes his head sadly "Tina, I am sorry you have had such a terrible time with this. You are probably in the 10%, possibly 5%, of people who have everything happen to them." He adds wryly, "You are skewing our statistics."

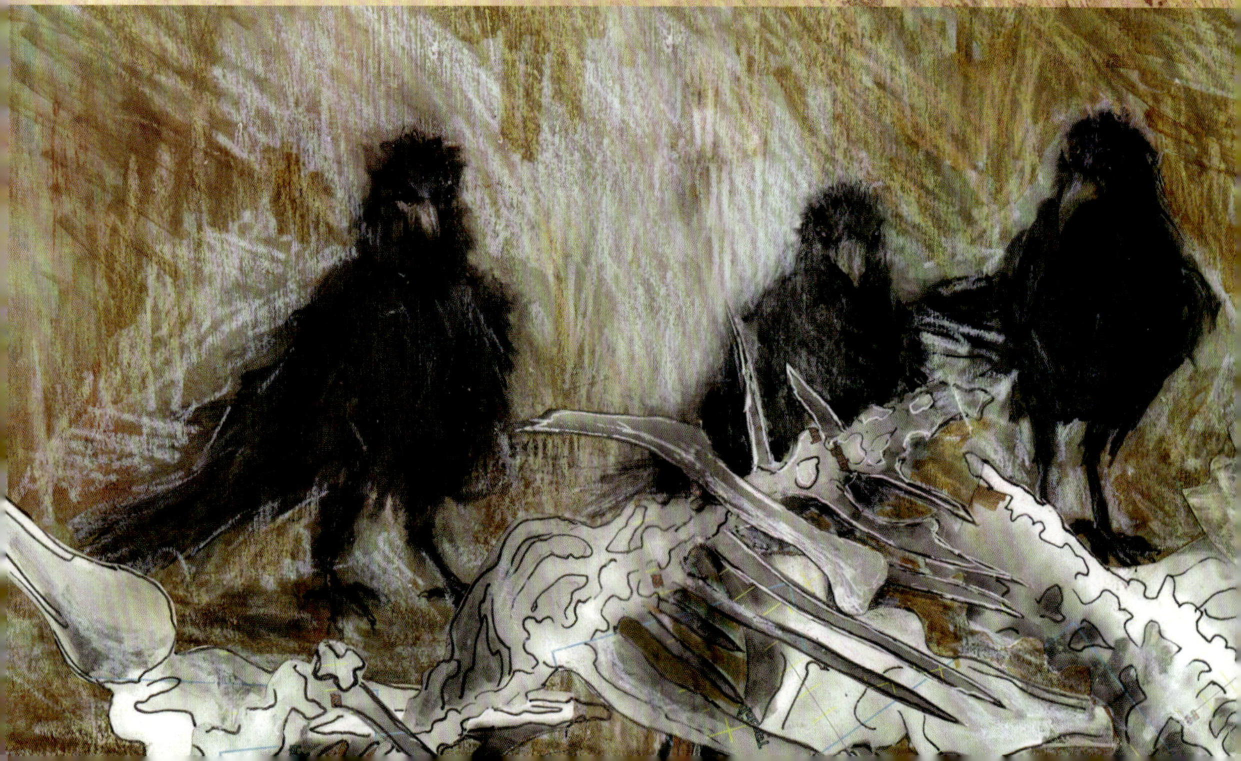

As if all of this were not quite enough I have found another large lump in my left breast.

I go for a mammogram and ultrasound and as soon as the radiologist on call receives the results she examines me. The lump is the size of a golf ball. I watch on the screen as she inserts a needle and it shrinks before my eyes. After two weeks of waiting for the appointment worrying that I had an aggressive and fast growing cancer, it is dealt with in a few minutes. She tells me it is nothing more than a nasty cyst, albeit one for the record book.

That night, at the end of my yoga practice, I decide to apologize to my broken and shattered body for the agony I have subjected it to. As my breath slides easily in and out I search for unity between body and mind. Stillness settles over me and I send a sincere and heartfelt I am sorry. I wait and listen. The reply comes back loud and clear:

"FUCK YOU LADY!"

I sense distrust and leave it for now.

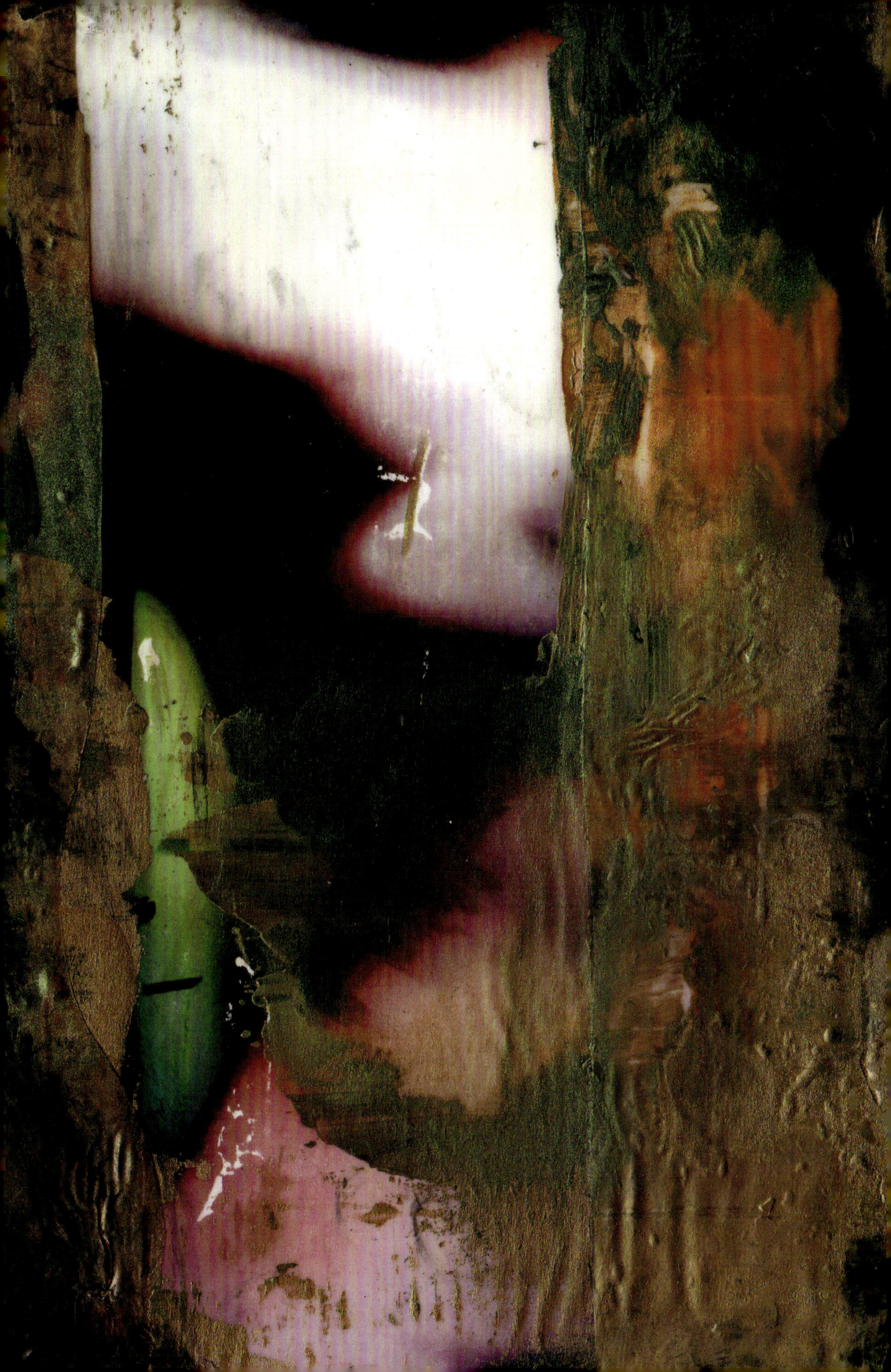

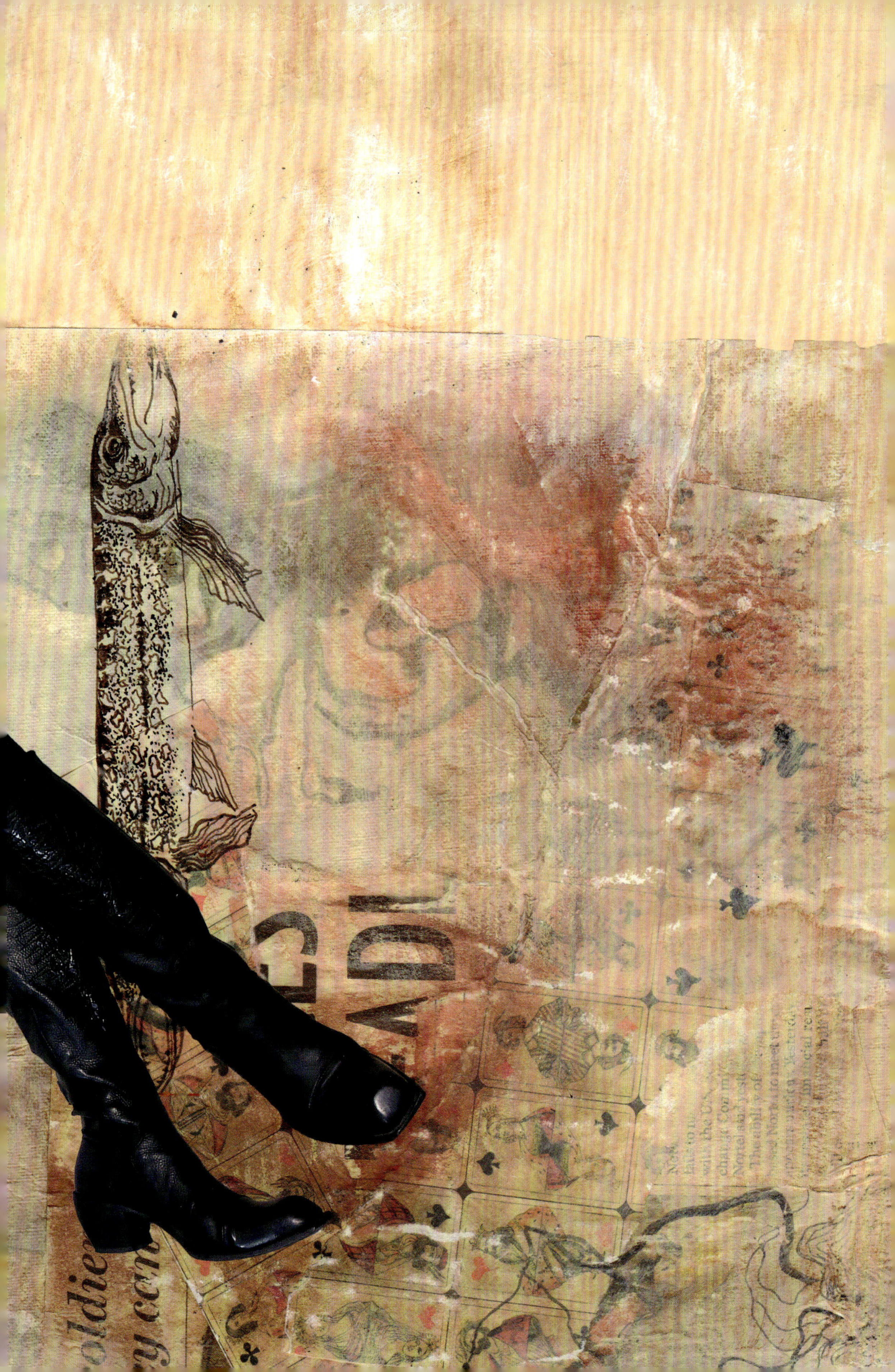

changing minds

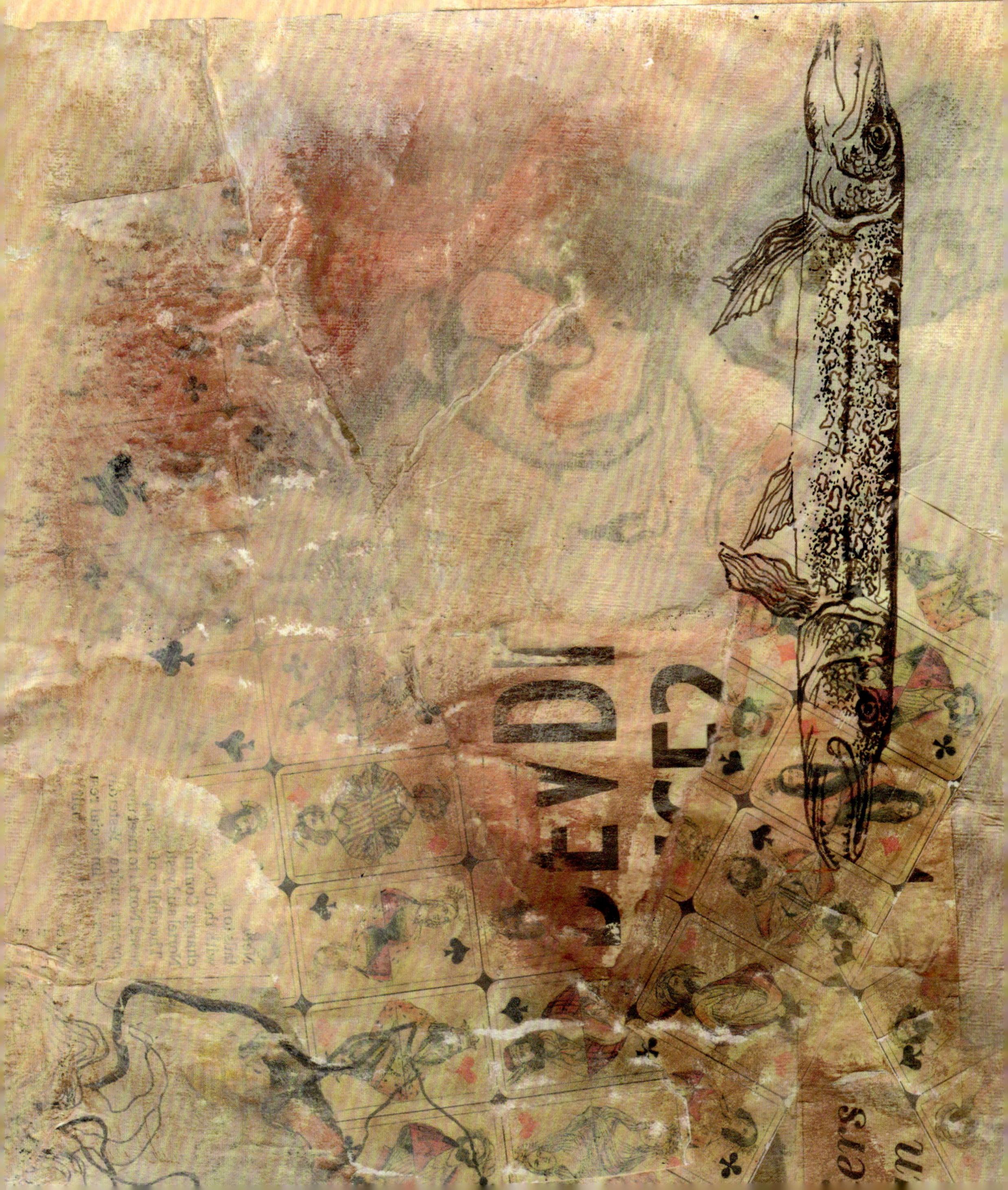

My friend Candace warned me that people would say the craziest things. And they did.

Some of my favourites:

Listing all the people you know who have died. I understand you are attempting to relate to what I'm going through. But somehow, telling me about your aunt, your sister or your neighbour and how they lost their struggle isn't particularly comforting at the moment.

"This will be over in no time." For you. Not for me. The days are endless when your bones ache, your hands hurt, food smells bad and tastes worse, and it is hard to lift your throbbing head off a pillow for longer than a couple of hours at a time. Yep, the next few months should just fly by.

"You look like your husband's twin." My husband is a handsome man. Did you catch the last part of that? M-A-N! Is this helpful to what is left of my fragile self-esteem? I have had a quarter of my breast removed, I am thin as a rail, completely hairless, exhausted, I have been pushed chemically into menopause and de-sexualized to the point of looking like a 14-year-old boy. Or so I thought. Now, apparently I look like a 54-year-old bald man. Do you wonder why I am not joining in the general hilarity?

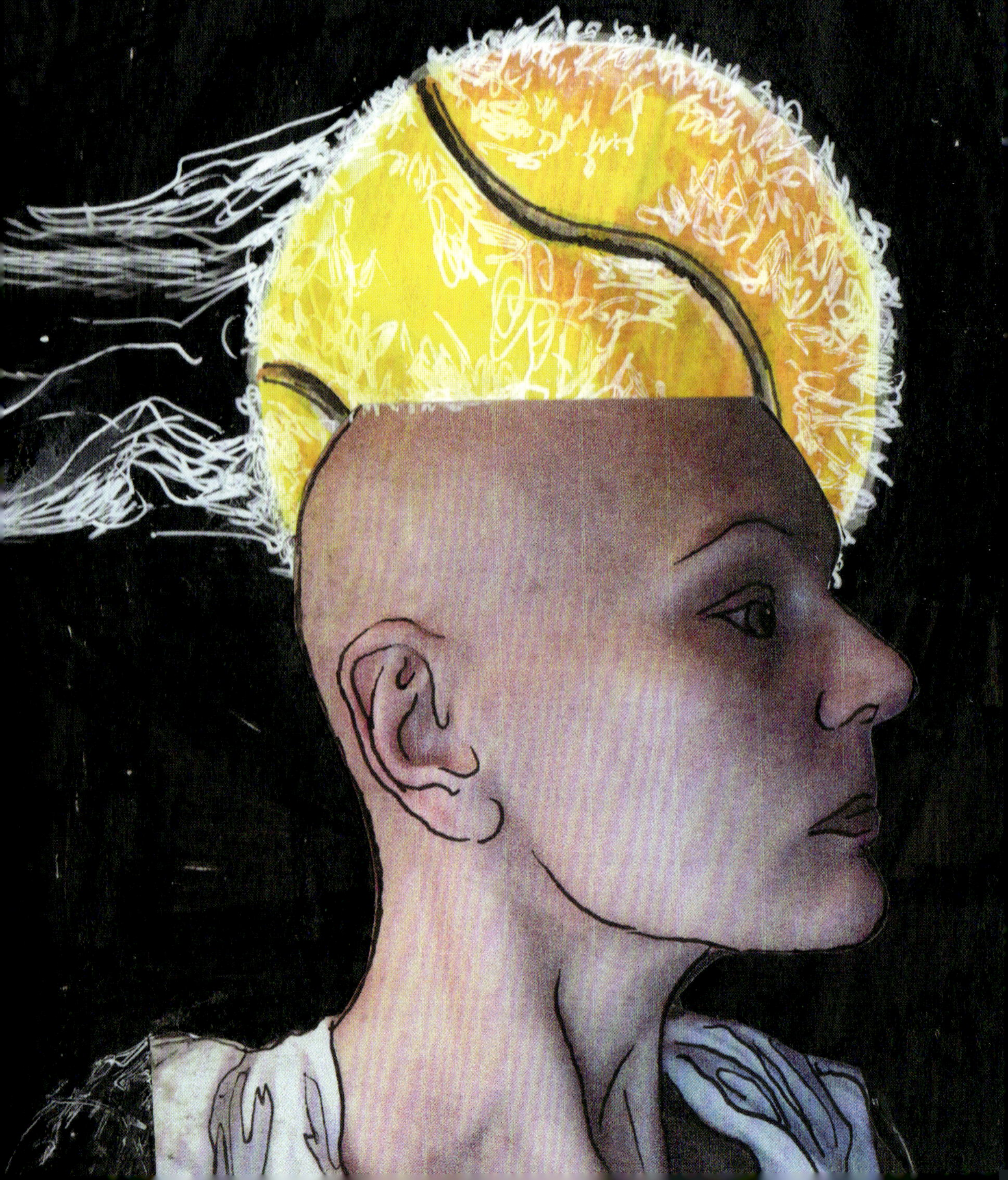

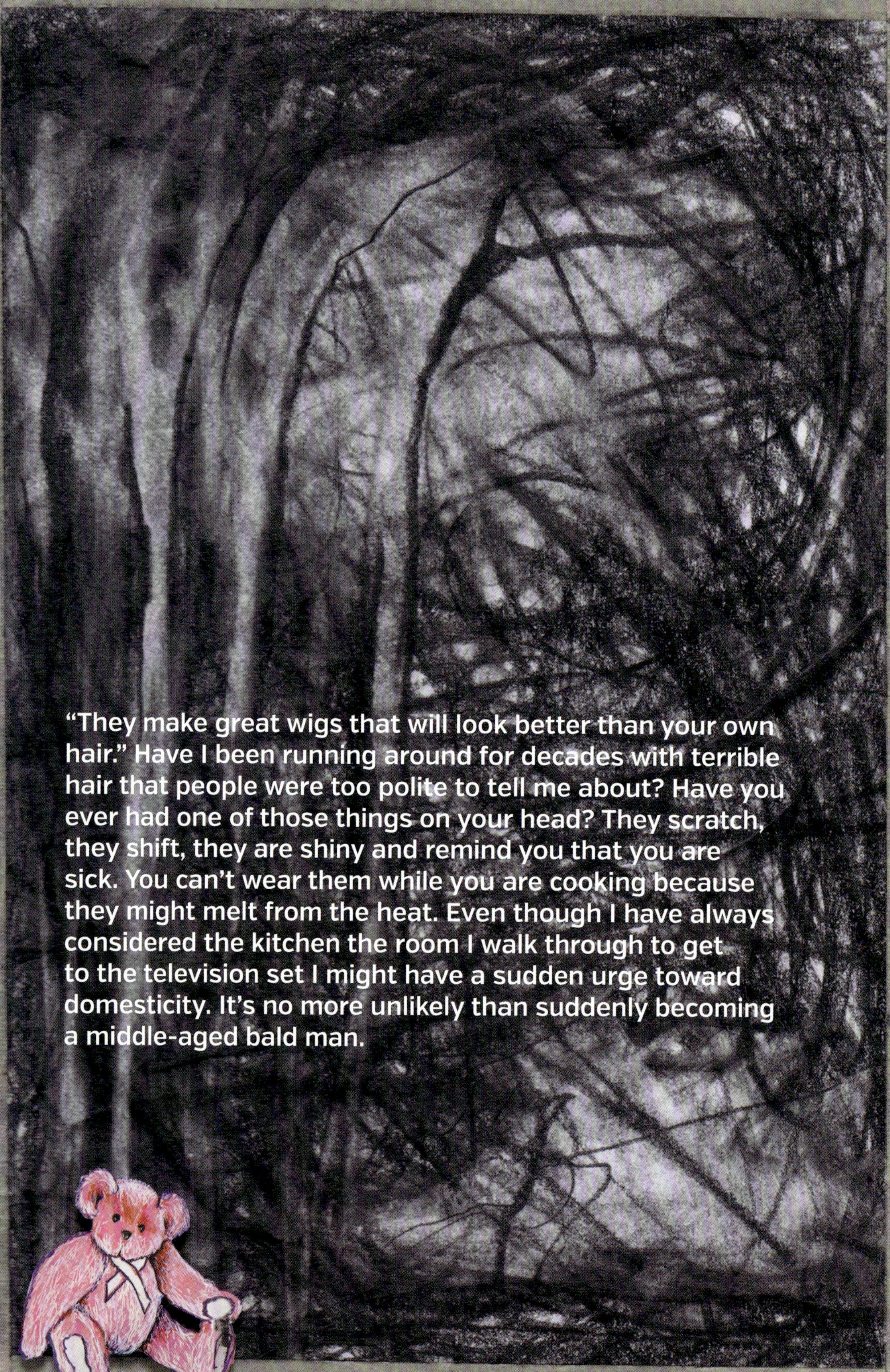

“They make great wigs that will look better than your own hair.” Have I been running around for decades with terrible hair that people were too polite to tell me about? Have you ever had one of those things on your head? They scratch, they shift, they are shiny and remind you that you are sick. You can’t wear them while you are cooking because they might melt from the heat. Even though I have always considered the kitchen the room I walk through to get to the television set I might have a sudden urge toward domesticity. It’s no more unlikely than suddenly becoming a middle-aged bald man.

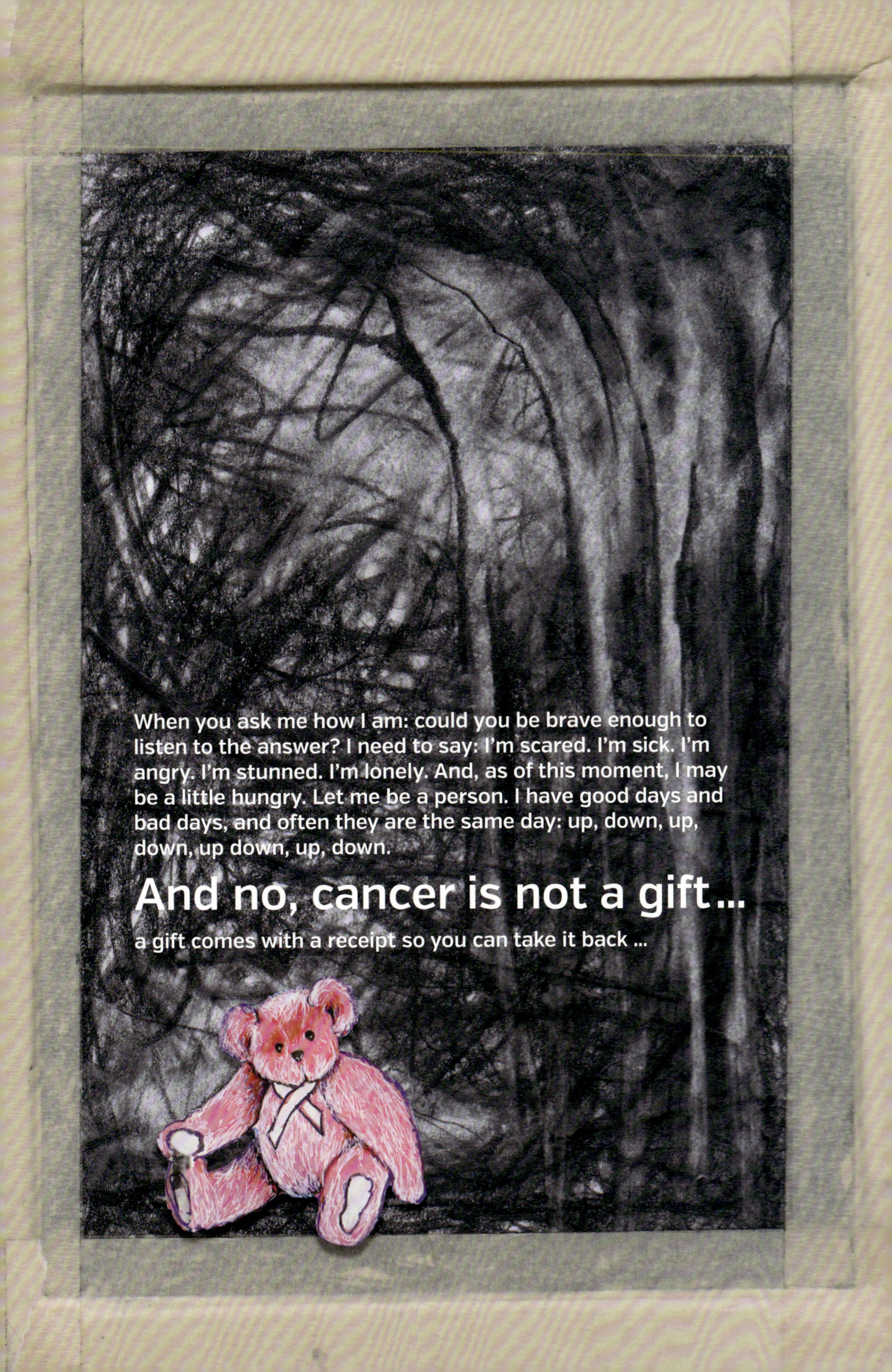
When you ask me how I am: could you be brave enough to listen to the answer? I need to say: I'm scared. I'm sick. I'm angry. I'm stunned. I'm lonely. And, as of this moment, I may be a little hungry. Let me be a person. I have good days and bad days, and often they are the same day: up, down, up, down, up down, up, down.
And no, cancer is not a gift...
a gift comes with a receipt so you can take it back ...

"You will survive this if you have a positive attitude." Keep a sunny disposition. Wear funky hats. Smile. Really? Now, in addition to dealing with a potentially fatal disease, I am supposed to become Rebecca of Sunnybrook Farm? Perhaps the next time I purchase a latte, a hat, or a great pair of boots I'll buy a small box of positive attitude. Tied up with a pink ribbon.

One of the biggest myths surrounding cancer is that positive thinking can not only cure it, but prevent it. I am in a high-risk group: late menopause, childless, and my mother had breast cancer. However, I am not overweight. I am not a drinker. I eat well. I exercise. But because I am not permanently upbeat I have given myself cancer. If I had been more highly evolved and self-aware, this never would have happened. If I had found Jesus, meditated, been one with the universe, balanced my chakras and eaten a paleo/vegan/vegetarian or possibly nothing-that-casts-a-shadow diet, this disease would not have occurred. Not only do I have a potentially deadly cancer - I shoulder the heavy burden of knowing it is my fault.

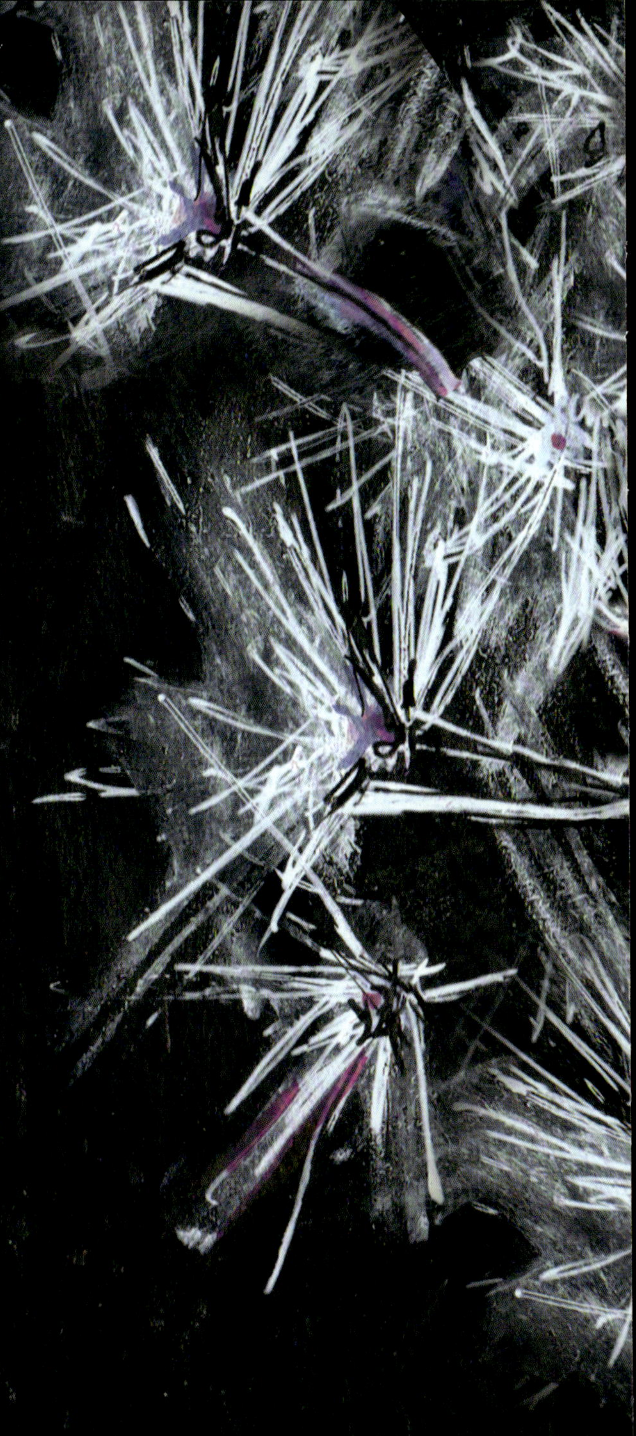

I carry enough guilt as it is. I have interrupted everybody's life: I've let my husband, my colleagues, my students, my friends and my family down. My artist's career is at a stand still. And now I am on the ticket for refusing to become Yoda, mainly because it is hard to be a beacon of enlightenment when you are ill most of the time. Candidly, now is probably not the time to search for my place in the world or find my true path, as was cheerily suggested I do with all the time I have on my hands. Currently, I am using that time to search in my bag for wherever I put the rice crackers. And using every positive thought just to keep them down.

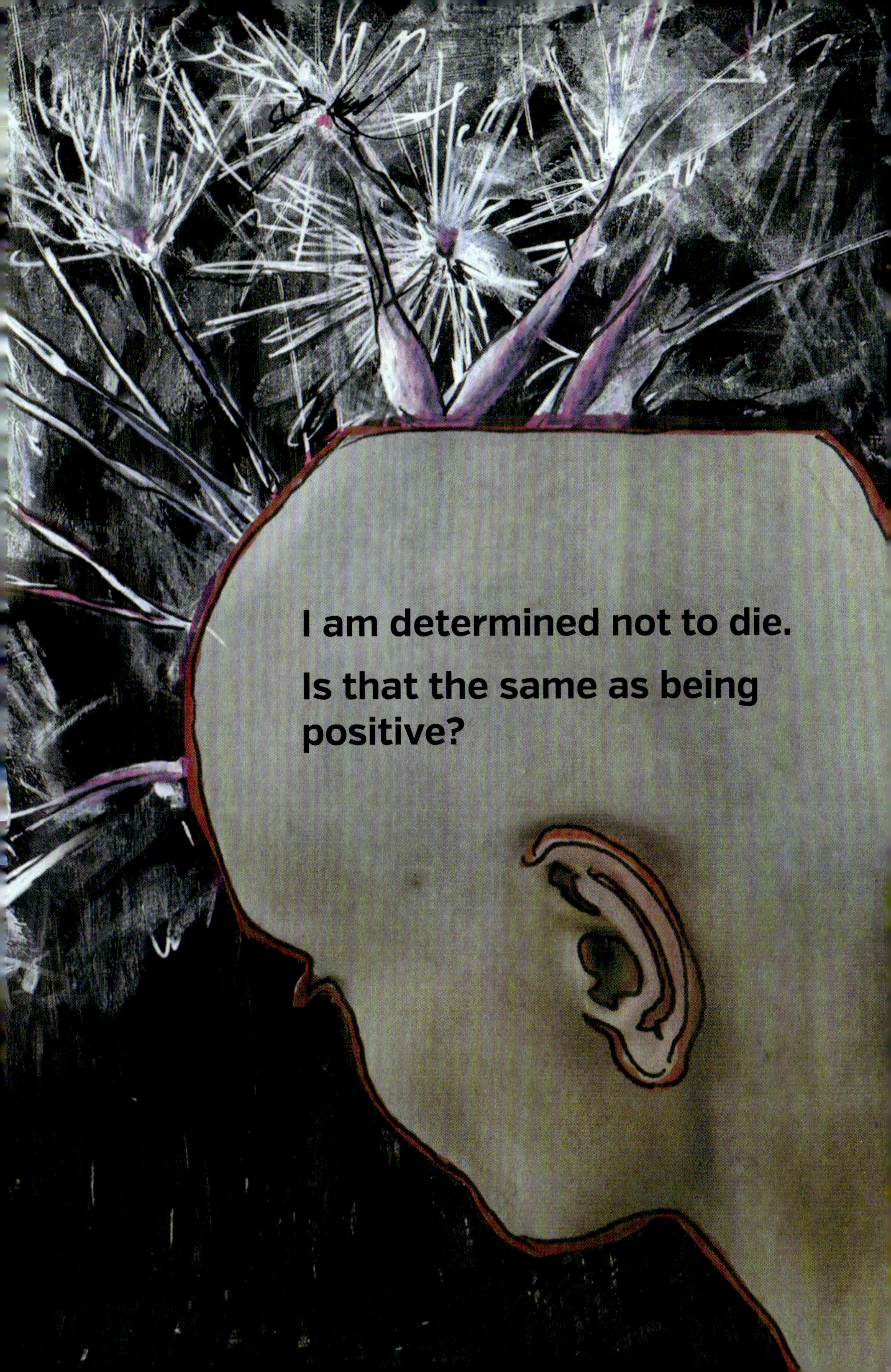
I am determined not to die.
Is that the same as being positive?

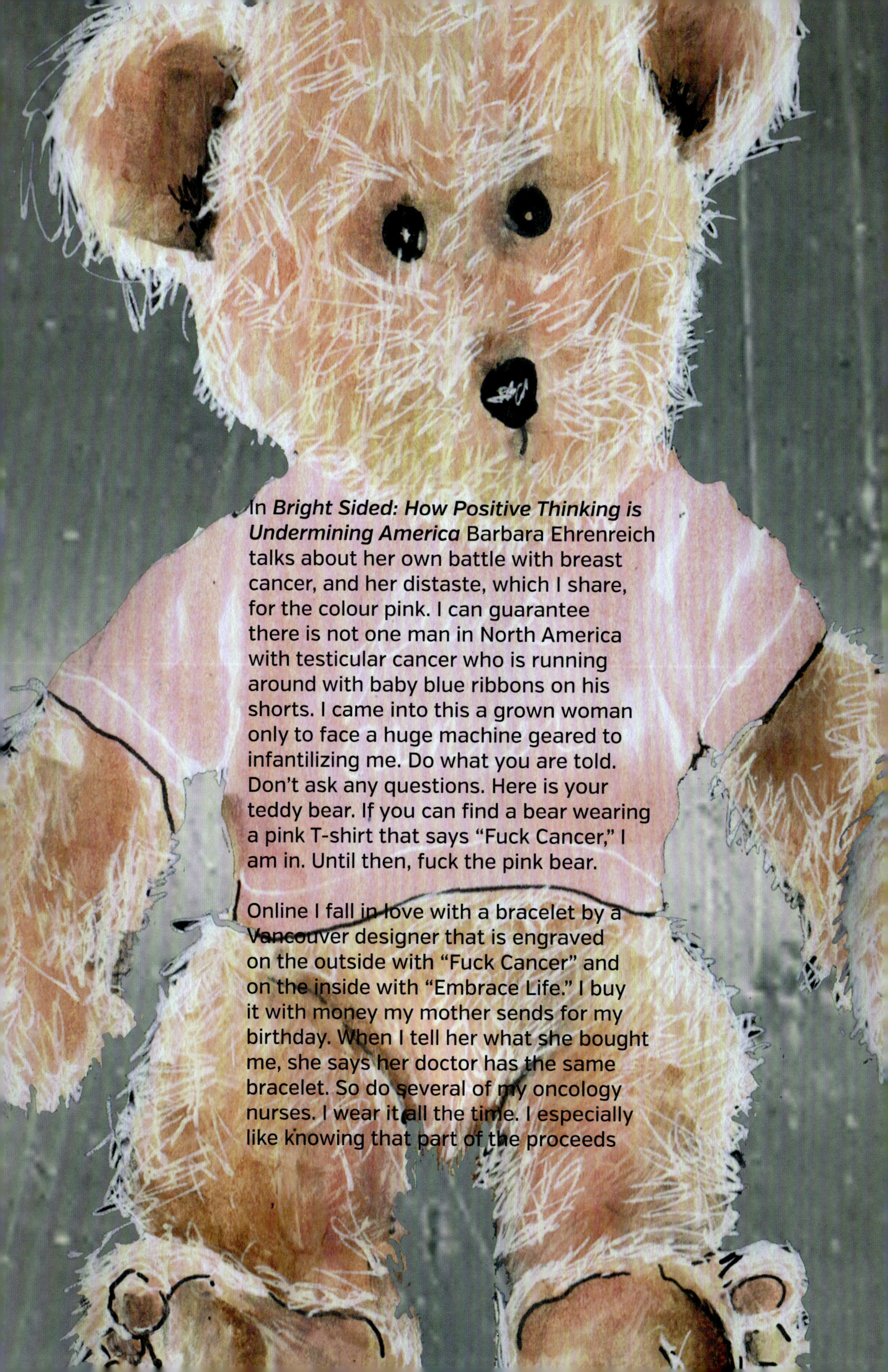

In ***Bright Sided: How Positive Thinking is Undermining America*** Barbara Ehrenreich talks about her own battle with breast cancer, and her distaste, which I share, for the colour pink. I can guarantee there is not one man in North America with testicular cancer who is running around with baby blue ribbons on his shorts. I came into this a grown woman only to face a huge machine geared to infantilizing me. Do what you are told. Don't ask any questions. Here is your teddy bear. If you can find a bear wearing a pink T-shirt that says "Fuck Cancer," I am in. Until then, fuck the pink bear.

Online I fall in love with a bracelet by a Vancouver designer that is engraved on the outside with "Fuck Cancer" and on the inside with "Embrace Life." I buy it with money my mother sends for my birthday. When I tell her what she bought me, she says her doctor has the same bracelet. So do several of my oncology nurses. I wear it all the time. I especially like knowing that part of the proceeds

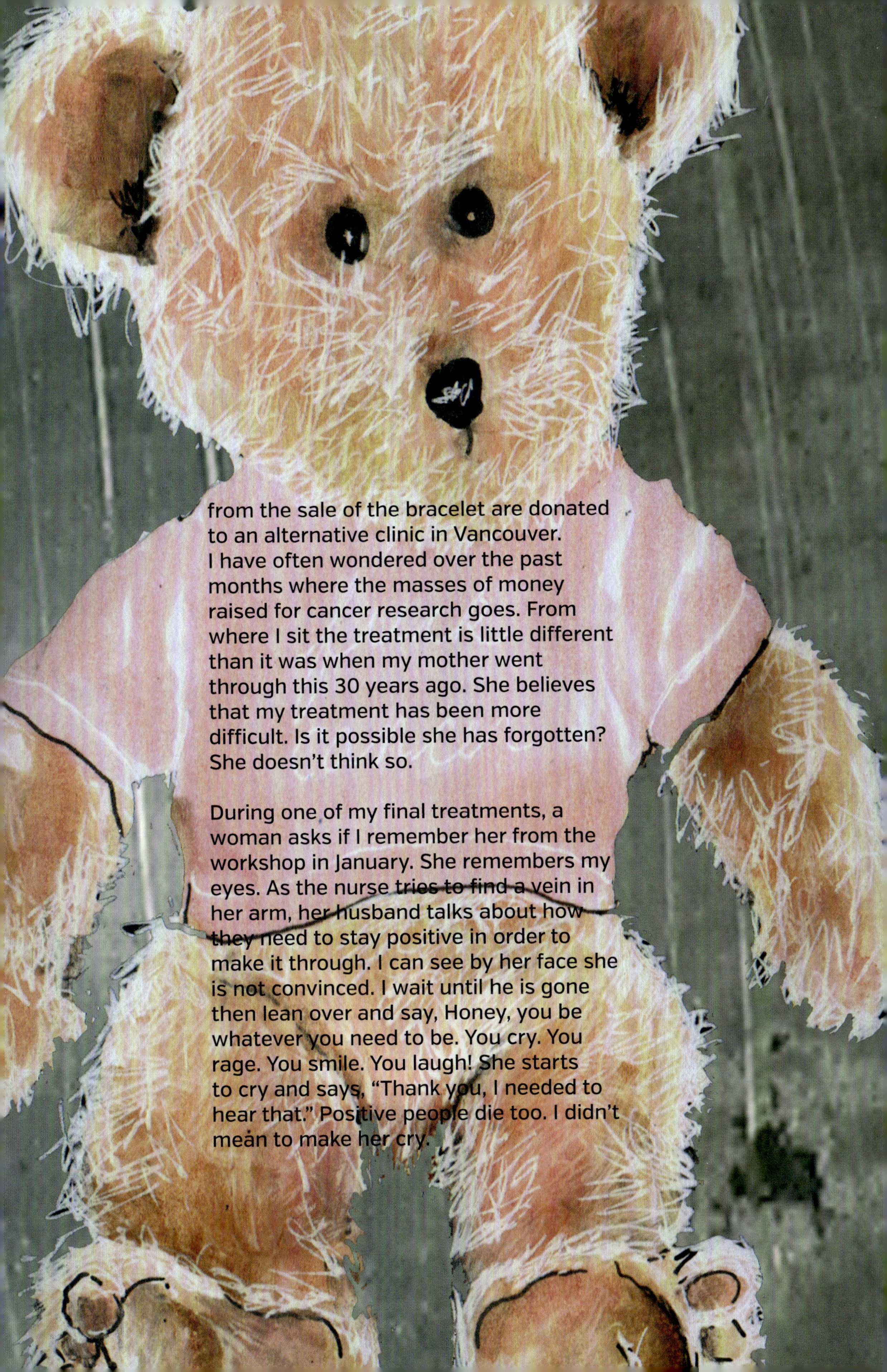

from the sale of the bracelet are donated to an alternative clinic in Vancouver. I have often wondered over the past months where the masses of money raised for cancer research goes. From where I sit the treatment is little different than it was when my mother went through this 30 years ago. She believes that my treatment has been more difficult. Is it possible she has forgotten? She doesn't think so.

During one of my final treatments, a woman asks if I remember her from the workshop in January. She remembers my eyes. As the nurse tries to find a vein in her arm, her husband talks about how they need to stay positive in order to make it through. I can see by her face she is not convinced. I wait until he is gone then lean over and say, Honey, you be whatever you need to be. You cry. You rage. You smile. You laugh! She starts to cry and says, "Thank you, I needed to hear that." Positive people die too. I didn't mean to make her cry.

On my stronger days I say bullshit to all of this!! I want a personal apology from the Universe. I imagine others do to. Something we can frame and hang on our walls. Because the Universe is undoubtedly very busy I have written up the document so all that is left is to fill in the blanks and sign it.

The Universe would like to take this opportunity to personally and profoundly apologize to Fill in Name Here for making her/him feel guilty during her/his recent bout with cancer. It has been determined by a panel of experts that it was in no way, shape or form your fault. Any inconvenience will be made up to you in the form of good health for the remainder of your life. Now go eat your cookies.

Sincerely,

The Universe.

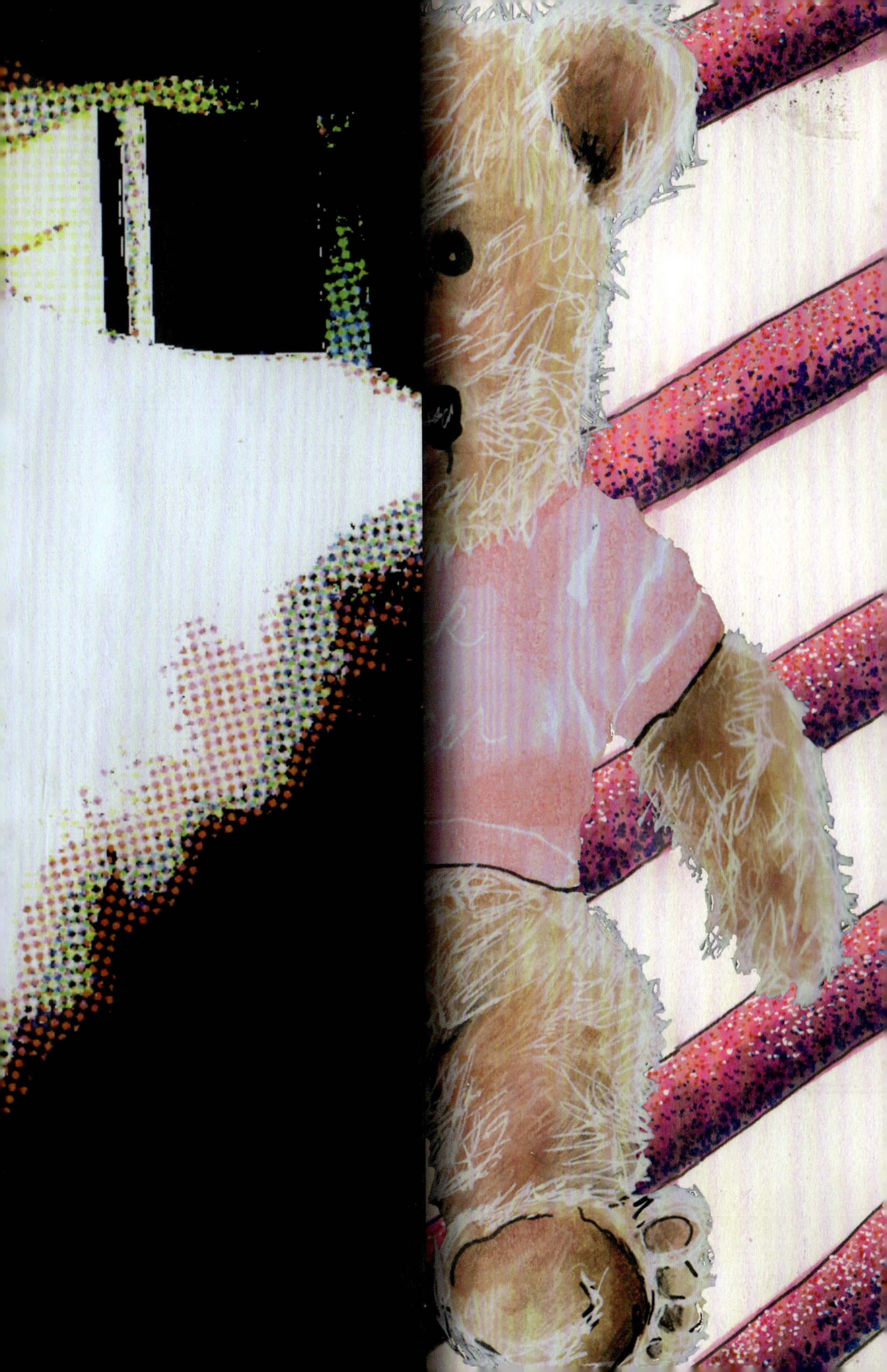

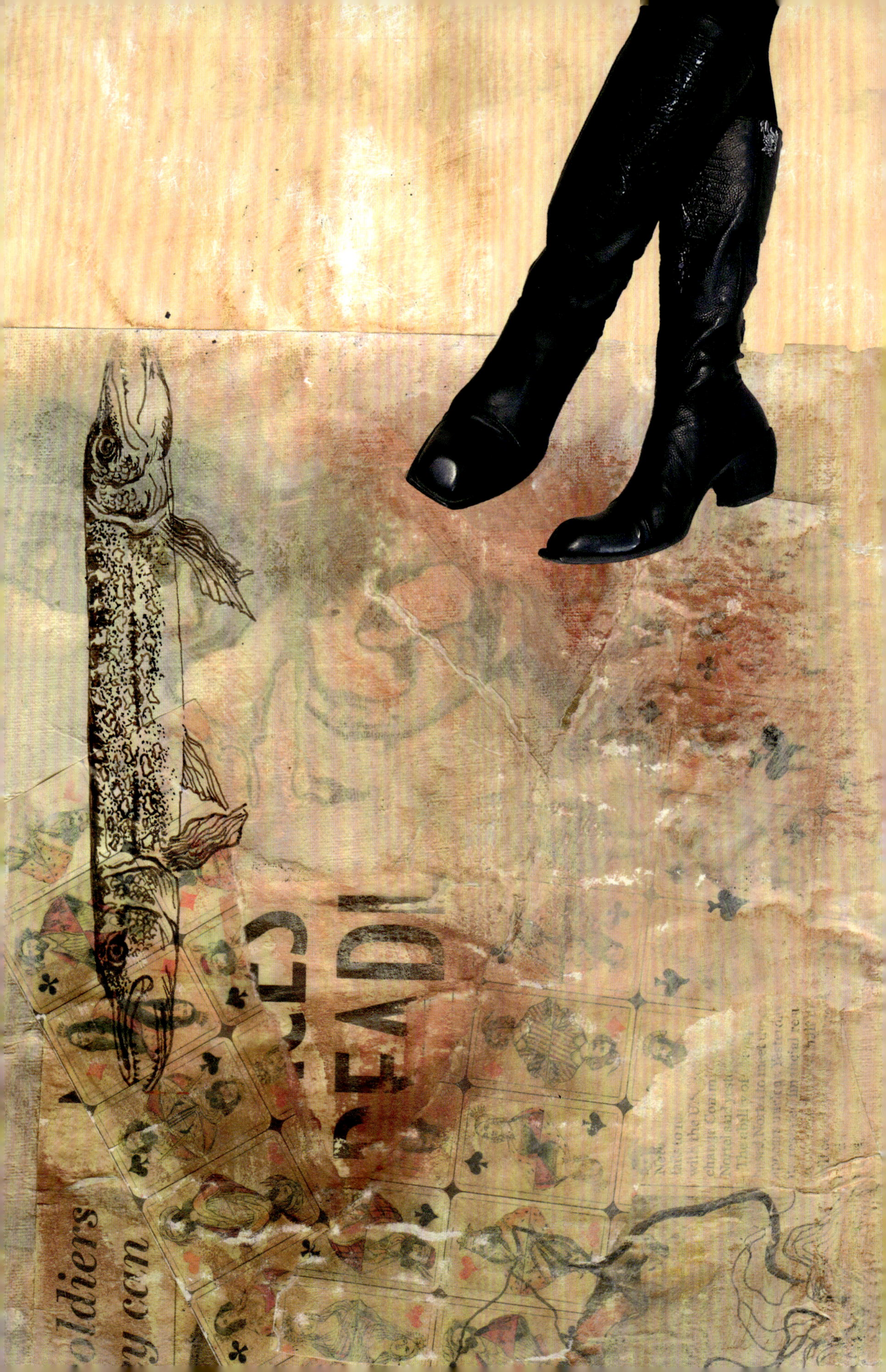

last stage chemotherapy

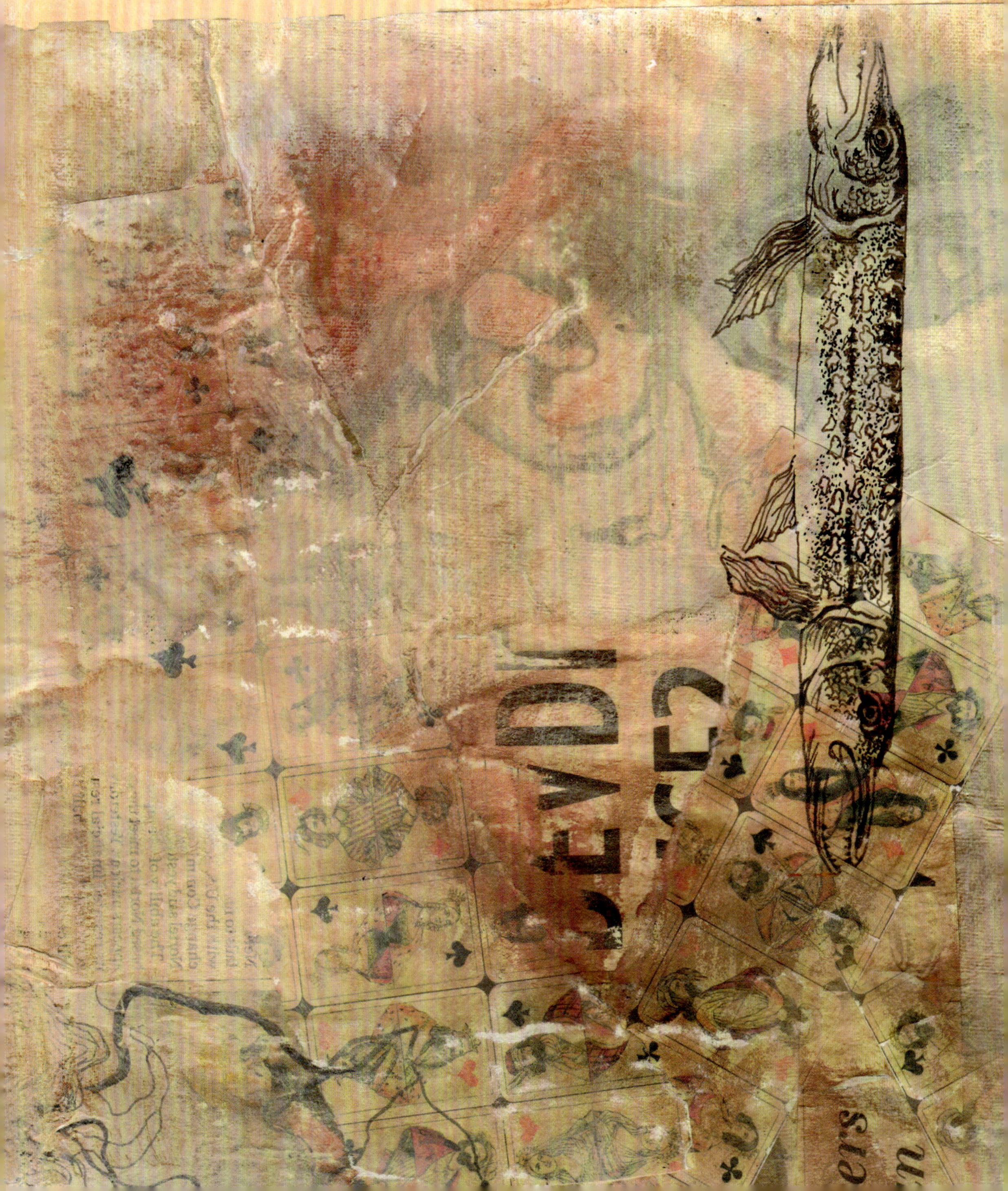

I am icing my hands and feet in the hope it will save my nails. 20 minutes on 20 minutes off. The Centre does not have ice mitts on their chemo wards. Ordering online requires too long. Doug and I buy all the varieties of ice packs we can find at the drug store and haul them in a cooler to my treatments. I traveled to Italy with less luggage. Also had a much better time.

To no avail. My nails lift off their beds. They ache. When I call the triage nurse for advice, her curt reply is "They are not supposed to hurt." I am feeling a little snarky myself and answer, I am sorry. I am obviously not doing this right. There is silence. I have a brief flash of my mother reminding me to be quiet if I have nothing nice to say. Oops. Too late.

I lose the first one when I am pulling off a sweater. After that I can't stop staring at them counting them off as they go. I am sitting on Doug's knee as he works on the computer when my last fingernail falls to the floor. It must be alarming to watch bits of your wife dropping off.

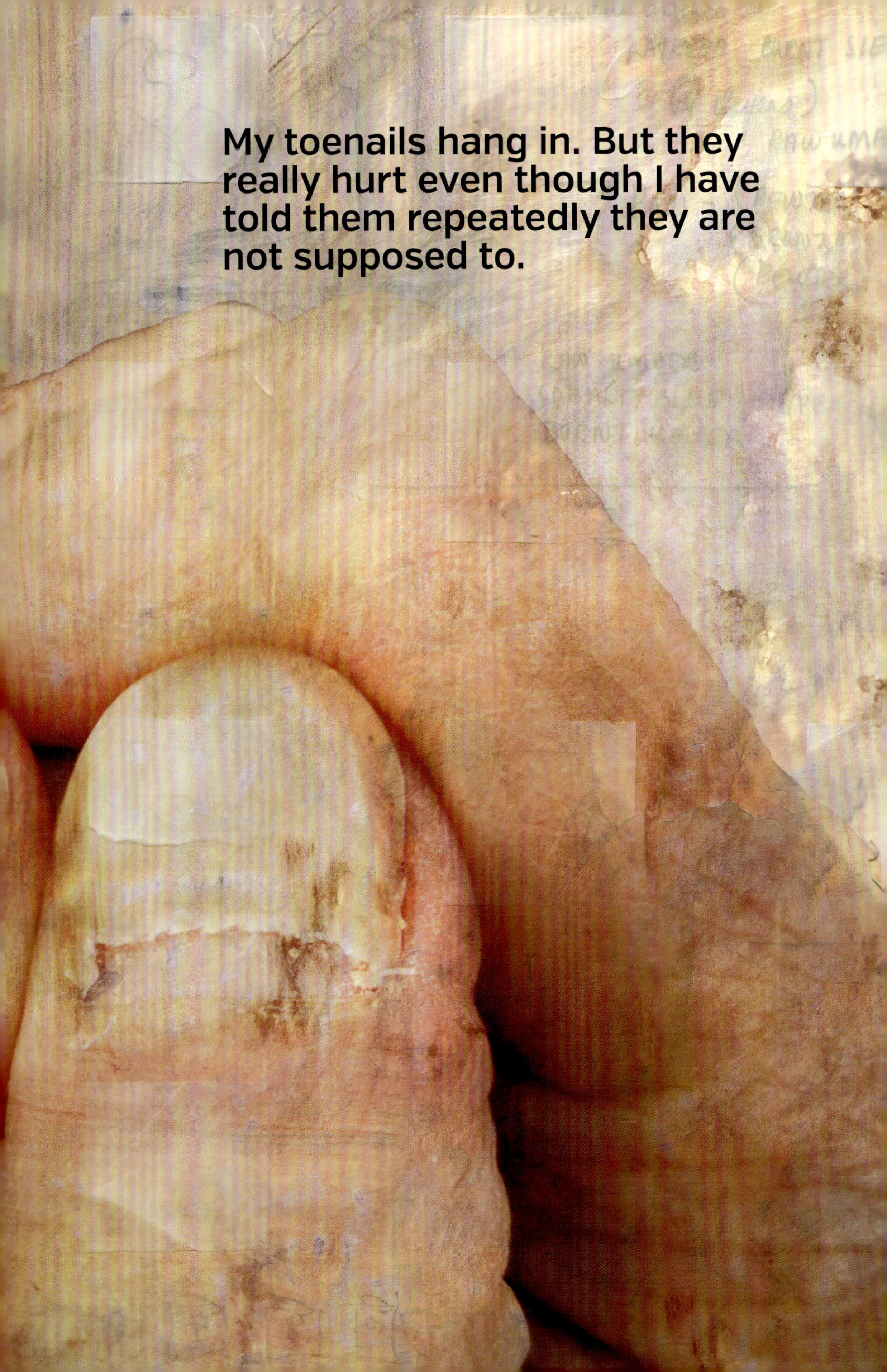

My toenails hang in. But they really hurt even though I have told them repeatedly they are not supposed to.

My days cycle through acupuncture, infusions, oncology appointments, blood tests, treatments, sleep, nap, walk, sleep, yoga ... rinse, repeat ... My uncooperative veins are now in full rebellion and they collapse on more than one occasion. I know how they feel. I get huge lumps on my arms that have to be taken down with ice, then heated again ... rinse, repeat ...

I am reduced to watching mindless television and loll on the couch watching reruns of ***Buffy the Vampire Slayer***. Repeating after her, I was always brave and kind of righteous ... now I find I'm wavering ... My feet are elevated in an attempt to battle the swelling. I go through a period of being unable to read or write on the computer; even drawing in my sketchbook is an effort. My eyesight deteriorates, a side effect of chemo as the fluid in the eye alters its shape. Apparently it is not permanent.

I remind myself there are people in far worse shape then I am. I see them every week. People who are on the third or fourth round of battling this disease. And losing. Damn that enlightenment is elusive. I am waiting for the other shoe to drop ...

Even though I spend most days alone I feel surrounded by people who love me. For all of my frustration with some of the thoughtless things people say those closest to me are my bulwark. Doug is always here. Strong, patient, nurturing. Ready to do anything for me, as are my friends. Learning to sit still and let others do for me has been a challenge. Not to mention the fear of going out with my compromised immune system. I am used to going all the time. The Energy Battery bunny. Now it is a massive feat when I drive to the train station by myself and pick up a friend. We lunch. I come home exhausted and exhilarated. Small steps ...

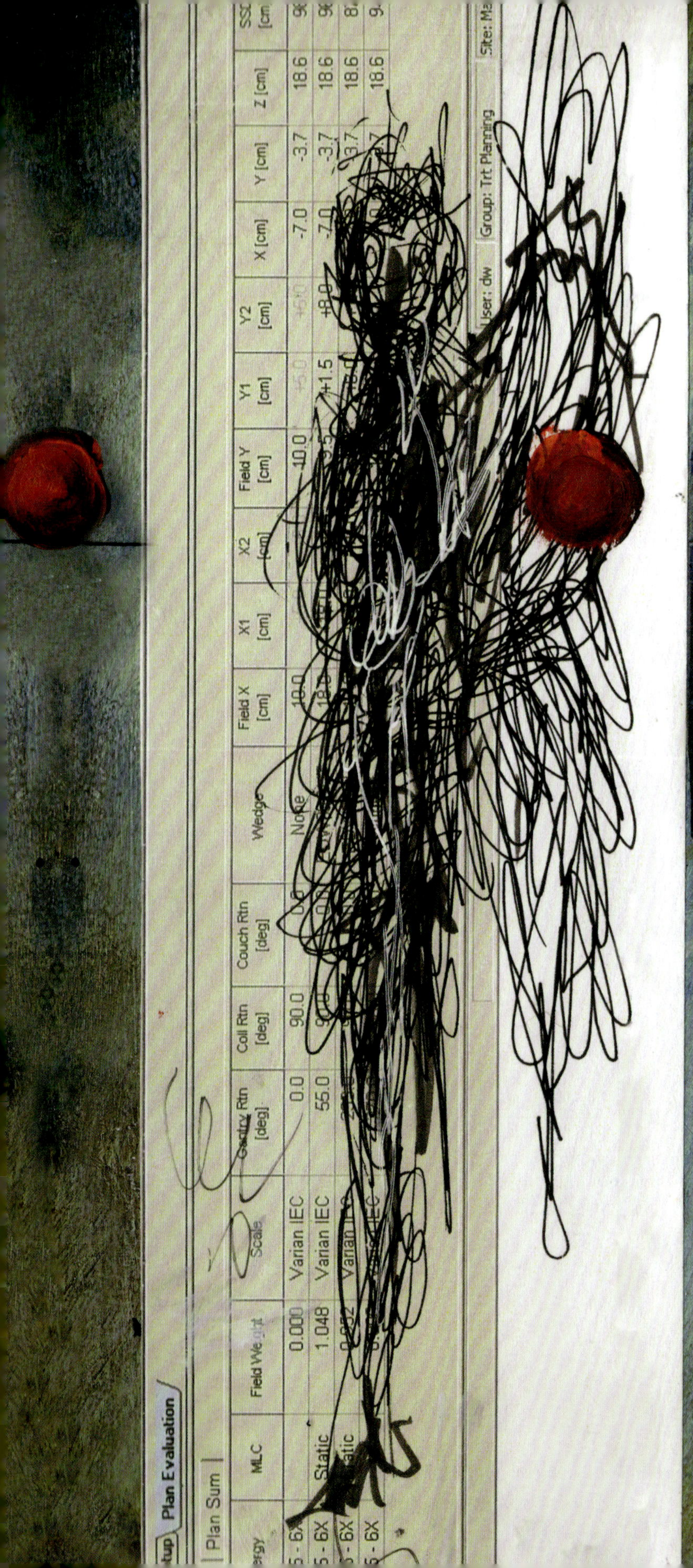

I am scheduled to start radiation. Fifteen sessions, five days a week over a three-week period. Naively, I thought only the tumour area would be targeted, not a large square that stretches from the scar under my arm to the lymph nodes in the centre of my chest. Potential side effects include permanent damage to the lung, the bones and the

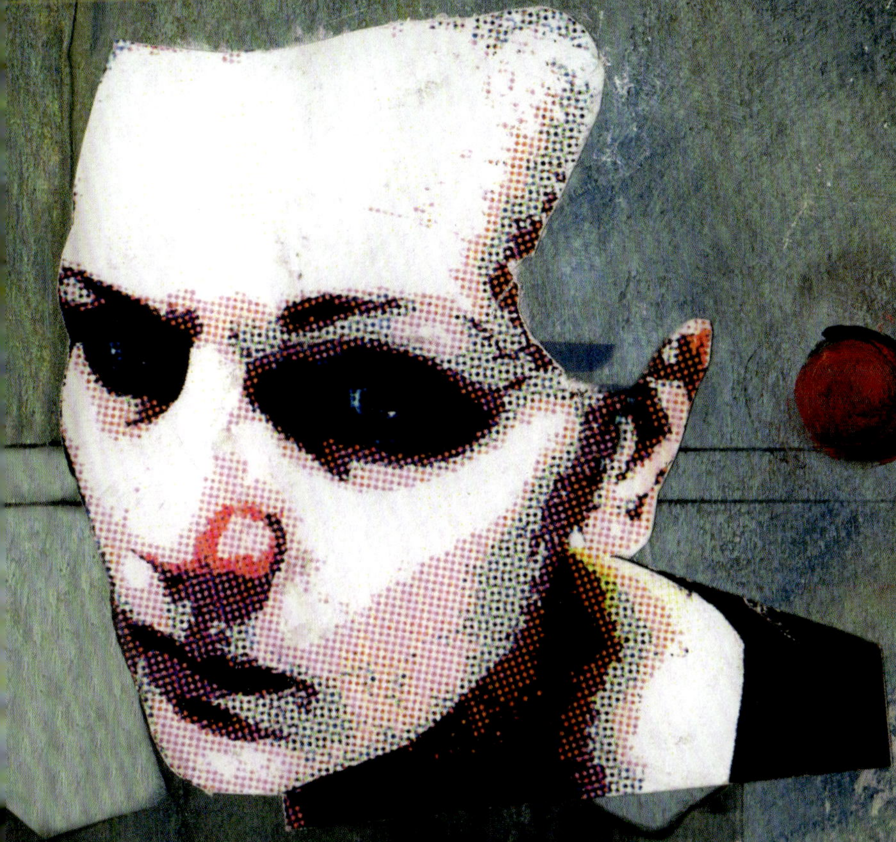

skin; the breast tissue may harden and require re-constructive surgery. For the umpteenth time I say, Really? Dr. R seems to think that anyone would want new breasts. Mine may not be much, but I have fought to keep them and had no idea that I might not be able to. I opt not to have the lymph nodes under my arm radiated. It would add another week to the treatment and possibly more complications. She is not pushing. It is my choice.

For the radiation staging, I am on a table, arms over my head, hands wrapped around two posts, in the position I will be in for the actual treatments. I need to have three tattoos, all about the size of a pen tip, two on either side of my rib cage and one located centrally under my breasts. As I lie there the technicians discuss their concern the tattoos will be lost as my skin is already so marked. I resist reminding them that I am right here and can hear everything they say. My chronic nasal drip kicks in. Immobile, I ask if someone will wipe my dripping face. No one does. I leave embarrassed. Insignificant and ugly to boot.

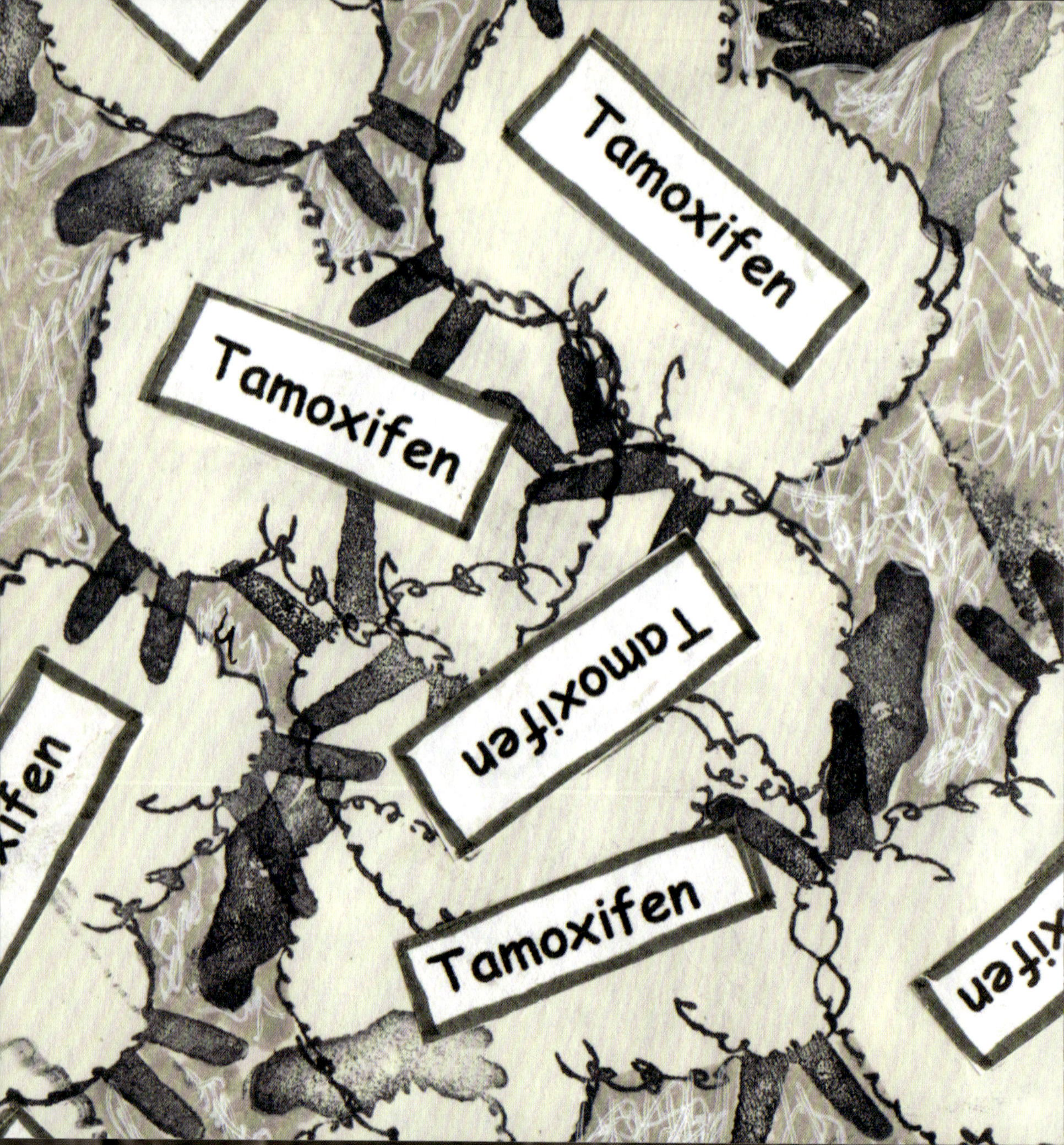

Dr. O is urging me to take Tamoxifen but I am still reluctant. The side effects frighten me: hot flashes, vaginal dryness, low libido, mood swings, depression, anxiety, nausea, cataracts, an increased risk of blood clots and cancer of the womb. In lab tests some rats on Tamoxifen developed liver cancer. Dr. O tries to reassure me by saying that Tamoxifen is no more difficult than the pill for most women. He could not have come up with a worse analogy. I was crazed during my three months on the pill. I was working as a florist and once drove two hours through a storm to return a poor batch of flowers that a supplier had sent me. I stalked into the room, tossed them dramatically into his garbage can and stalked out again without saying a word. Later in the week I found myself eying my

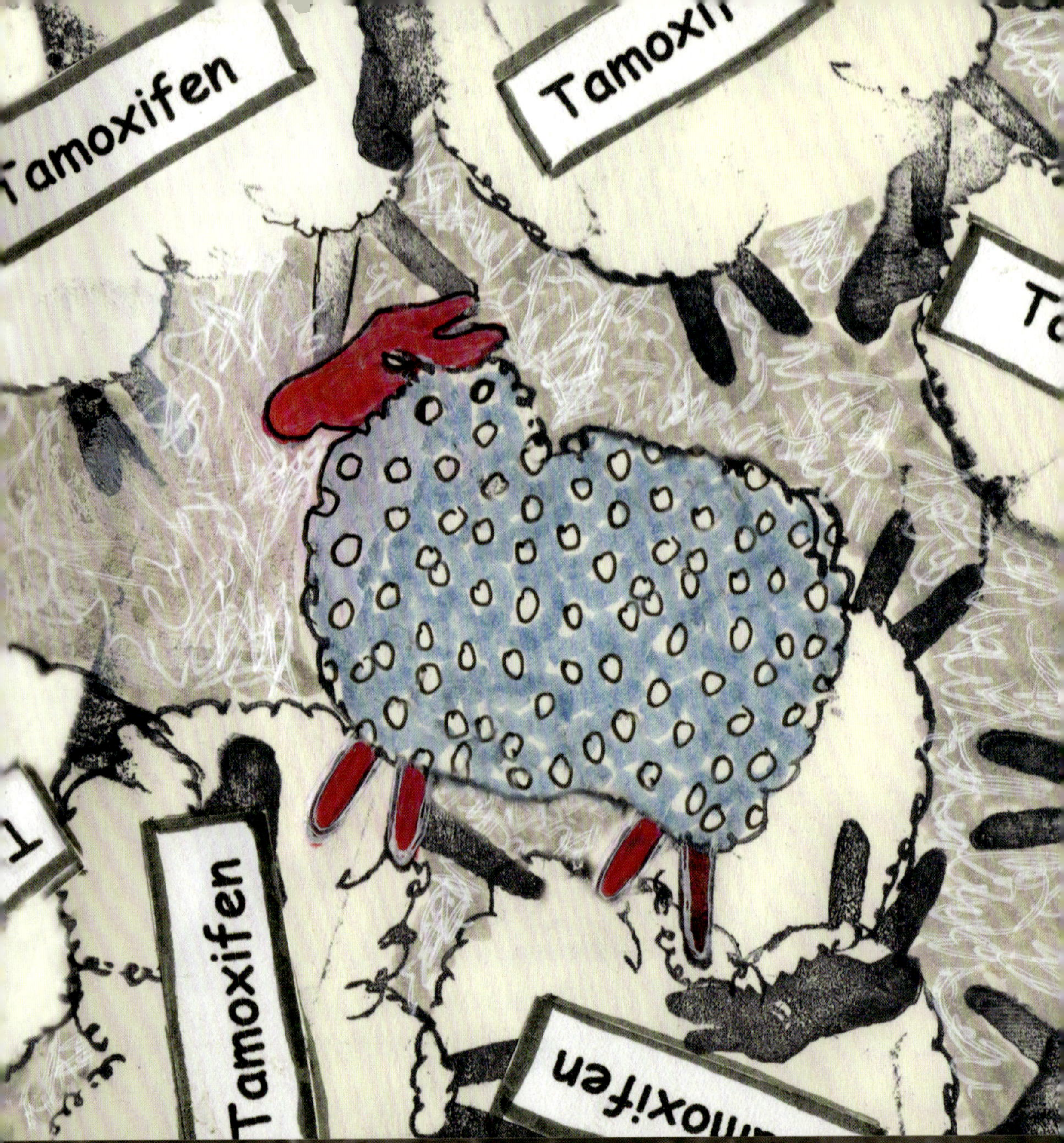

father's shotgun and figuring out roof angles. No more difficult than that???

I agree to have the prescription filled. The rest of the world can duck.

I ask the pharmacist about building up to the dose Dr. O is recommending. "Why would you want to do that?" she says. I confess my reluctance to take it at all. She chastises me "If you go in with that attitude of course you will have trouble. Besides if you fill the prescription and don't take it, it will mess up our system." There it is again, it is not the drug but my attitude that is the problem. My refusal to be compliant, the good patient … I pick up the pills and the information and elect not to strangle her.

I never take them.

It is my last day of chemo. I have taken to pausing on the stairs as I walk to the ward. Not because I'm tired but because I love the acoustics in the stairwell. I sing a few lines of whatever is running thorough my head. Sometimes it is a musical, sometimes it is a pop tune. It is silly but it makes me smile.

I bring a stack of my temporary "courage" tattoos to the ward. One of the nurses goes from bed to bed handing them out to anyone who wants one. I want to share my symbol. I have survived ... battered, bruised and not always courageous. More often defiant, cocky. My anger the equivalent of a child whistling in the dark pretending not to be frightened.

There is a tradition on the ward. A small bell sits on the nurses' counter. When it is your final treatment you ring the bell as you leave. I hit it so hard it skitters across the surface like a rat.

Doug and I leave immediately and travel to a group exhibition in which I am participating, my celebration for finishing one more stage of treatment. I need a chair half way through but otherwise it is a pretty good afternoon. We head home for the first time in four months. I have a month before radiation begins.

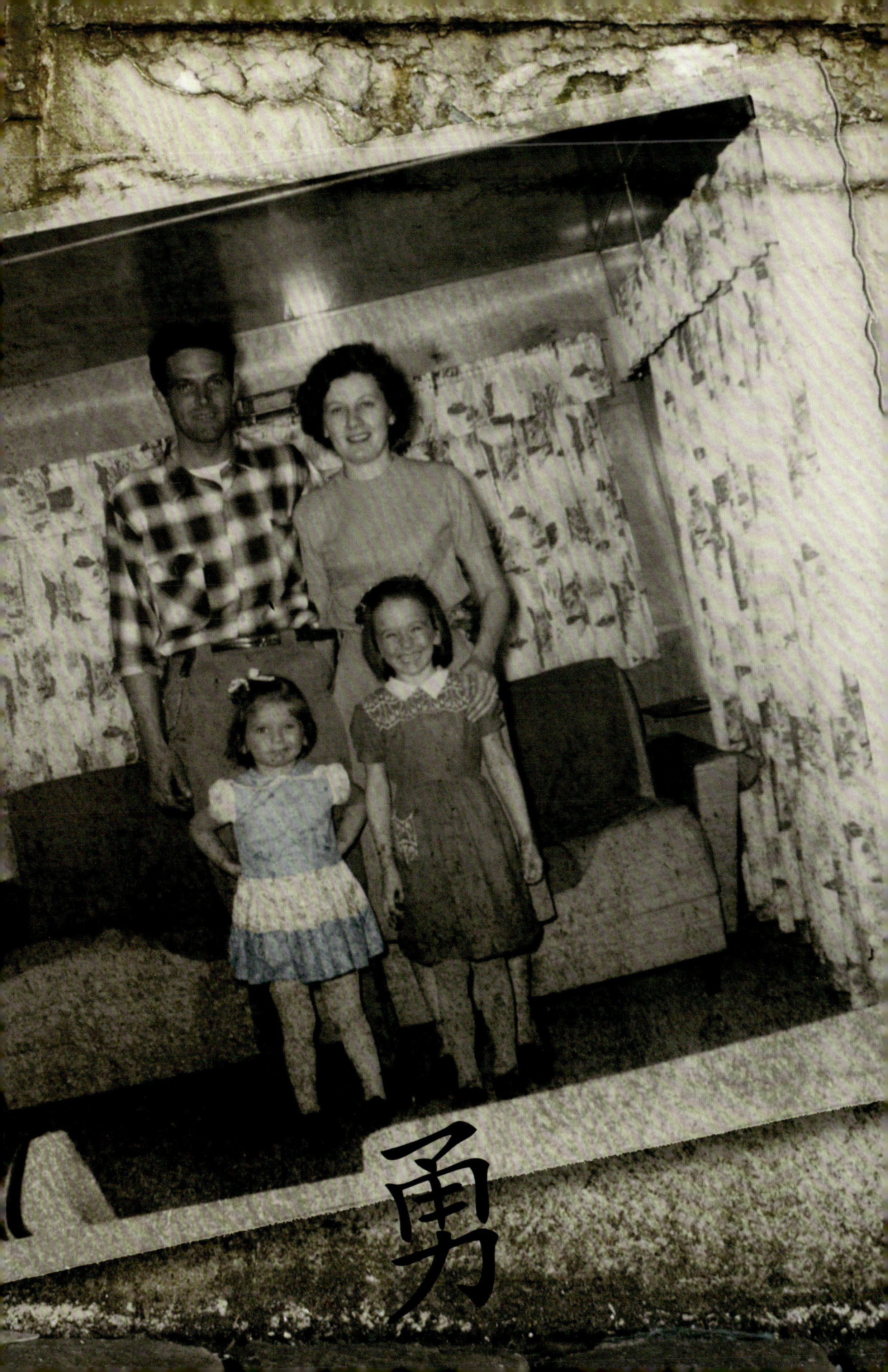
勇

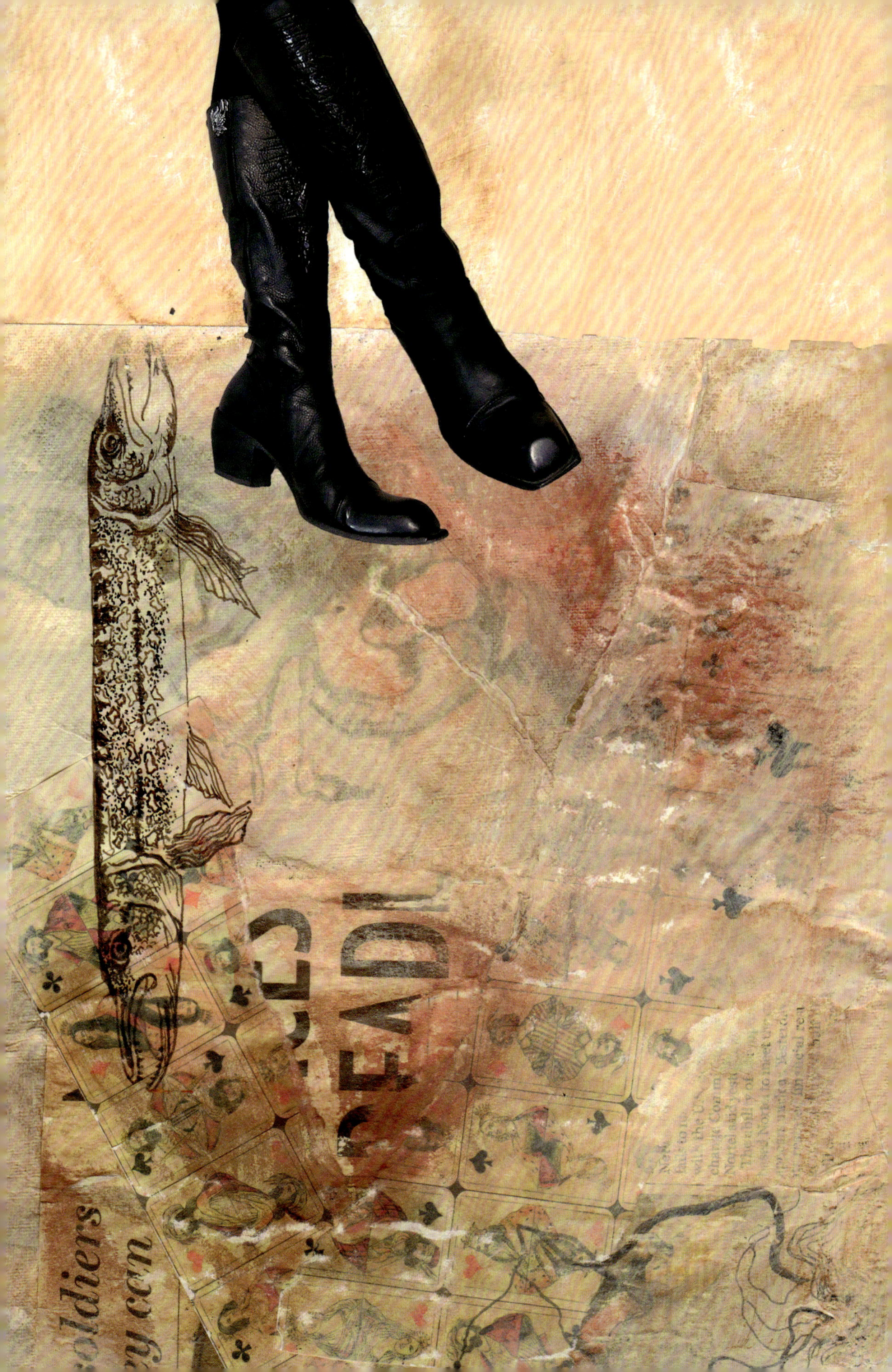

radiation

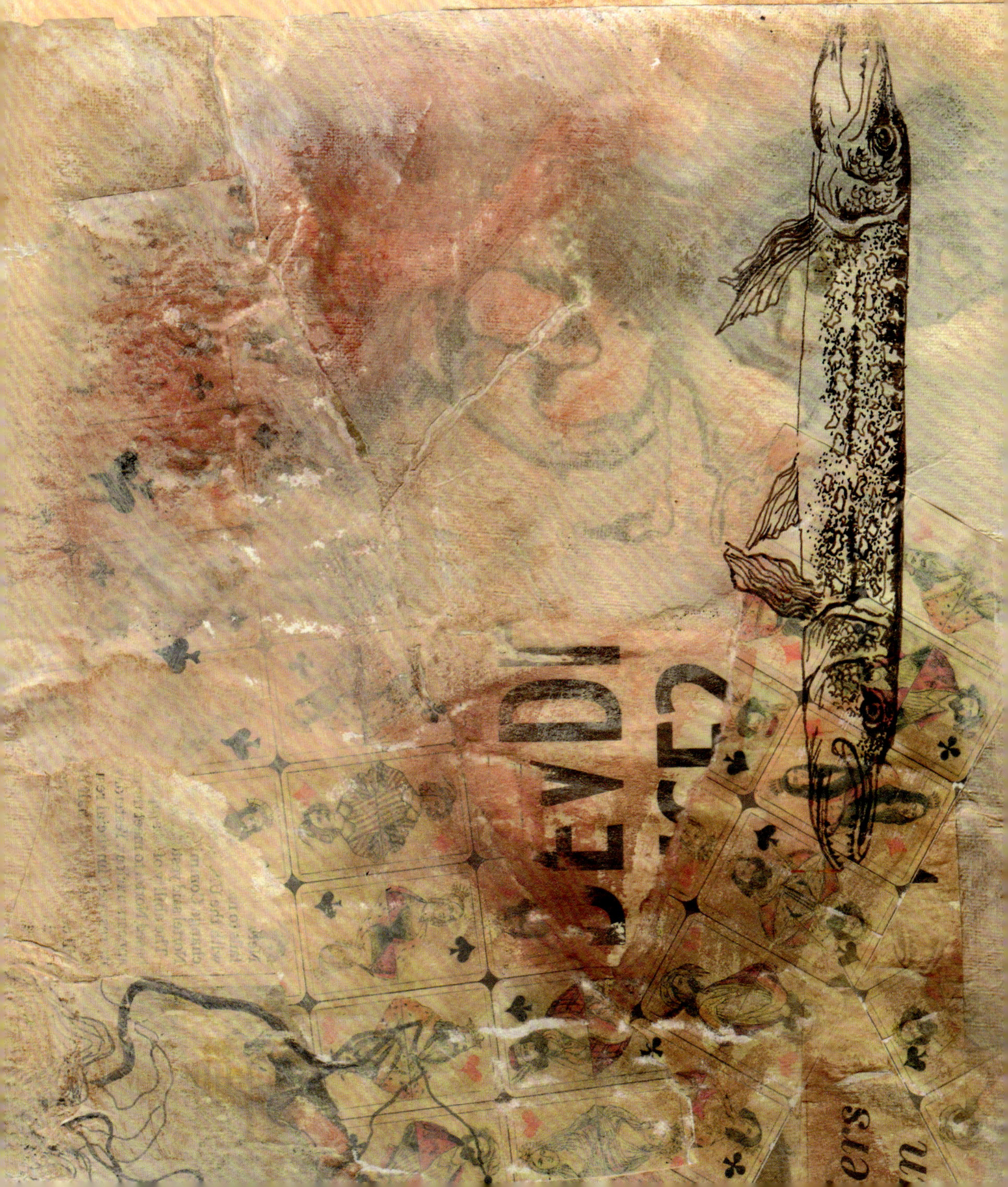

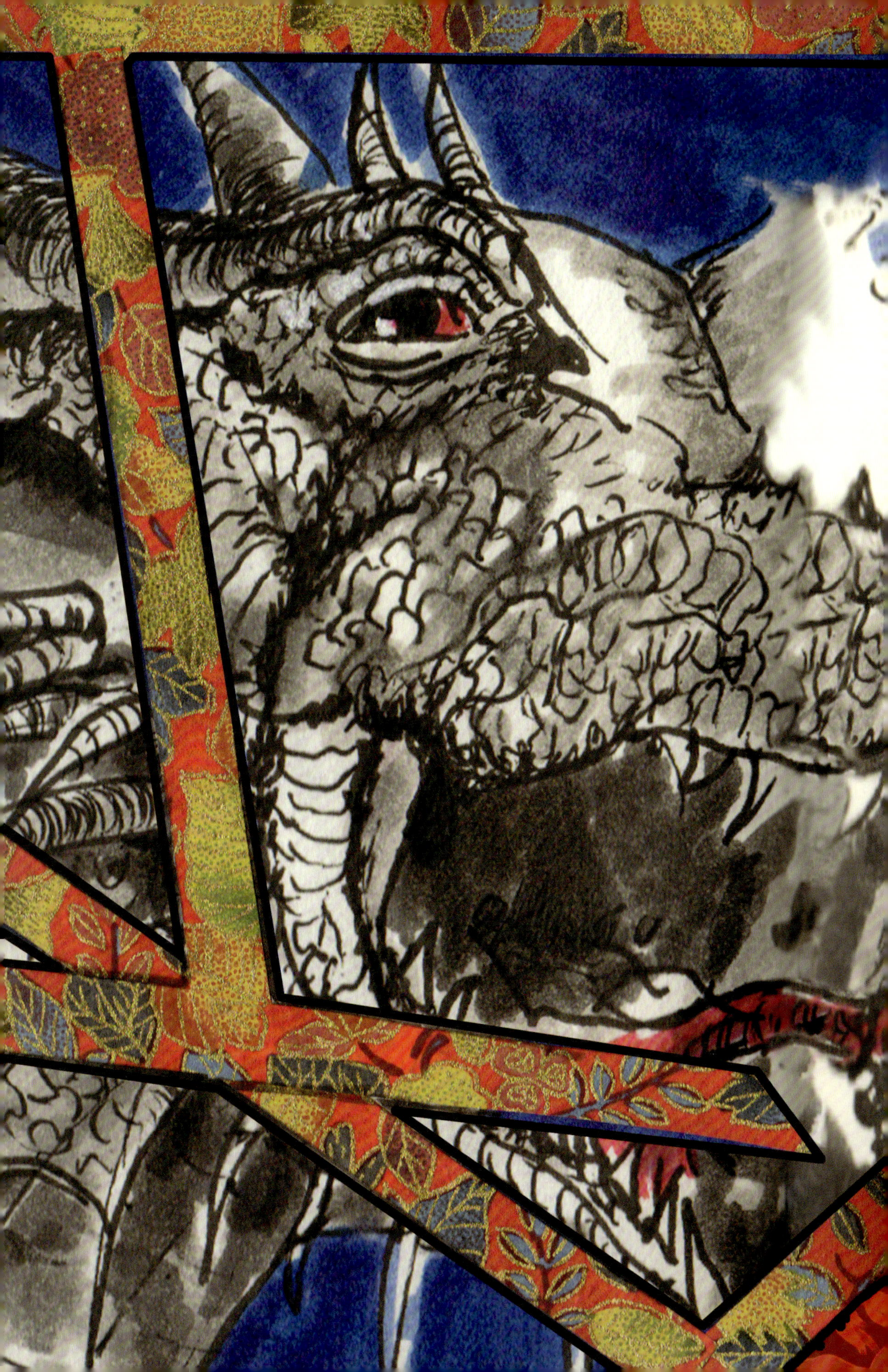

One night I dream that I am in a restaurant: a large, formal, space with linen tablecloths, candles, sparkling crystal and china. The walls are covered with ornate gilded mirrors. I am on the phone, not my cell, an old-fashioned cord phone. I am talking to someone. Sometimes it is my mother. Sometimes an old friend who for some reason is wearing camouflage pants. Sometimes it is the Marlboro Man. Whoever it is, I am promising them that I can show them all the best spots in town.

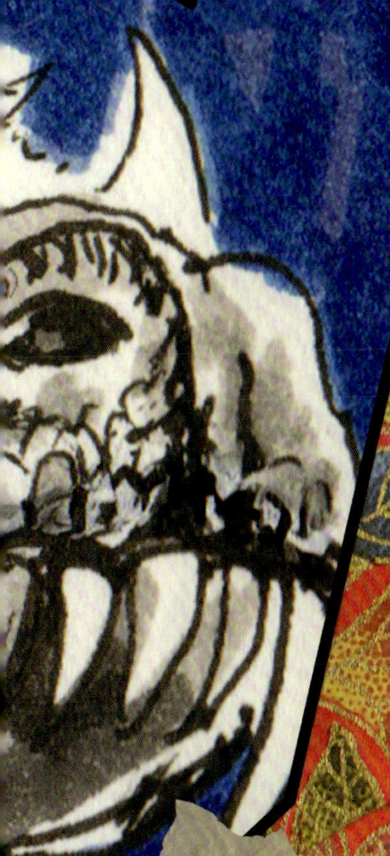

There is a commotion outside: screams, crashes, chaos. An enormous fire-breathing, smoke-belching dragon squeezes through the door. People flee. I scramble to hide on the other side of a wall that separates the back of the restaurant from the main dining area. Through the mirrors I watch the creature make its ponderous way through the room. It stops and pokes its head around the corner. I flatten along the floor trying to be as small as possibles knowing my only chance is to not move or breathe. When its leathery feet lumber level to my head I look up into lurid red eyes. He is searching for me. This is my dragon. I wake up.

During my chemo treatments we lived in my father-in-law's basement. After being in my own home for a month, I realize how starved I am for light and air. Though I am grateful for my father-in-law's kindness, when I return for radiation we decide to stay with our friends Peter and Linda. They have a lovely garden. The trees are blossoming. I can no longer sit in the sun – this will be a lifetime ban – but I spend as much time as I can on the back deck under the umbrella. I have purchased a hat so large it should have its own postal code.

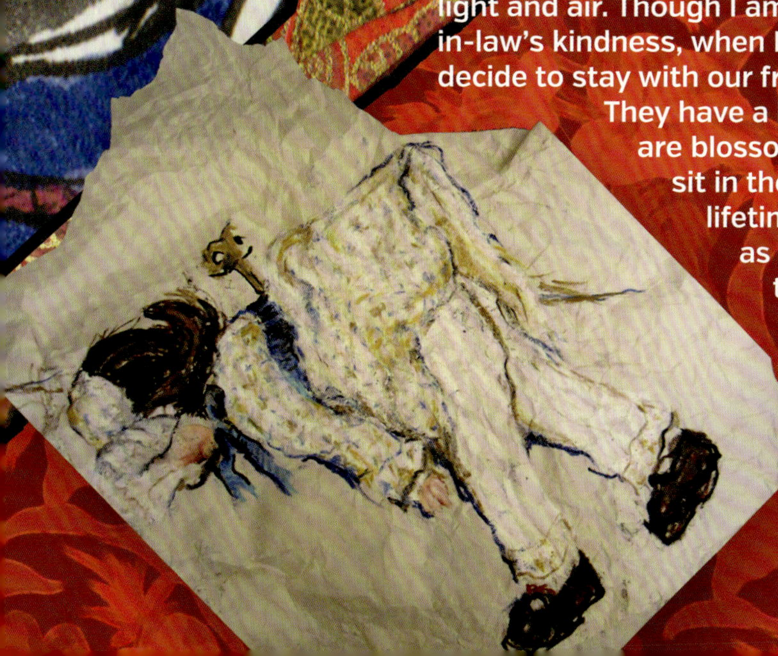

Day one of radiation. Even though everyone has said radiation is a piece of cake after chemotherapy, I am apprehensive. The room is warehouse sized and refrigerator cold. A rock-hard strip of metal passes as a bed. My neck and head are locked into a curved piece to keep me motionless. My arms stretched overhead and my hands curved around two posts. Above my body is a large machine with a disc in the centre. The technicians wrap me in warm blankets then move me back and forth, a millimetre at a time, lining up the tattoos they gave me earlier. Overhead I can dimly see my body's reflection criss-crossed with green lines and what resembles a bar code across my chest. The technicians yell out numbers at random. "94" "98" "96.7" Like quarterbacks calling plays in a game known only to them. After the X-rays, an alarm sounds, a red light flashes on the

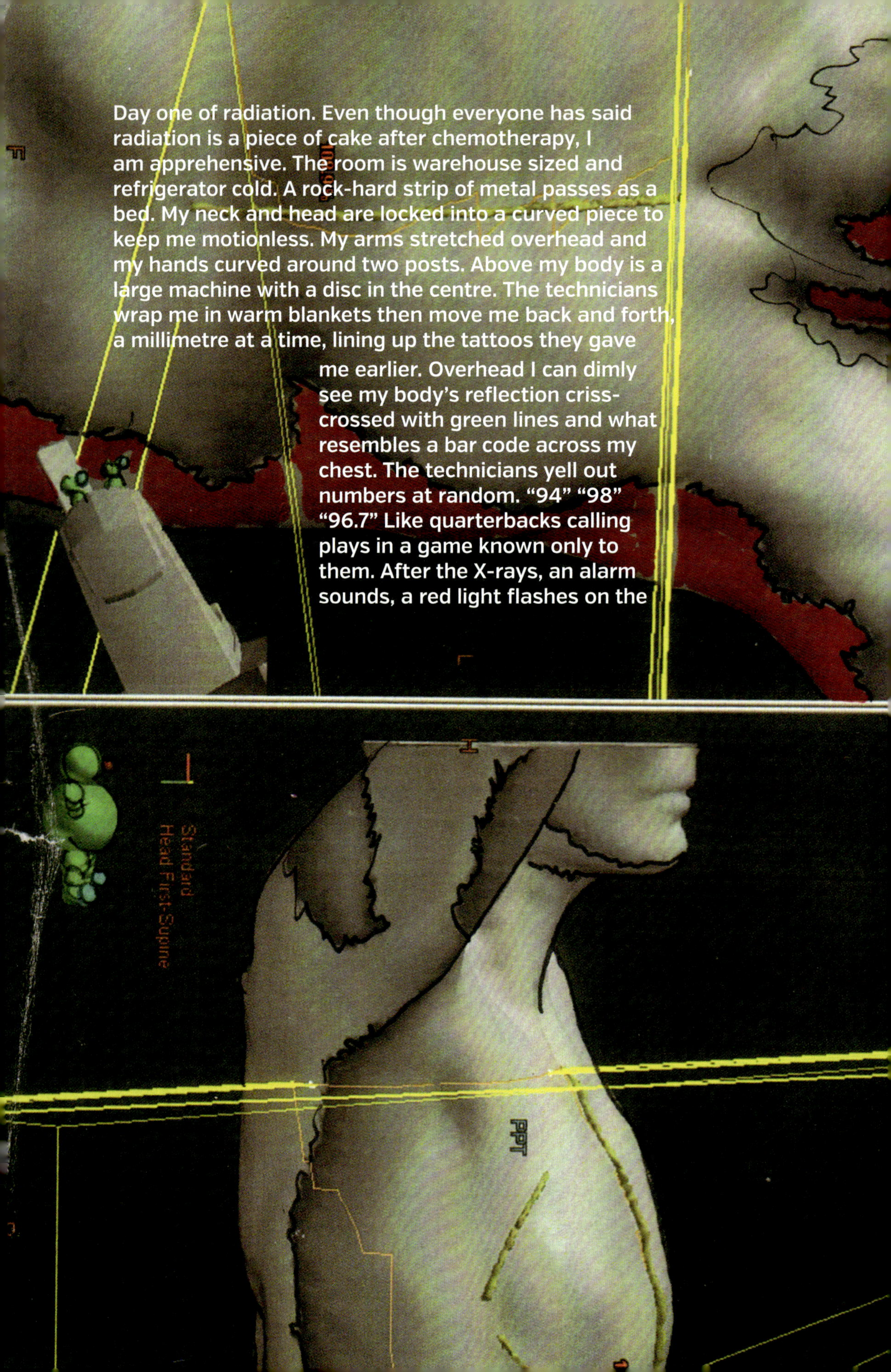

ceiling and everyone scatters. Like rats deserting a sinking ship, I can't help thinking. I am probably being unfair. Nonetheless, I am the only one left in the room. The machine emits an angry, buzzing sound and I count fifteen seconds. The disc swings right and all but disappears. From my locked-in head forward position I can only see it out of the corner of my eye. The whole process is repeated on the other side. The technicians return when the red light stops.

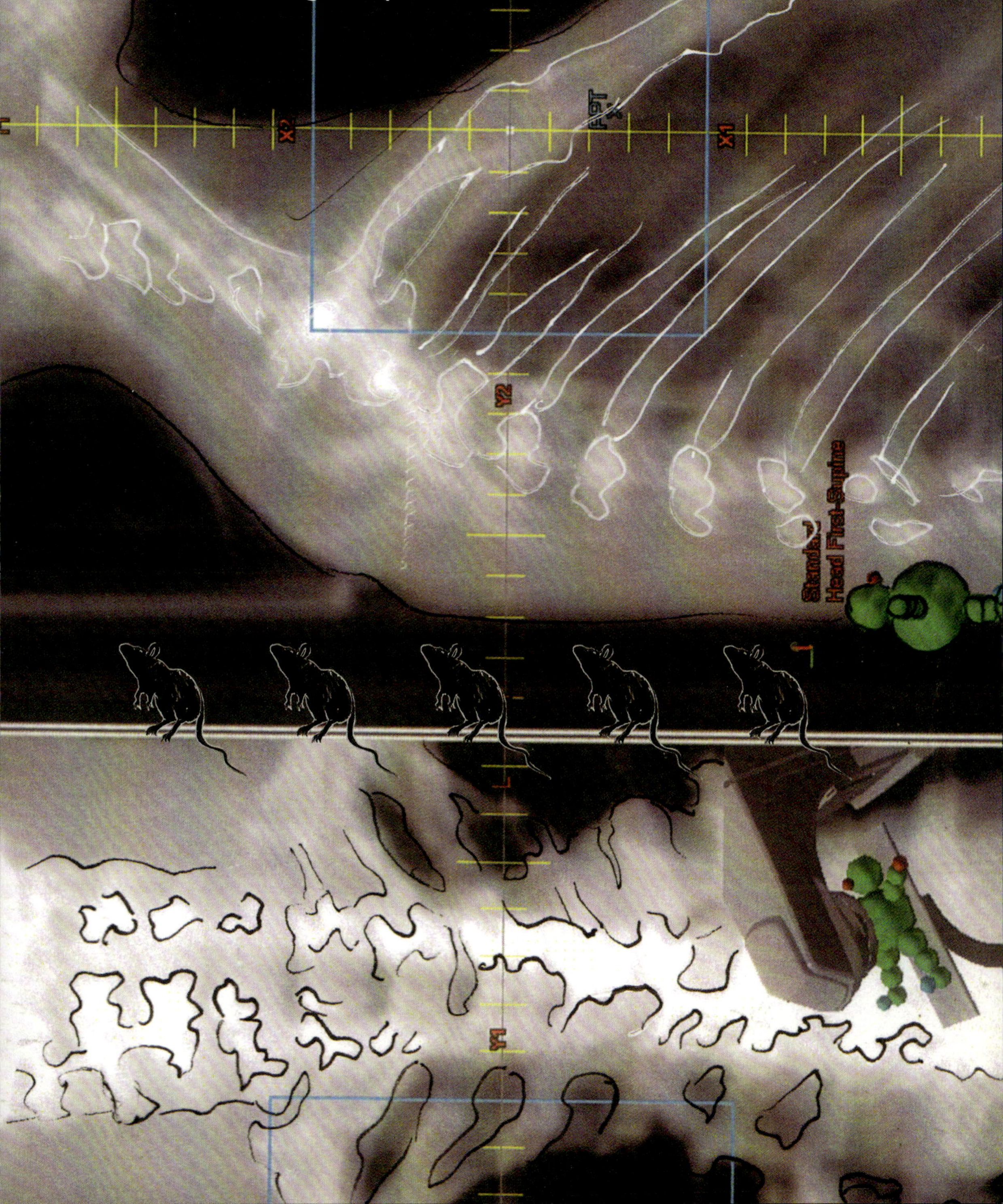

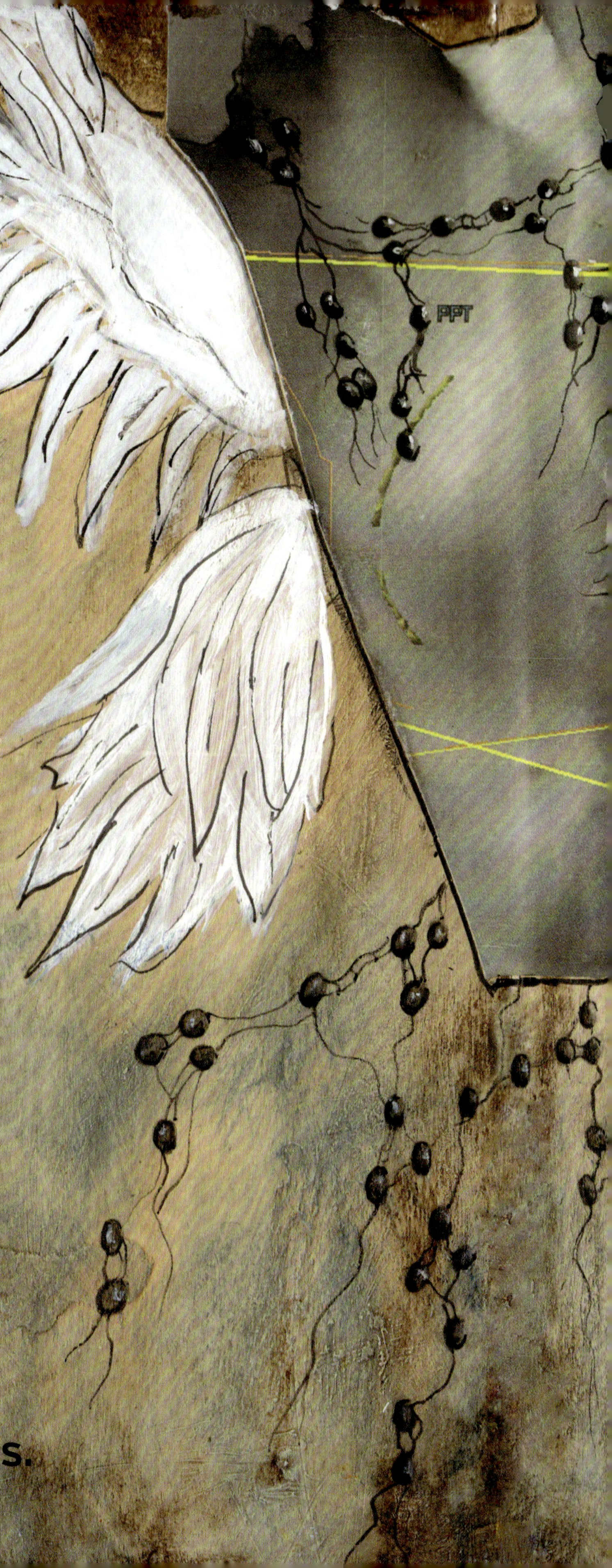

What would happen if I bolted? Has it ever happened? Would they chase me down the hallway or let me run? I picture a half-naked woman dashing through the waiting room past open-mouthed patients, fluorescent lights flashing off her bald head, yelling, "Start the car! Start the car!"

I have to admit to a total meltdown. It is so ... strange. I manage to hold myself together until the end of the radiation session when the head technician mentions casually that I'll need another tattoo but not to worry, it's no big deal. Barely holding it together, I say I am sure it is not a big deal to you but I have been poked, prodded, sliced and marked as much as I am going to be and I do not want one more FUCKING tattoo.

She apologizes.

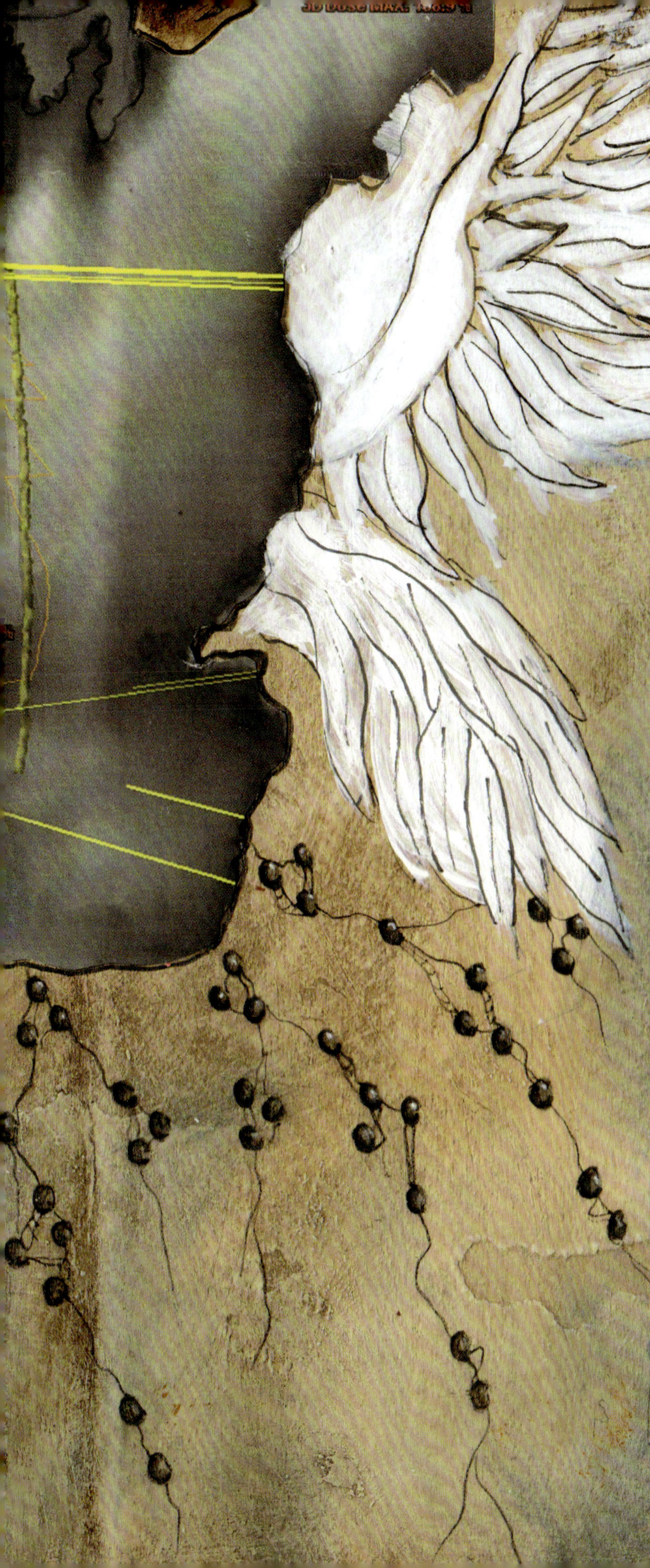

"It is easy to forget how stressed people are during this time." At her sympathetic tone I melt into uncontrollable sobs.

The short version: I don't have to get the extra tattoo. Apparently there is an alternative, involving a large red X and a see-through plastic bandage. It is not pretty but it is not permanent.

She must have wondered why such a little thing should push me over the edge. I blame my temporary courage tattoo. Half of it had rubbed off and left me with what I believe to be rage. For everyone's safety I must remember to re-apply them before I go for treatments. Although my guess is that everyone in the ward has already been warned I am a wee bit unstable. So things are normal.

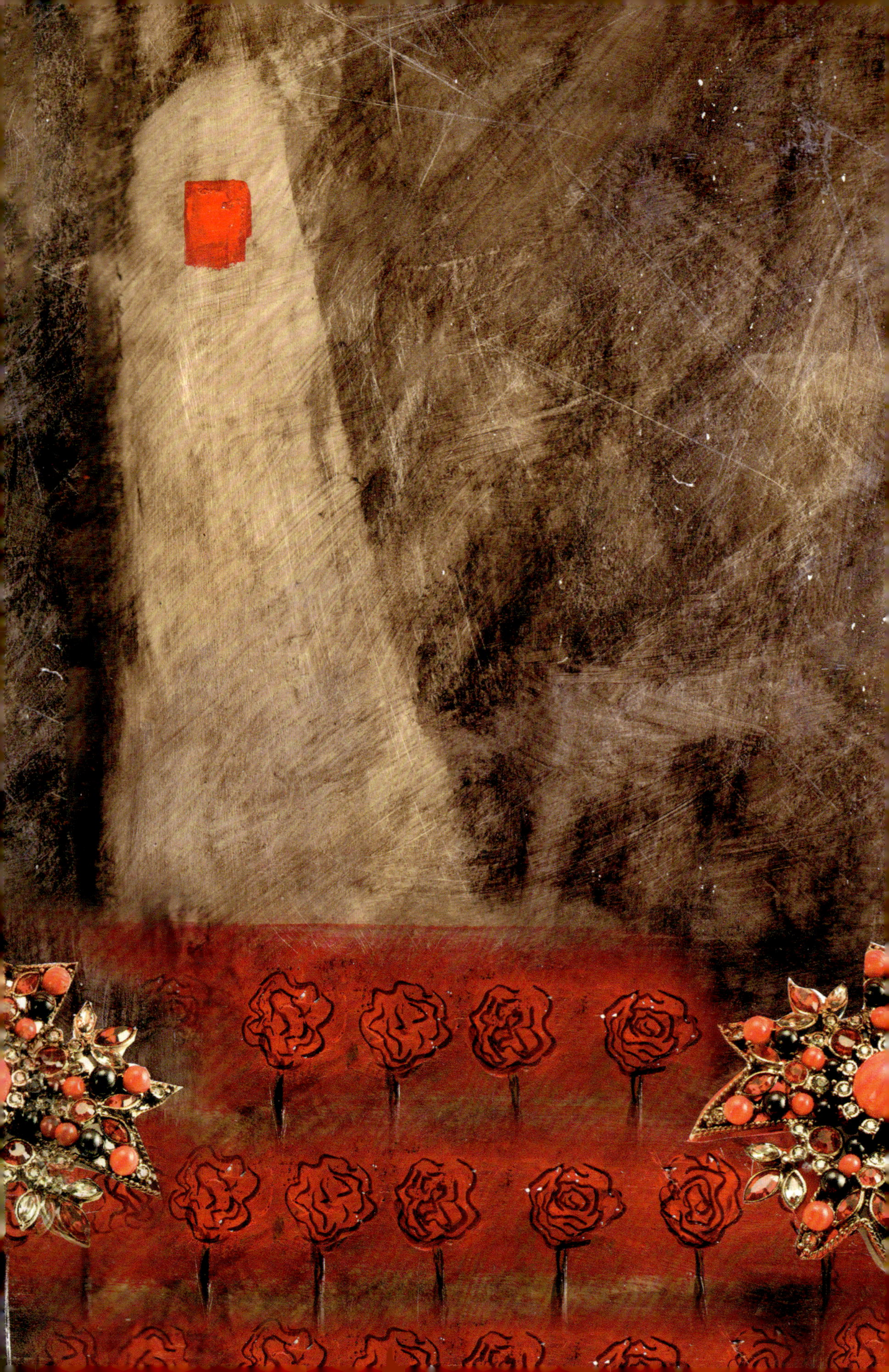

I discover that as much weight as I lost through chemotherapy I'm about to lose more during radiation. It burns huge amounts of calories. Our host Peter, is an amazing cook who is personally affronted that I am refusing to put on weight. He puts bacon on everything. Doug comes up to our room one morning asking if I would like Eggs Benedict made with last night's leftover salmon steak. I am in the kitchen in under 15 minutes and dig in. I have gone from being almost a vegetarian eating only raw foods to consuming as much protein as possible. My friends find it very entertaining.

I say just pass the bacon.

It takes several days for the cumulative radiation treatments to have an effect. When they do I find it difficult to stretch without pain. Ants crawl under my skin. Biting ants. The burns could be compared to a bad sunburn – if you were sunning yourself at Chernobyl. I take to sitting half naked in front of a fan to cool my skin.

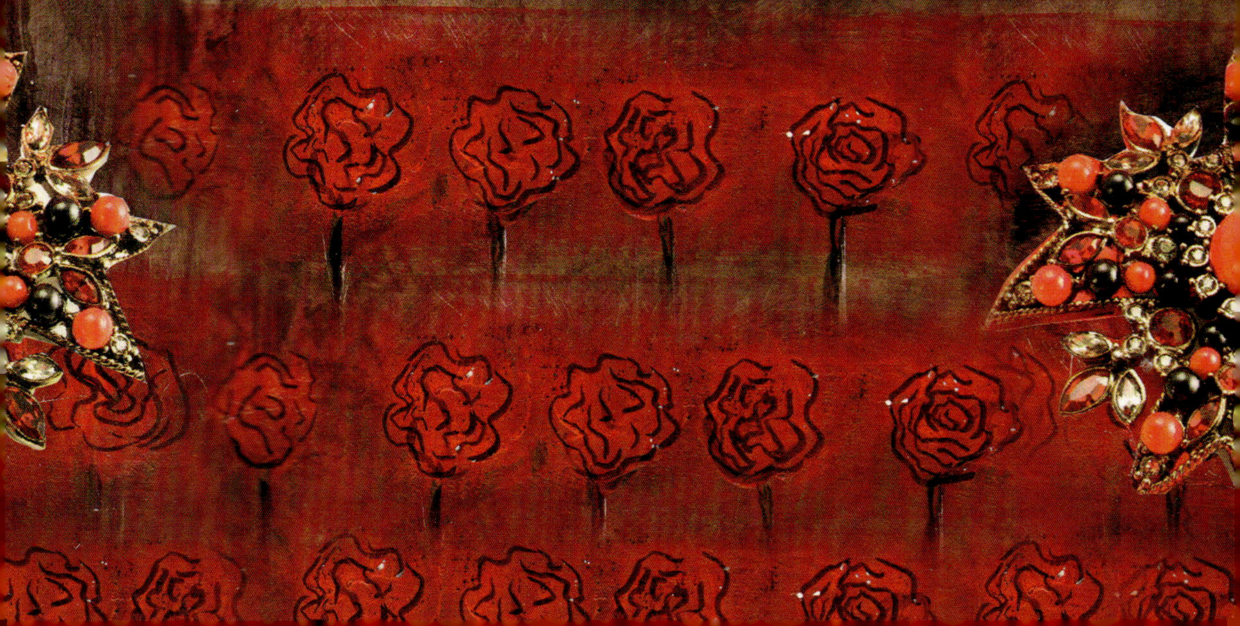

Halfway through my 15 doses I am at the Wound Treatment Centre to have my poor burned breast dressed. I am not keen on having anyone handle a wound that can't even bear the weight of light cotton, but the gods are with me and send an angel in the form of Nurse M. She lathers up gauze with Glaxol, like spreading peanut butter, and applies layer after layer, smothering the entire right side of my chest while enthusiastically giving directions on how to do this at home. She tops it off with a net stocking into which I slip my arms. It holds the cooling layers snug against my chest wall. I feel distinctly mummy-like but comfortable for the first time in days. I breathe a sigh of relief as the cold cream soothes my aching skin. Doug repeats this process several times a day.

Later that week as I'm trying on a dress the sales clerk admires the net top I have on underneath it. She asks me where I got it. I tell her the Wound Treatment Unit at the Cancer Centre, but say she probably doesn't want to go through what I had to in order to get one. She looks confused. For about the millionth time I curse my sarcastic mouth and my penchant for shooting it off.

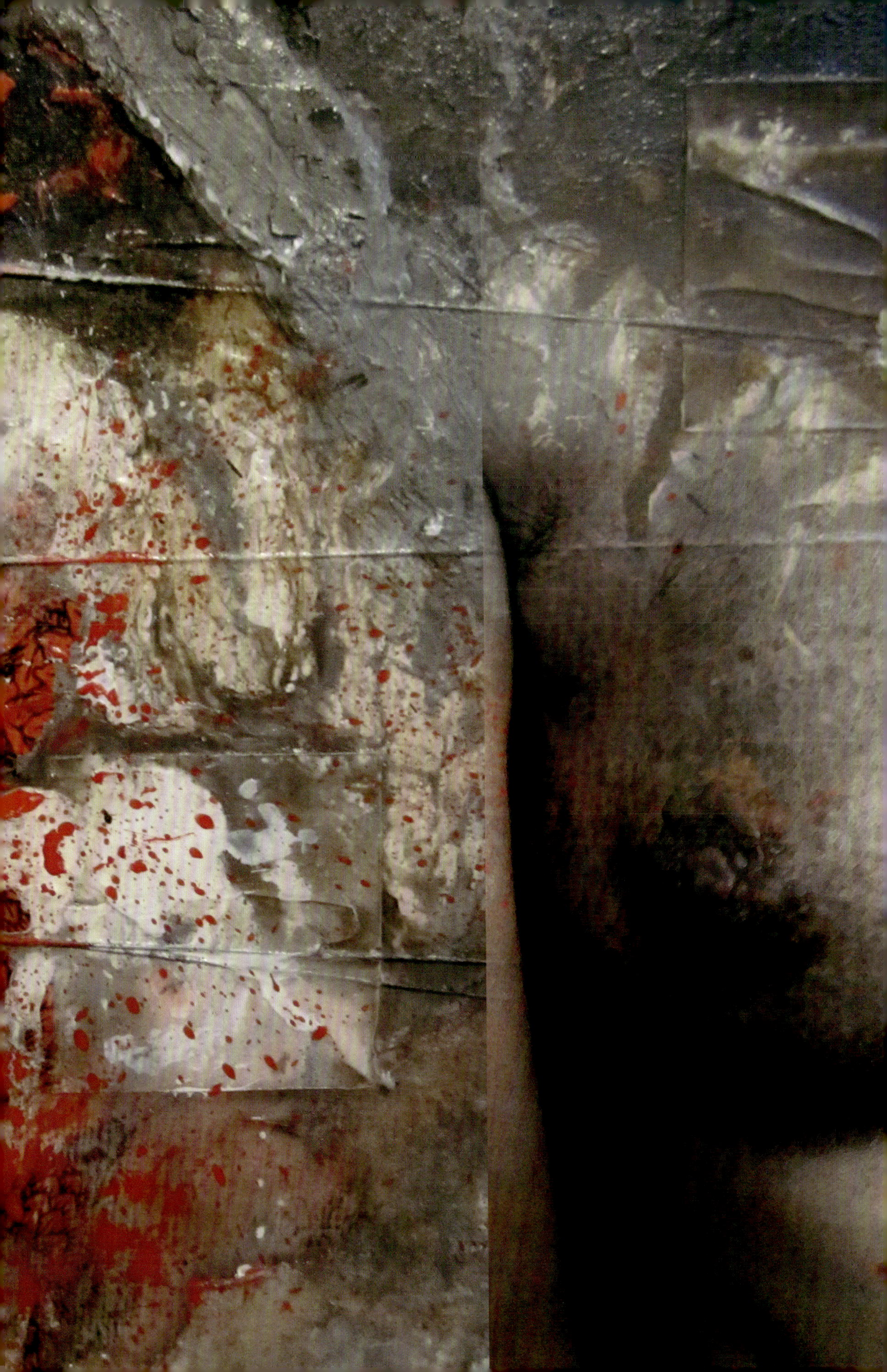

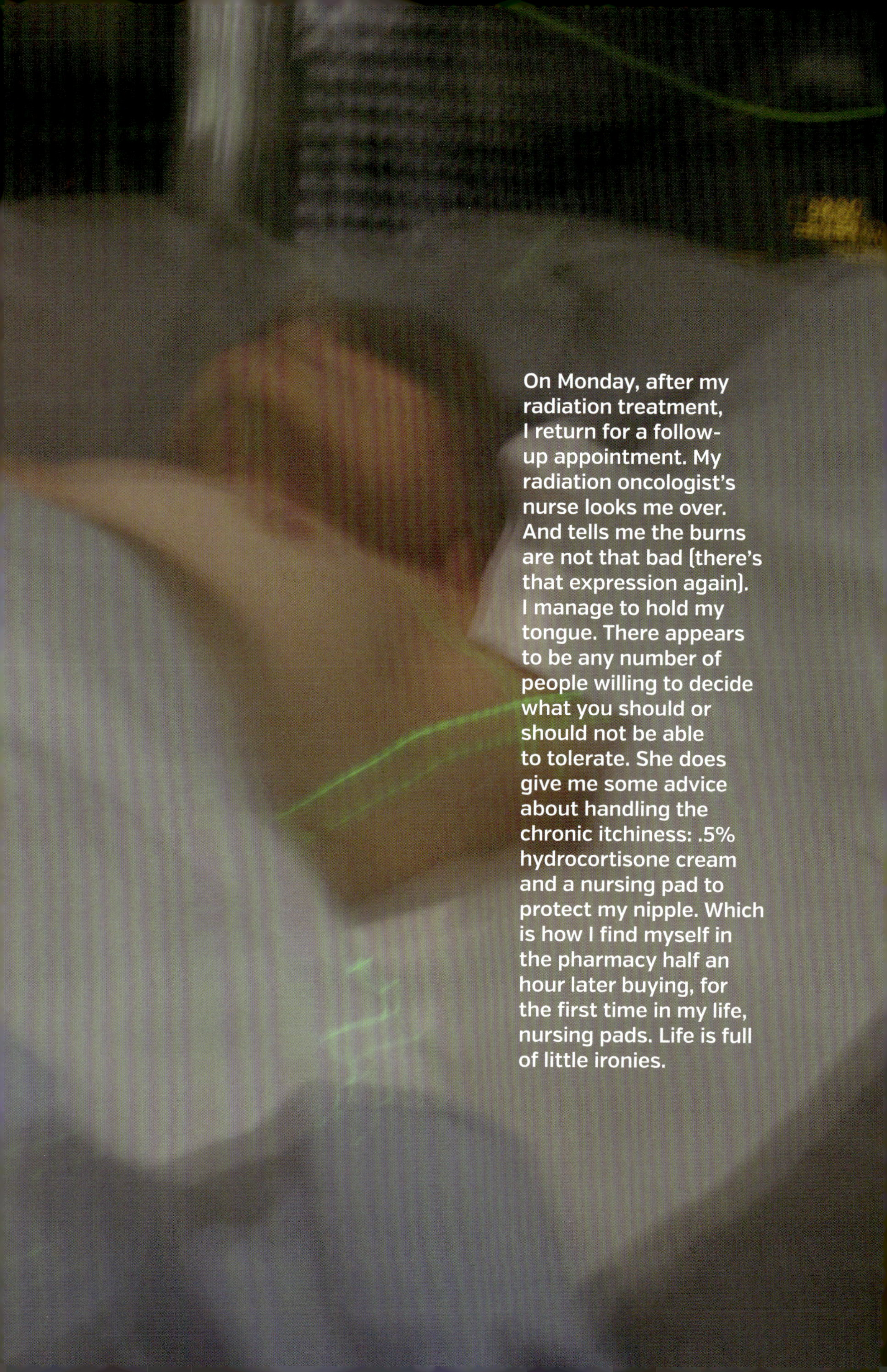

On Monday, after my radiation treatment, I return for a follow-up appointment. My radiation oncologist's nurse looks me over. And tells me the burns are not that bad (there's that expression again). I manage to hold my tongue. There appears to be any number of people willing to decide what you should or should not be able to tolerate. She does give me some advice about handling the chronic itchiness: .5% hydrocortisone cream and a nursing pad to protect my nipple. Which is how I find myself in the pharmacy half an hour later buying, for the first time in my life, nursing pads. Life is full of little ironies.

In the waiting room next to me is an older woman accompanied by her husband, a stoic Eastern European with a resigned expression. She is nervous, inquires about my chemotherapy treatments but really seems more interested in talking about her own. I understand completely and listen patiently. But when she says her nails are a disaster some of my patience slips. She shows me the white lines in her nails. I hold up my nail-less fingers informing her bluntly, Mine fell off. Without missing a beat, "Do you think mine will?" I am almost laughing, at her and myself. I recognize the self centredness that is a key part of this journey. I try to reassure her that if it hasn't happened yet it probably won't.

On the days when I have more energy, Doug and I lunch at a 50s style diner and remember what it is like to have a life outside of the hospital. I also occasionally indulge in a forbidden latte in my favourite coffee shop. I love these moments of warmth and hope.

I know I am not through the tunnel yet, but I march forward and toward the light.

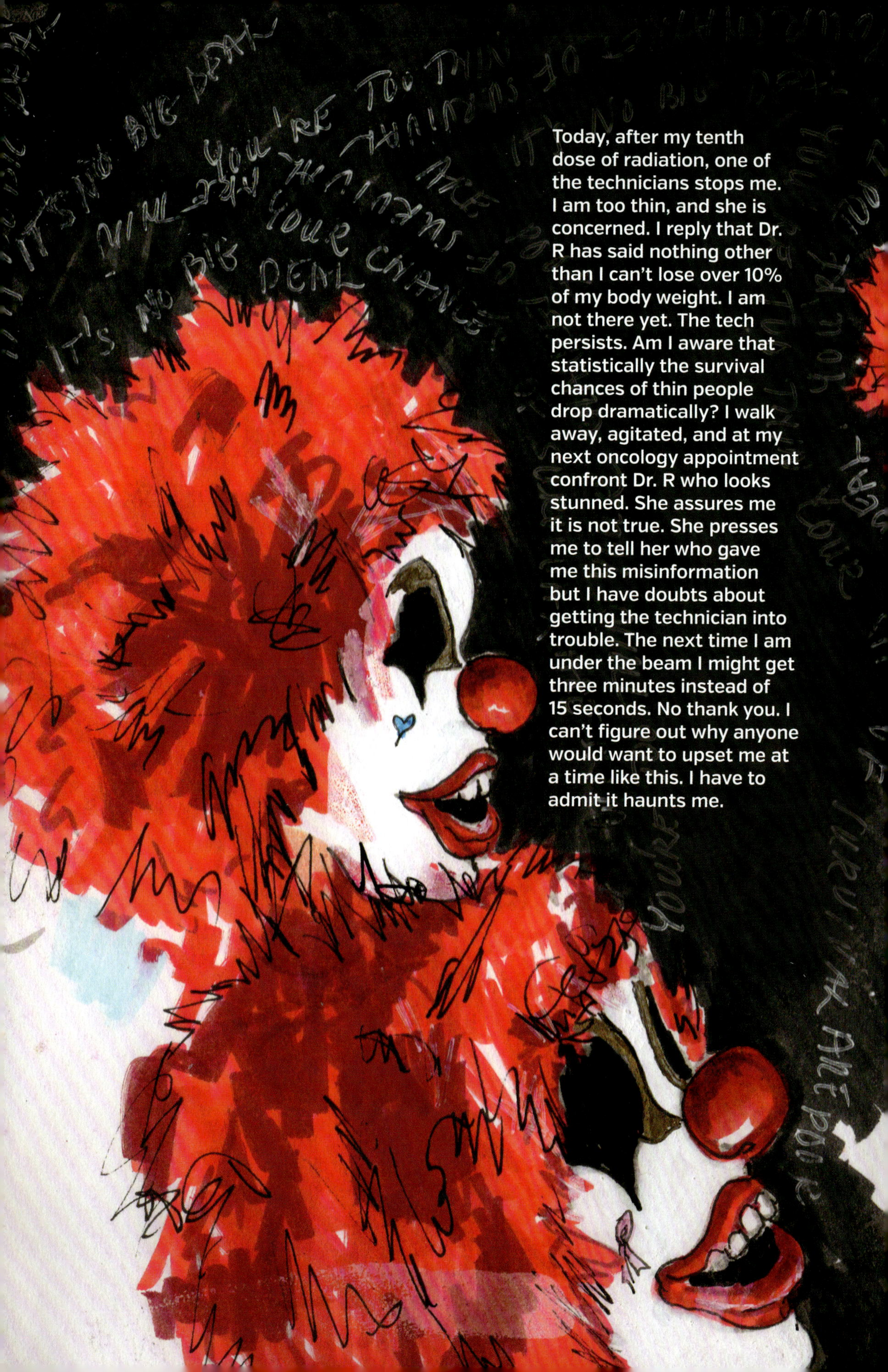

Today, after my tenth dose of radiation, one of the technicians stops me. I am too thin, and she is concerned. I reply that Dr. R has said nothing other than I can't lose over 10% of my body weight. I am not there yet. The tech persists. Am I aware that statistically the survival chances of thin people drop dramatically? I walk away, agitated, and at my next oncology appointment confront Dr. R who looks stunned. She assures me it is not true. She presses me to tell her who gave me this misinformation but I have doubts about getting the technician into trouble. The next time I am under the beam I might get three minutes instead of 15 seconds. No thank you. I can't figure out why anyone would want to upset me at a time like this. I have to admit it haunts me.

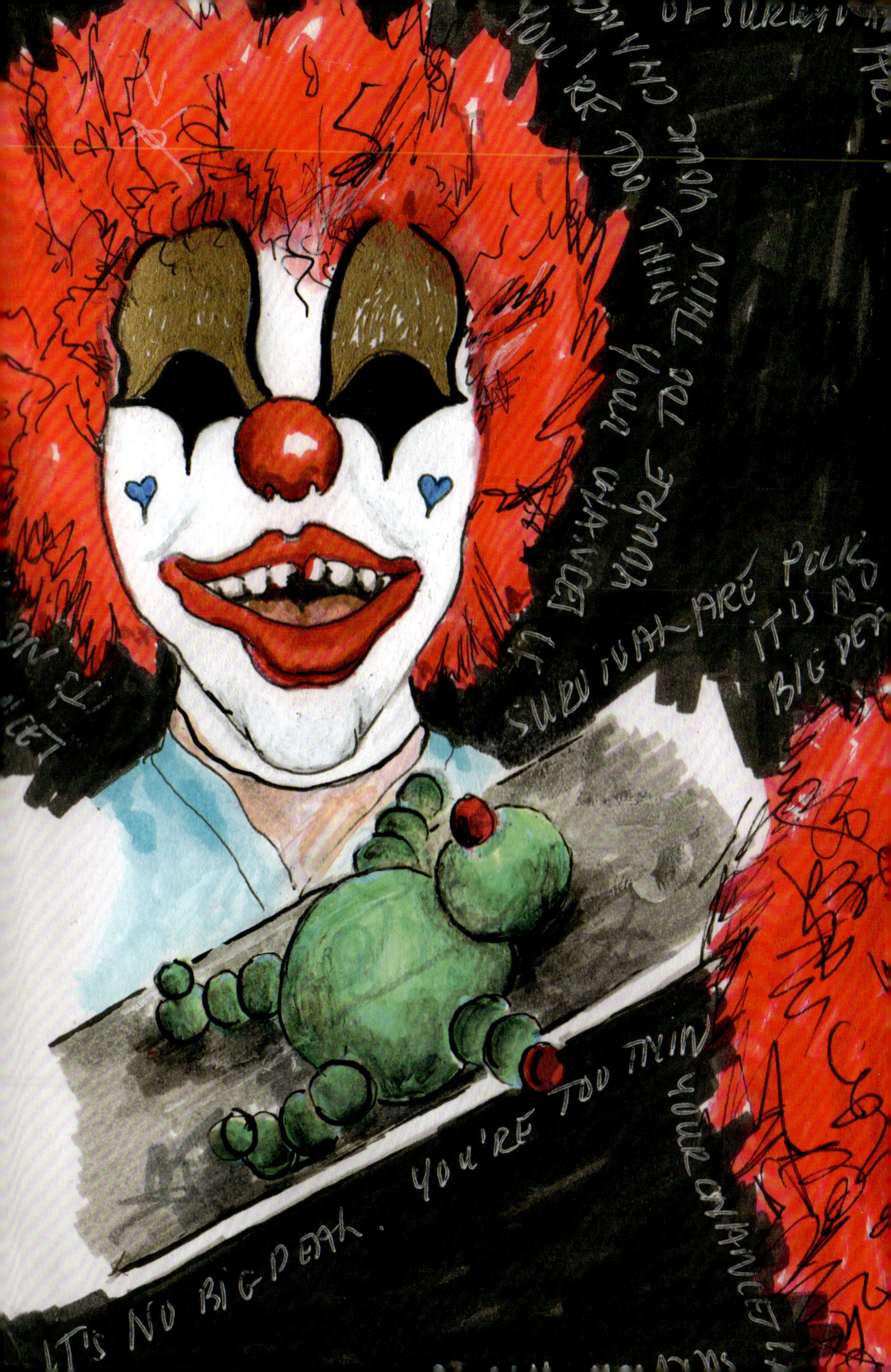
YOU'RE TOO THIN
SURVIVAL ARE POOR
IT IS NO BIG DEAL
IT'S NO BIG DEAL. YOU'RE TOO THIN

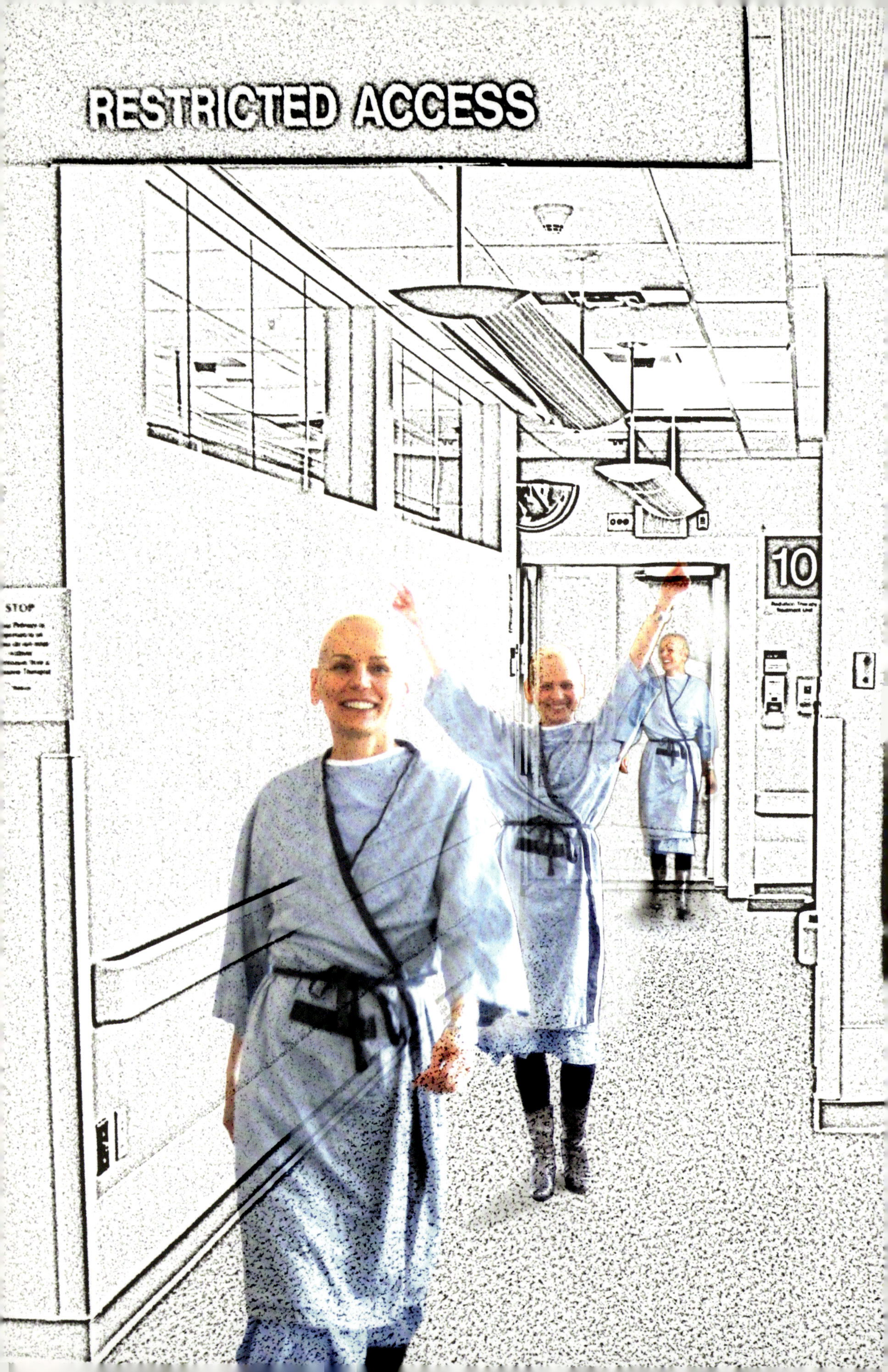
RESTRICTED ACCESS
STOP
10

It is my last day of radiation and I am thrilled. The ward is in chaos as one of the radiation machines has broken down. Patients are being moved from one room to another, tempers are short and the waits are long. The technicians ask Doug if he would like to come with me into the room. He has the camera with him. I have been trying to record as much of this journey as possible; although it may seem morbid to some, as an artist I need the visuals. He takes photographs of the machine, of me, of the technician setting up. Then we ask the technician to take our picture. I am lying on the table, half naked, he is crouched beside me smiling as if I am some kind of tourist attraction. I am laughing only slightly harder than the technician, who has never had anyone request a photograph like that.

I can't decide if she admires us or she thinks we are insane.

Possibly both. I walk out of the room and down the hallway for the final time. I sashay, maybe even shimmy.

I am done. Like an overcooked turkey. I celebrate with two teaspoons of 18-year-old Ardbeg Scotch. I don't even like scotch. Tonight, with all of this behind me, in the company of my husband and my friends, it is the best thing I have ever tasted.

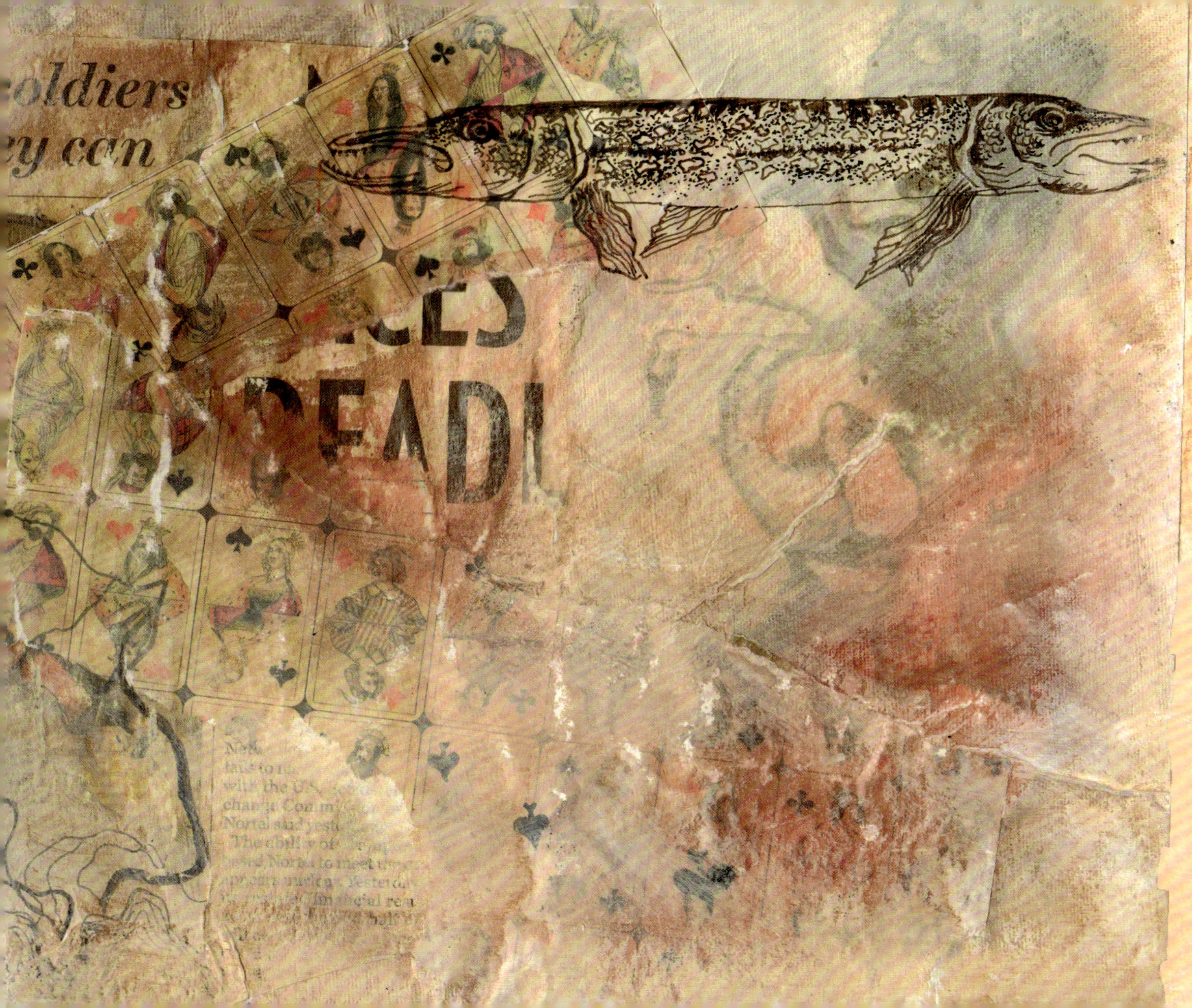
oldiers
y can

epilogue

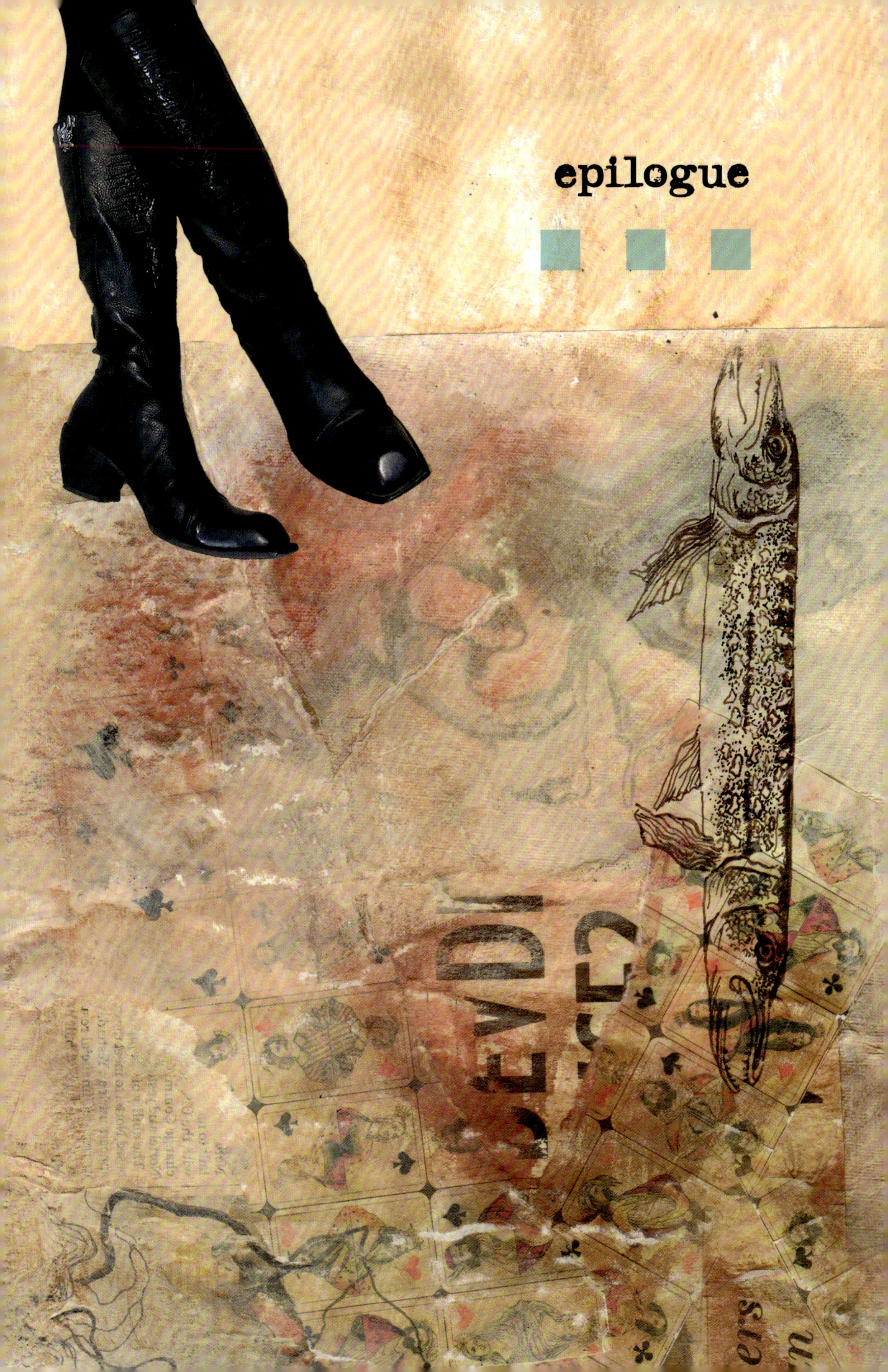

I am determined to walk the survivor's lap at the annual Run for the Cure. Every year my mother volunteers for the Cancer Society at the relay and this year my sister and I help her. The previous summer, I happened to be home and for the first time since my mother was diagnosed I walked with her. I had no idea that in less than a year I would return to walk my own lap.

When I register I am asked how long I have been a survivor. I finished radiation two days ago. I casually say since Wednesday. The registration woman seems a little miffed at my lack of seriousness. Plus there is no category. My mother tells her to put down six months. I walk with Doug, my family and my video camera. We shed more than a few tears. As this is my hometown, I see a lot of people I grew up with. Although I shouldn't be, I am stunned to see the number of people affected by this disease.

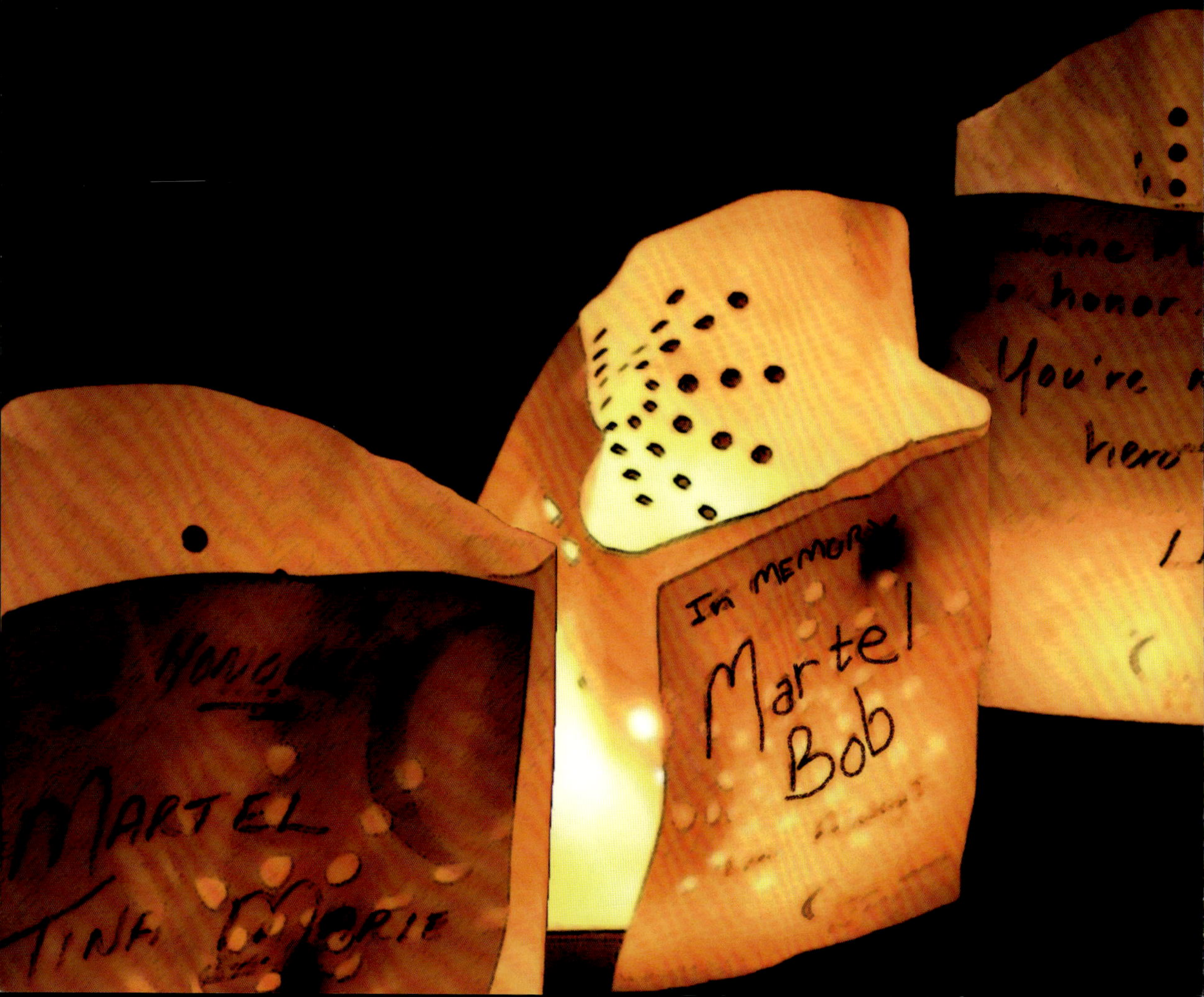

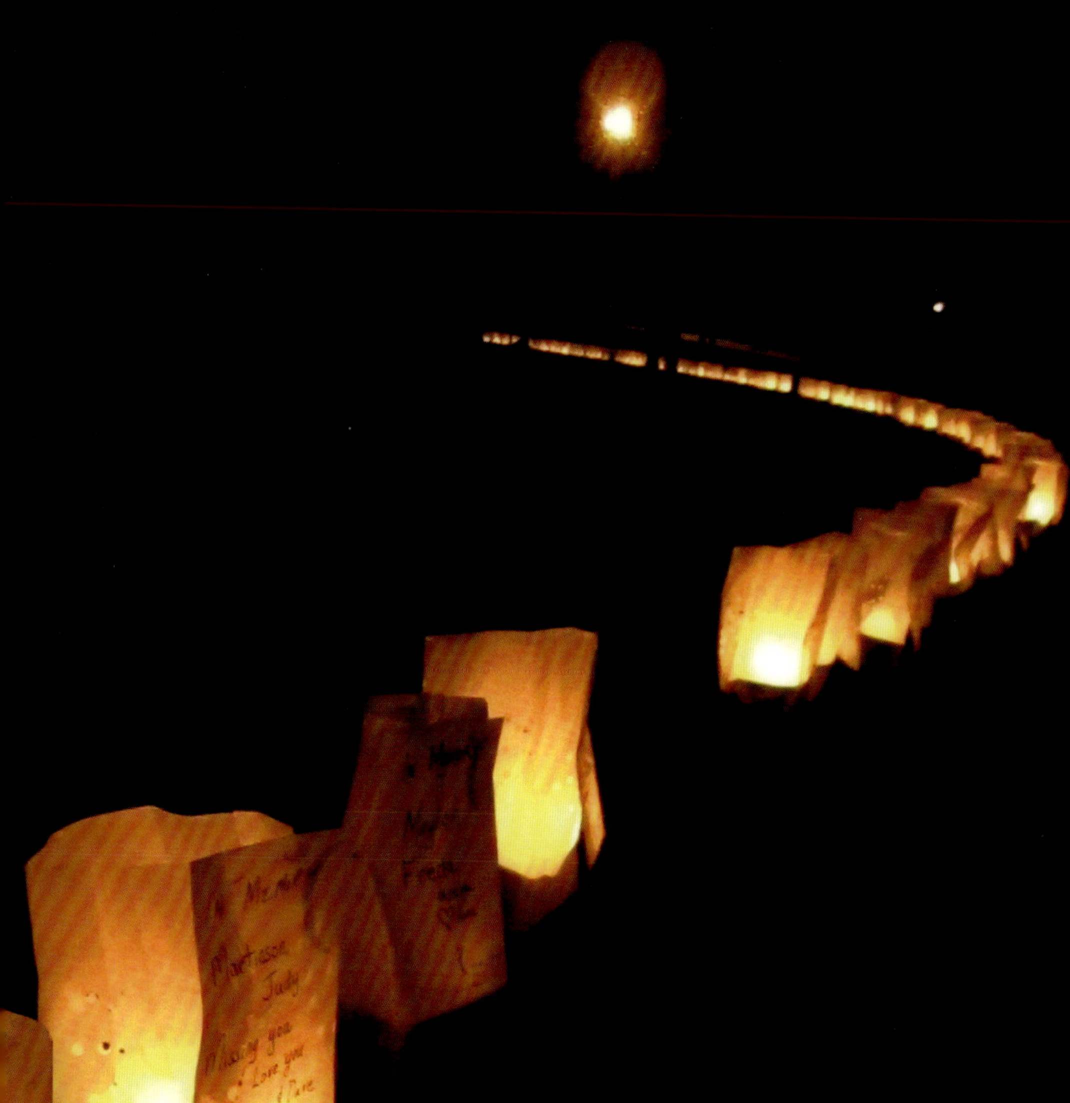

The entire field glows. Handwritten messages of sadness, triumph and hope. Doug and I light candles for his deceased partner, Janet, and for his dad, Arlo, who fought through pancreatic cancer. One for my Dad ... one for my Mom. Although I have my issues with fundraising and cancer research money, it is a moving event to attend.

I feel a bit hypocritical but mostly I am sad.

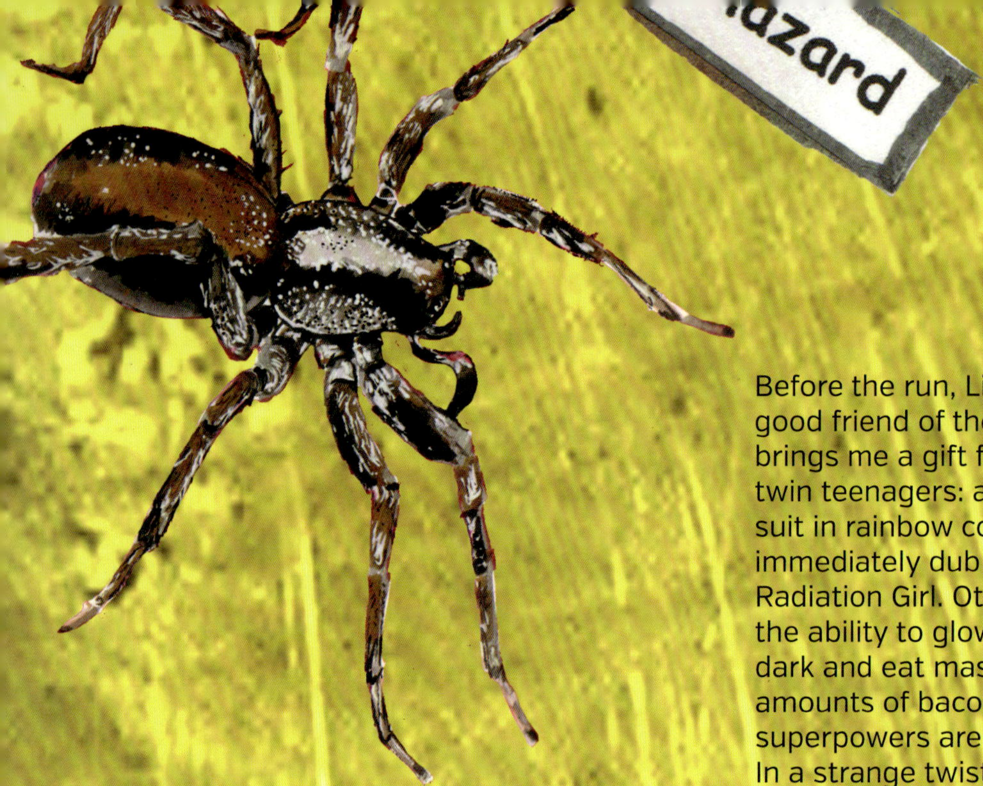

Before the run, Lisa, a good friend of the family, brings me a gift from her twin teenagers: a morph suit in rainbow colours. I immediately dub myself Radiation Girl. Other than the ability to glow in the dark and eat massive amounts of bacon my superpowers are few. In a strange twist of the classic Spiderman tale if I were bitten by a spider, it would become radioactive.

The effects of the radiation peak over the next several days. The itch is almost unbearable and even though I did not think I could become any redder, I do. Although I photograph the damage I can hardly bear to look. How is it possible to heal from this? I wear the burn dressings until the itch subsides. The square on my chest turns brown and flakes off.

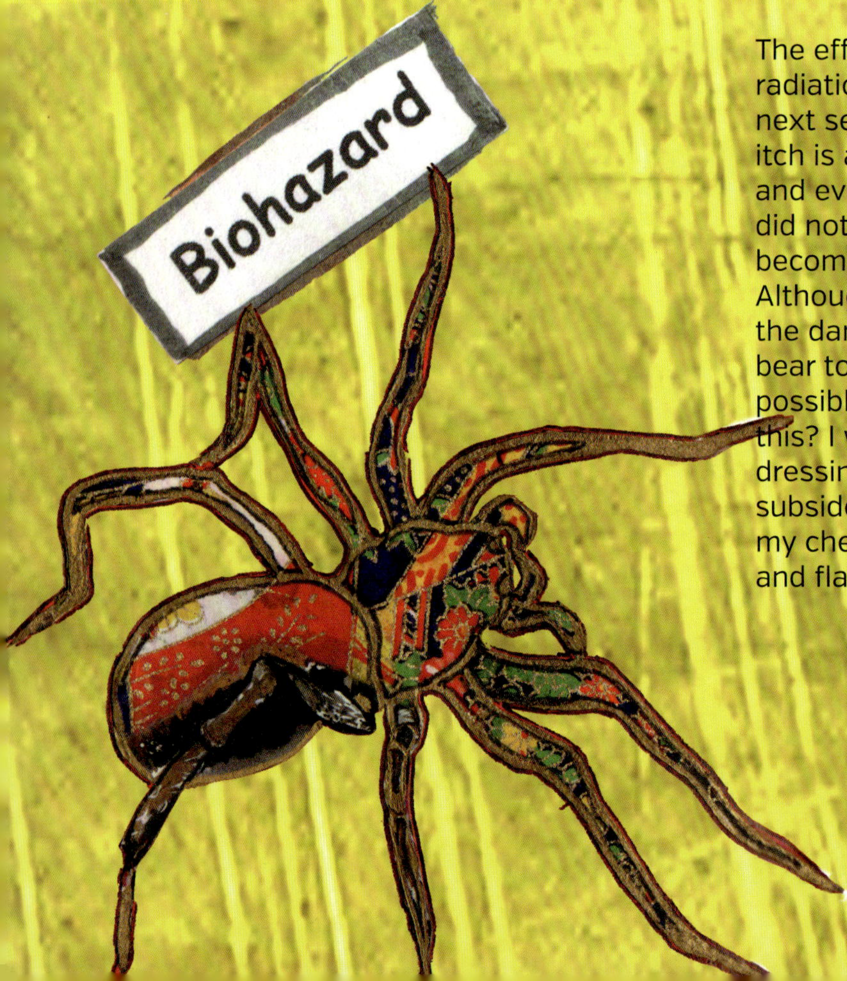

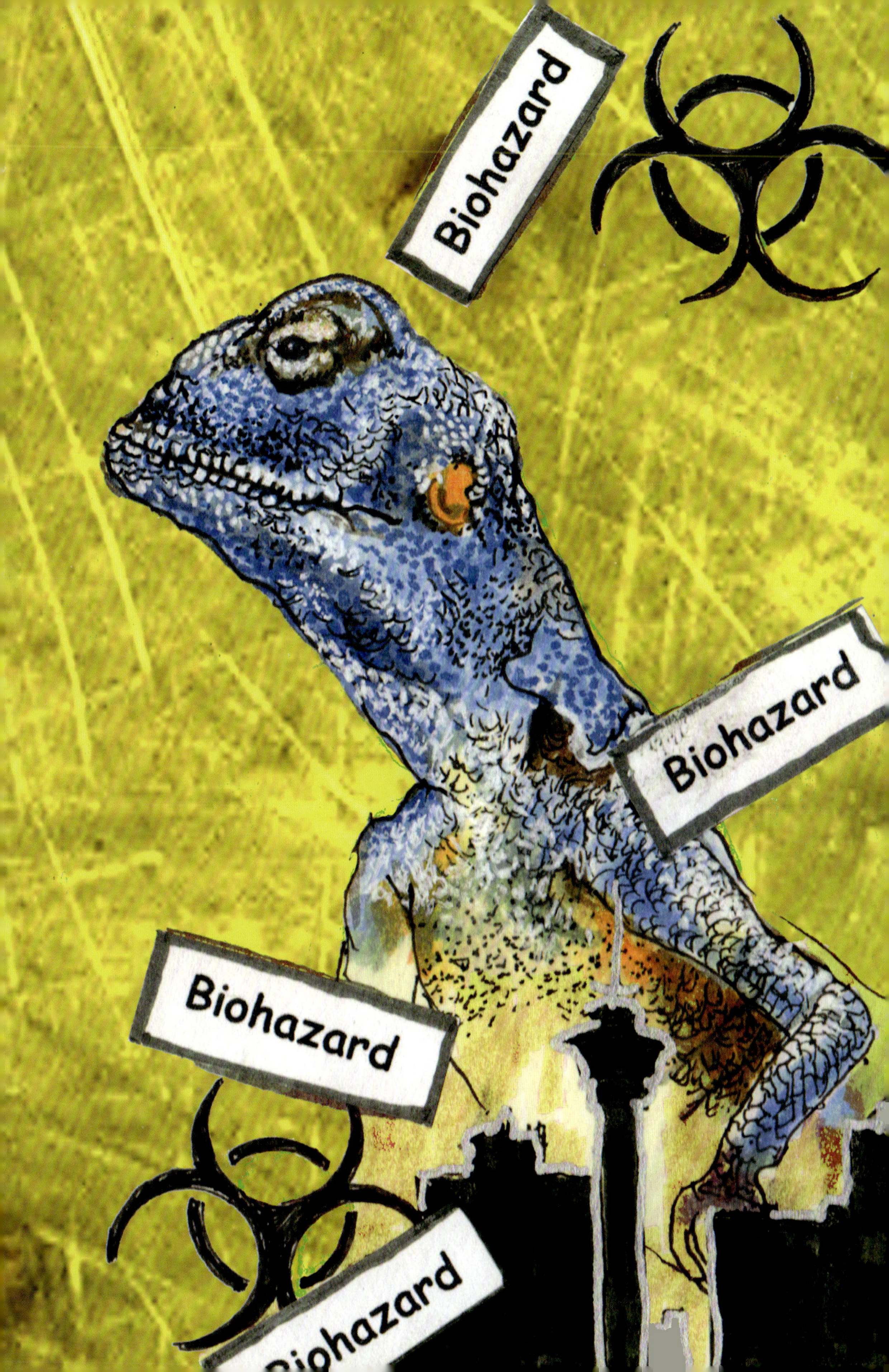
Biohazard
Biohazard
Biohazard
Biohazard

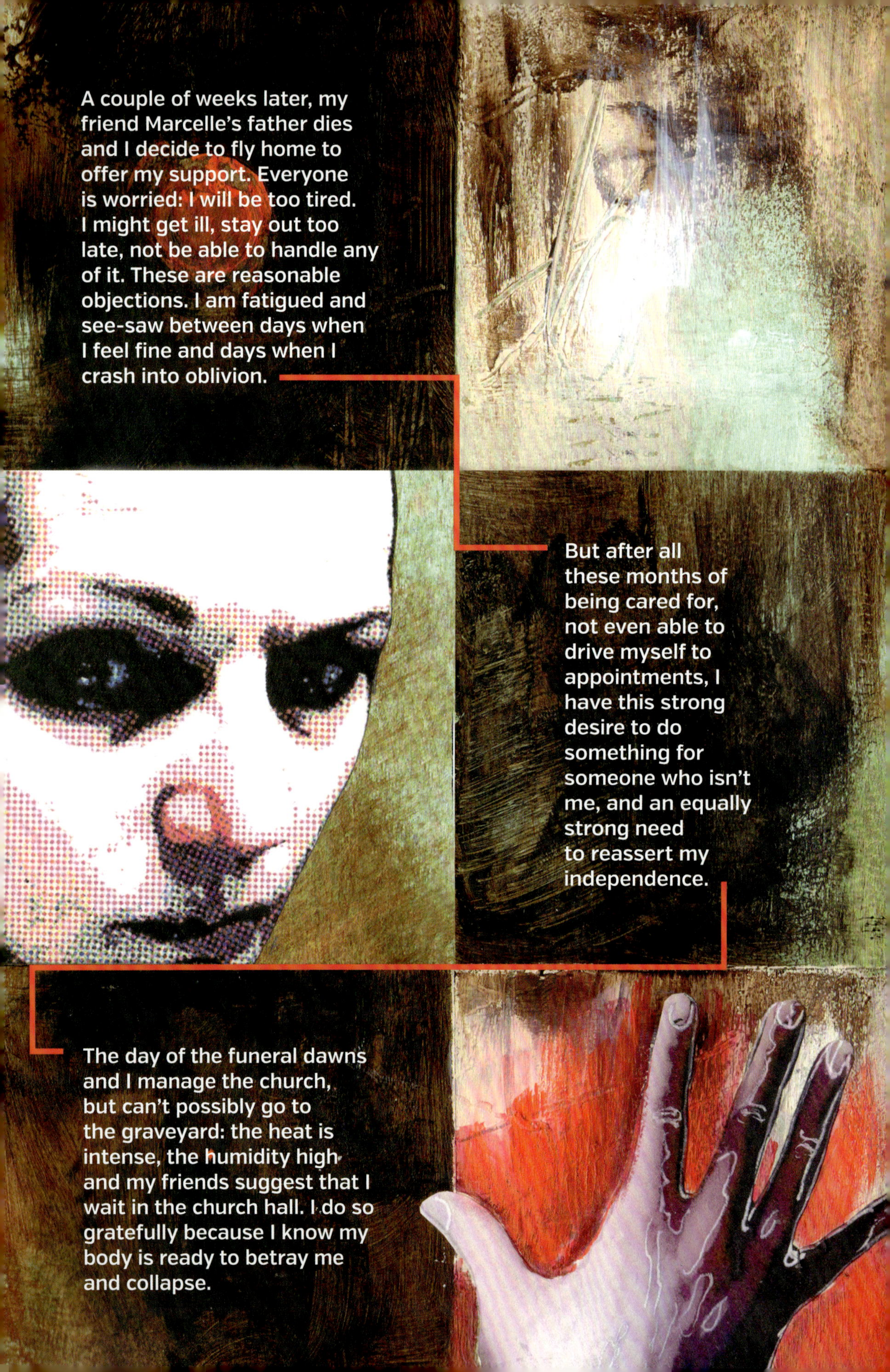
A couple of weeks later, my friend Marcelle's father dies and I decide to fly home to offer my support. Everyone is worried: I will be too tired. I might get ill, stay out too late, not be able to handle any of it. These are reasonable objections. I am fatigued and see-saw between days when I feel fine and days when I crash into oblivion.
But after all these months of being cared for, not even able to drive myself to appointments, I have this strong desire to do something for someone who isn't me, and an equally strong need to reassert my independence.
The day of the funeral dawns and I manage the church, but can't possibly go to the graveyard: the heat is intense, the humidity high and my friends suggest that I wait in the church hall. I do so gratefully because I know my body is ready to betray me and collapse.

I begin to ease myself back into life after treatment. My friend Lisa, a classically trained opera singer invites me to a "voice camp." She suggests I join the choir, which meets every day after lunch. I haven't sung in years. What a wonderful idea! On my first day, I meet Laurence, the über director, who has retired from the Vienna Boys' Choir.

He hands out the scores and I panic. What was I thinking??? I can't sight read, I am not a classically trained anything. I am an ex-rocker, country/folk singer who belly dances on the side. I am completely out of my depth … my sole hope is to put my head down and pray to stay invisible. I manage this for a couple of days but on day five, Über-director is telling us we have no rhythm. He stares me straight in the eyes. How did he even see me in the back row?

"You," he says. "Do you dance?"

It is out of my lips before I can stop it. A high pitched sound which remotely resembles a yes.

He says, "Then you know what I am talking about."

I have so much fun.

I visit a friend who lost her adult son a year ago in a terrible accident. We sit on the beach, our chairs partially immersed in the water to combat the overwhelming heat. I defy the no sun edict by wearing a bathing suit, but sit in the shade of the beach umbrella. We laugh. We cry. How we will ever be the same? She with her broken heart. Me with my broken body. I admire her strength. I will heal. Will she?

I go to a gig with friends who have a band. We're visiting before they go on, when one of the guys says, "That woman hasn't taken her eyes off you." I glance nonchalantly over to catch her quick turn away. At first I am flattered. Then in one of those strange perceptual flips I see myself through her eyes: dressed in black, skin tight jeans, sleeveless t-shirt, motor cycle jacket, skeletally thin, almost bald head and a couple of tattoos. Strange punk woman. Indeterminate sexuality. She's not attracted.

She's weirded out.

I get lost on the way home. Three in the morning. Pouring rain. I have no idea where I am and I panic. Burst into tears. This is not like me. Not like the old me. I stop, turn around, breathe, hope I am visible if someone flies around the corner. The only people on the road are driving home from the concert. Me and a whole boat-load of drunks. I briefly consider retracing my steps and spending the night at the party where I left my friend Jim, but I have my mother's car and she worries, still of the generation that thinks a woman shouldn't be out without her husband. Much less out all night. It is possible I shouldn't be out at all, but not for those reasons, and I am determined to reclaim my life. I try again and this time turn in the right direction.

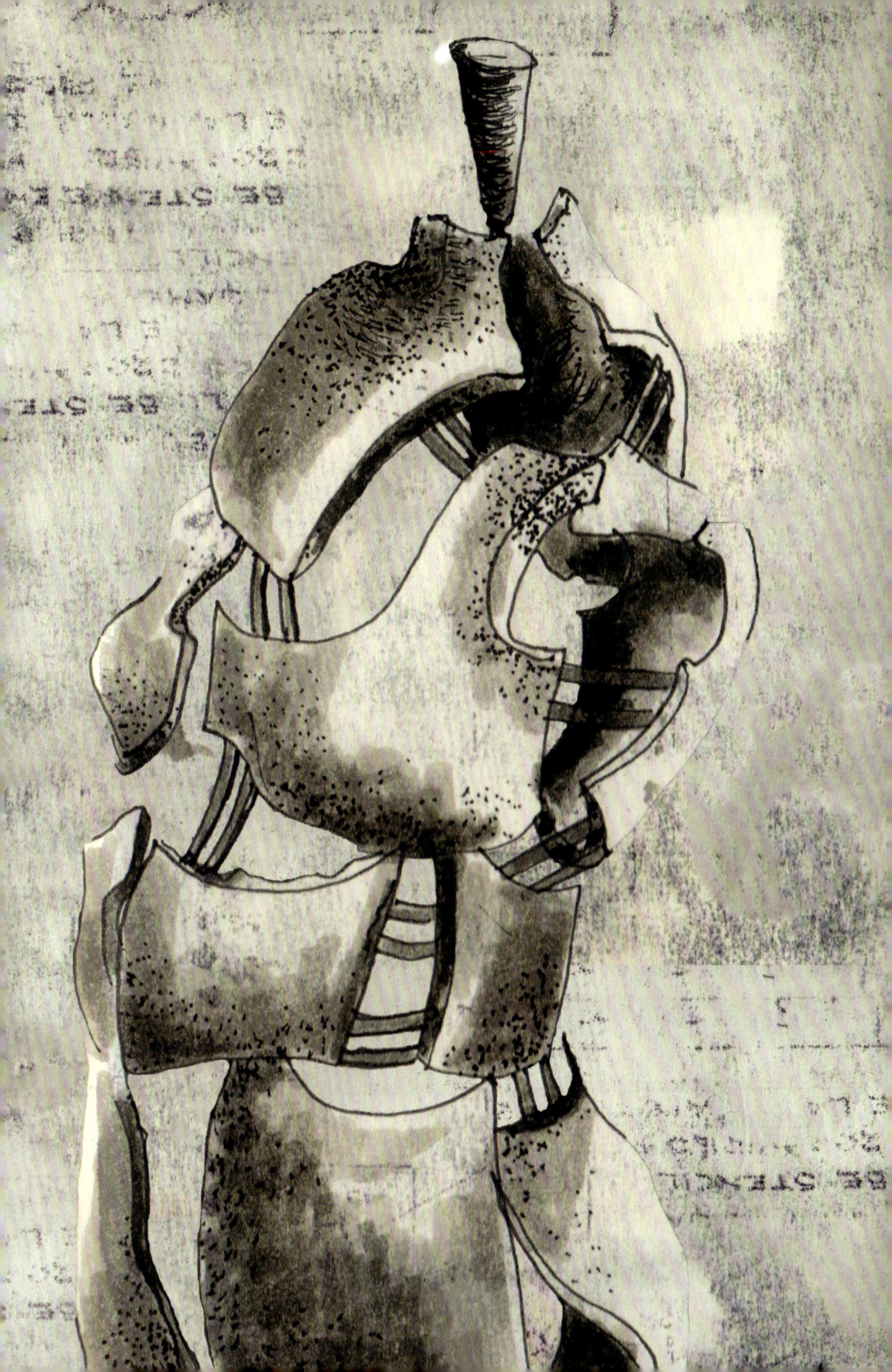

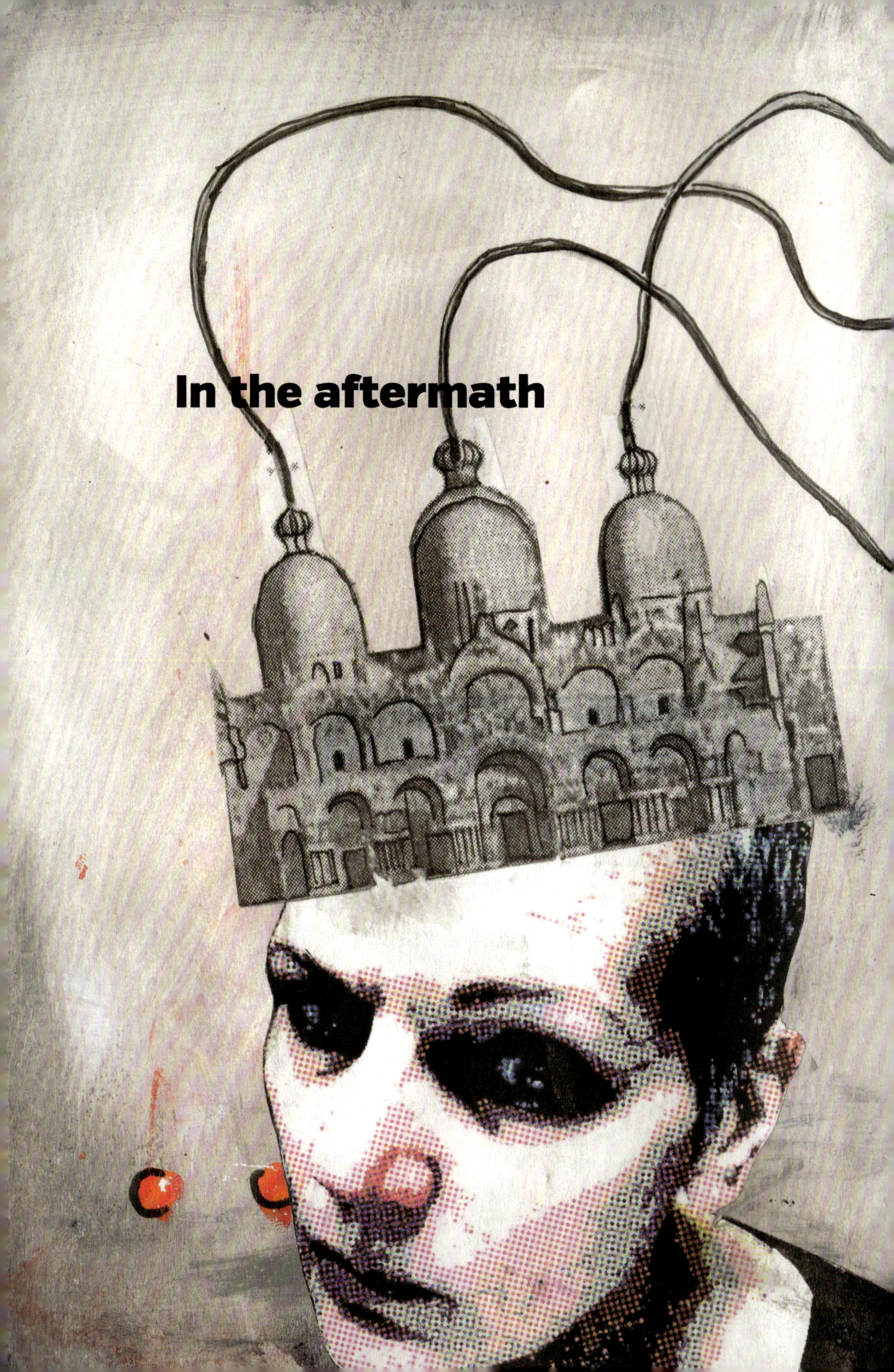
In the aftermath

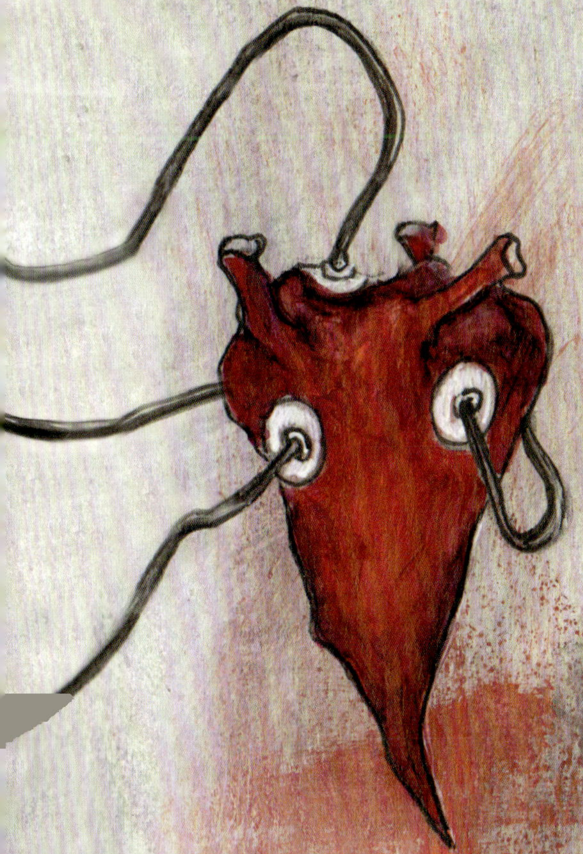

I return to work. Dr. O tells me bluntly that it is not a good idea but financially I am out of resources. My first day back I find the number of people who have tears in their eyes as they greet me overwhelming. My emotions are already high and theirs are wrenching for me. My friend Rob sends a text message wishing me "puppies, rainbows, dolphins and unicorns." HUH? Later I reply, Don't send me anything else. Two of the dolphins died, mumbling something about water. The puppies are needy little buggers, and I threw the unicorn out after he ate my Post-it notes. I chuckle as I hit send: I sound like myself.

The next day after work I am sobbing uncontrollably in the car. Hitting the steering wheel. I can't do this ... over and over again. Tasks I found effortless before are monumental now. My command of language is suddenly sketchy. Lectures grind to a halt as I search for the right word. I send a student into the woodshop with the directions to pick up a mirror in the thing under the window with the shelves and the door. She helpfully suggests, "The cupboard?" Yes. That's it. Often I have to look down at my hands to see what I am carrying in hopes it will give me a clue to what I am doing.

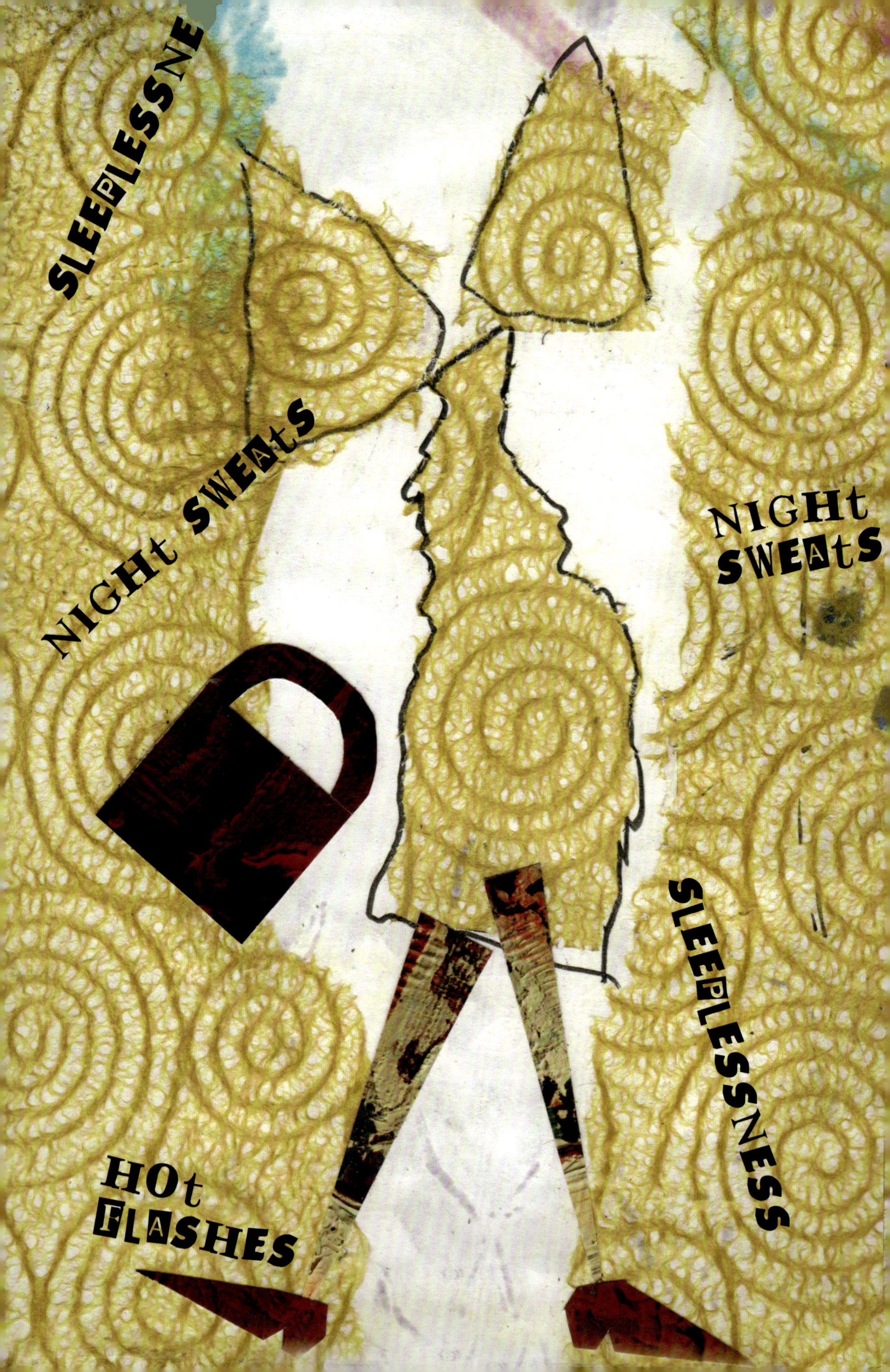
SLEEPLESSNE
NIGHt SWEAtS
NIGHt SWEAts
SLEEPLESSNESS
HOt FLASHES

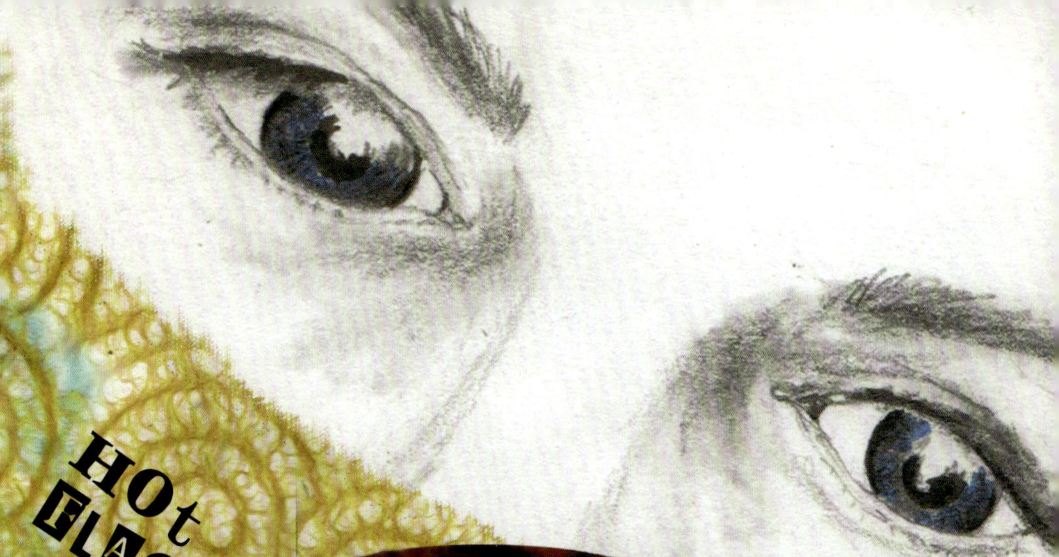

Each night before I leave I make stacks of what I will need for the next day. I top each stack with a Post-it note, my new best friend. On the one day I don't prepare, I break down before a lecture and my colleague Laura has to take me into my office to calm me down. I am discouraged, disheartened. "Chemo brain" continues.

My feet swell, I have severe joint pain. My eyebrows and eyelashes thin almost to the point of extinction every three months. My hair is patchy and wispy. Not mine at all. Menopause has arrived: hot flashes, night sweats, sleeplessness, not to mention the emotional backlash. I am more hormonal than a 13-year-old and I have disposable income. Dangerous combination.

Campus Operations finds a comfortable chair for my office and I curl up like a cat for a nap after lunch between classes.

I have a checkup every three months. I continue to see my homeopath. I find another cyst which this time requires a biopsy. It proves to be nothing but sends me into a panic. There is a problem with my liver enzymes and briefly there is a concern the cancer has metastasized. We spend a frightening week as we wait. The ultrasound shows nothing. The wife I have picked out for Doug won't be necessary after all.

But through it all I am alive. I have people who love me. I am in the studio painting like a mad woman. We implement new policies in my belly dance group: nobody gets pregnant; nobody dies. At work, I frequently shake my head at office politics and think,

You don't know what a bad day looks like. I try not to let the words leave my lips.

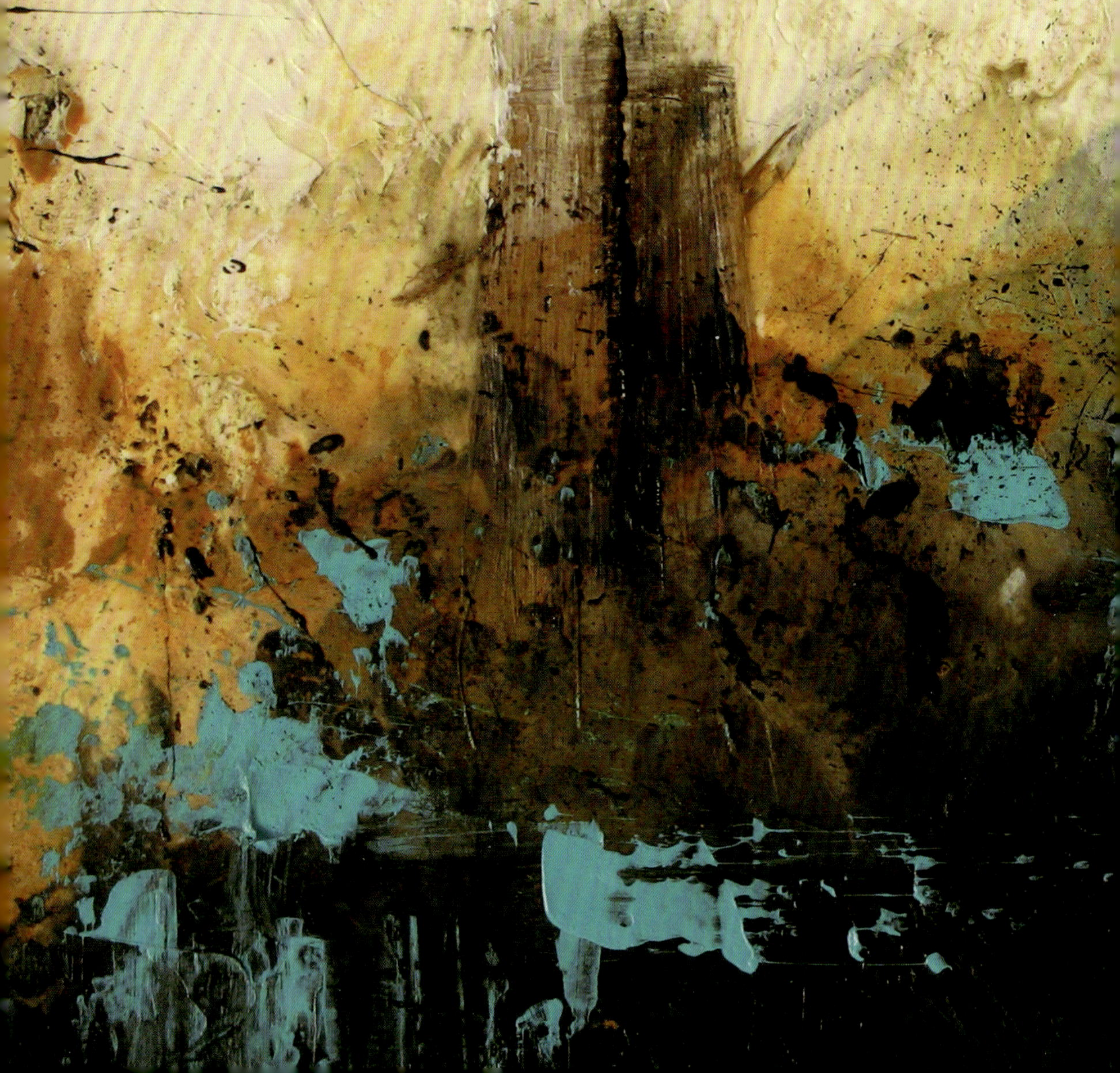

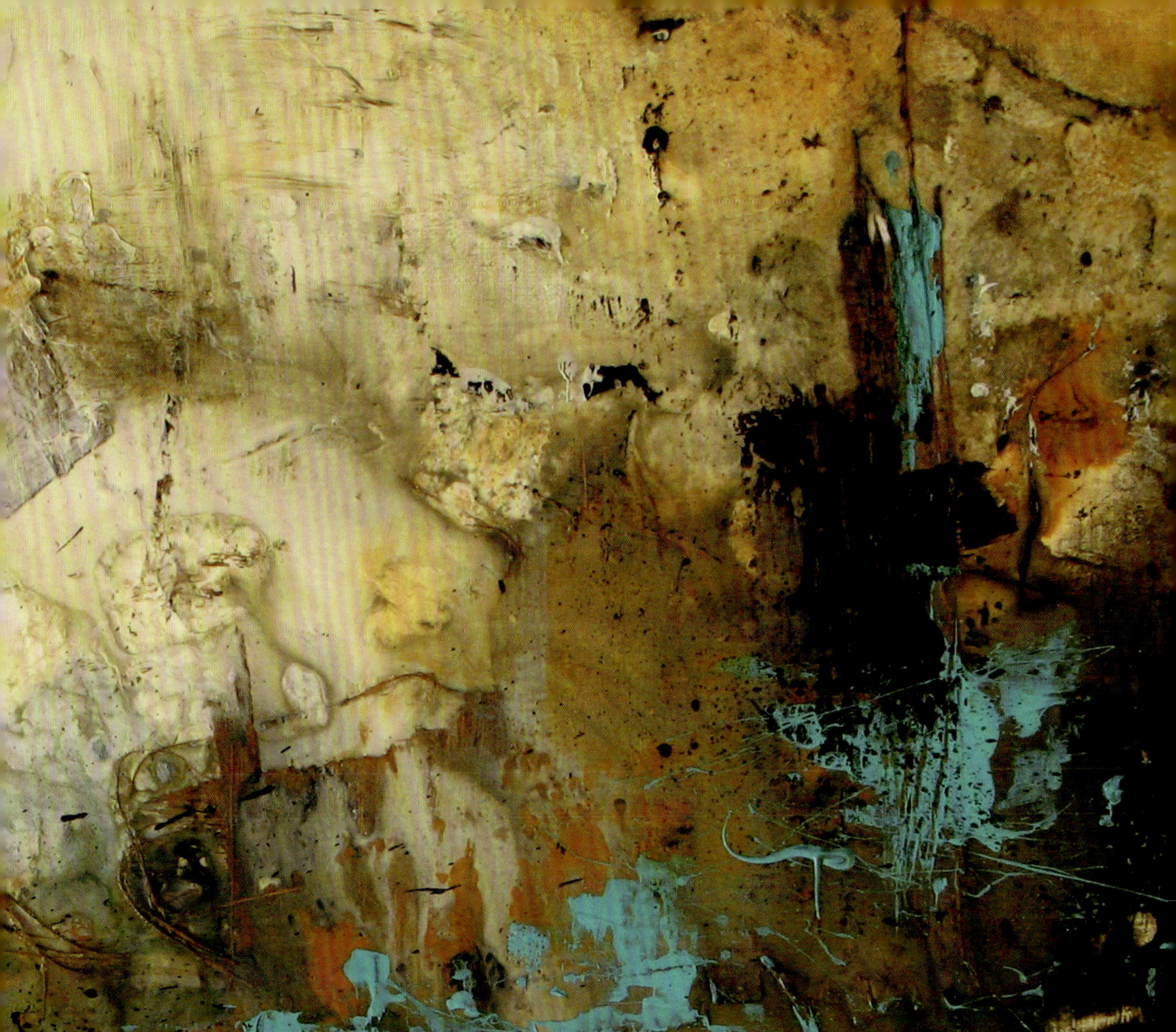

There are many times I am not sure who I am anymore. I do what I have always been taught. Keep moving. One day at a time. One step forward, two back. Two steps forward, one back. It is a dance. I am a dancer.

I think about all the women who have lived through this disease. All the women who didn't or won't. The people in their lives who are affected. I am lucky to be one of those who has survived. I wish I could have been more enlightened, more even tempered, could leave a better message of hope. I wish I had been stronger. More admirable. Less like one of those TV reality-show participants who makes you want to throw something at the screen. I wish I could worry less. I waver between taking everything in stride and being wound into a tight ball of grief and impatience.

At such times I hold on to these wise words offered by a kind friend:

"You need to be patient with yourself, Tina. After all, you didn't have the flu."

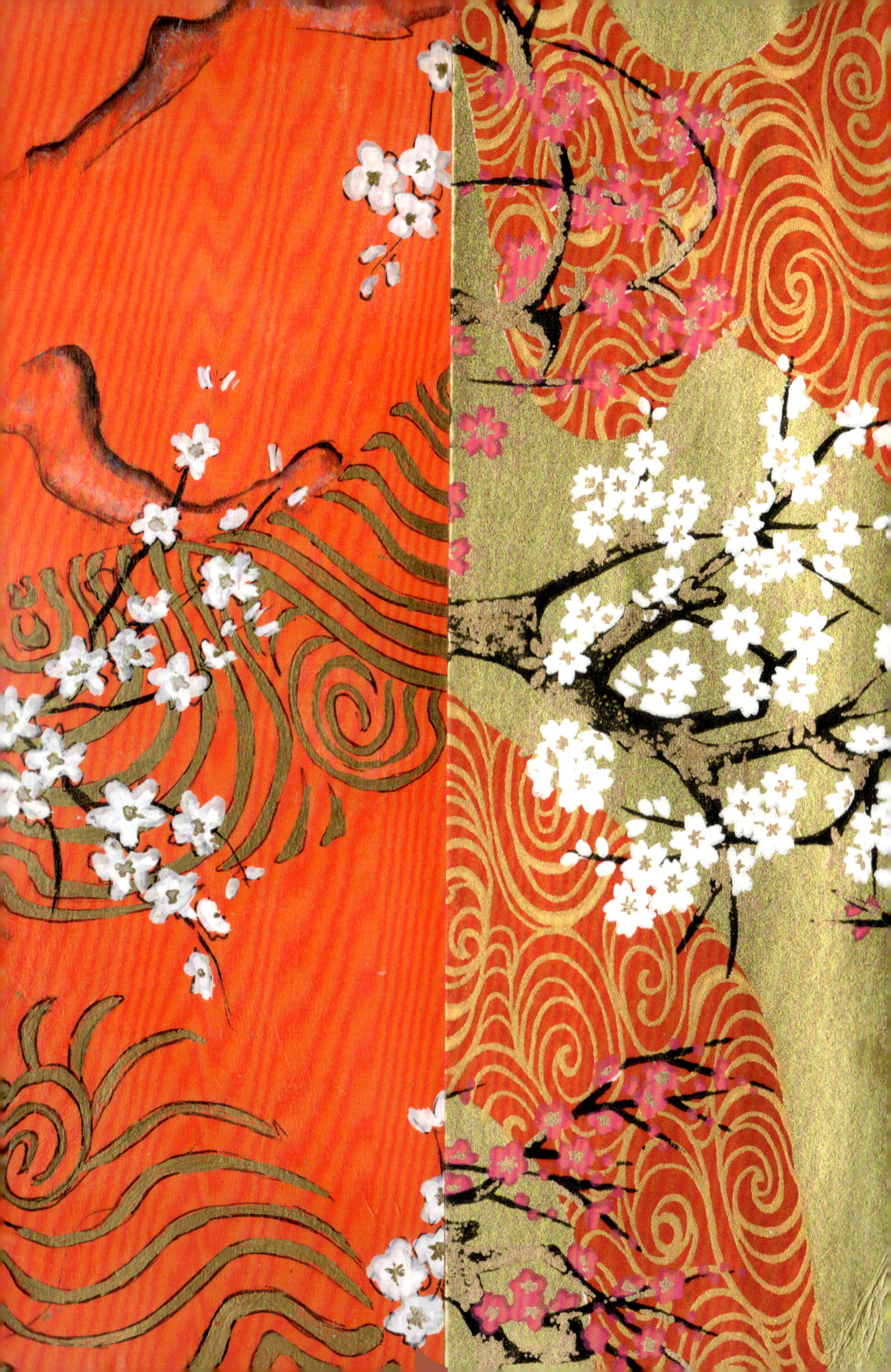

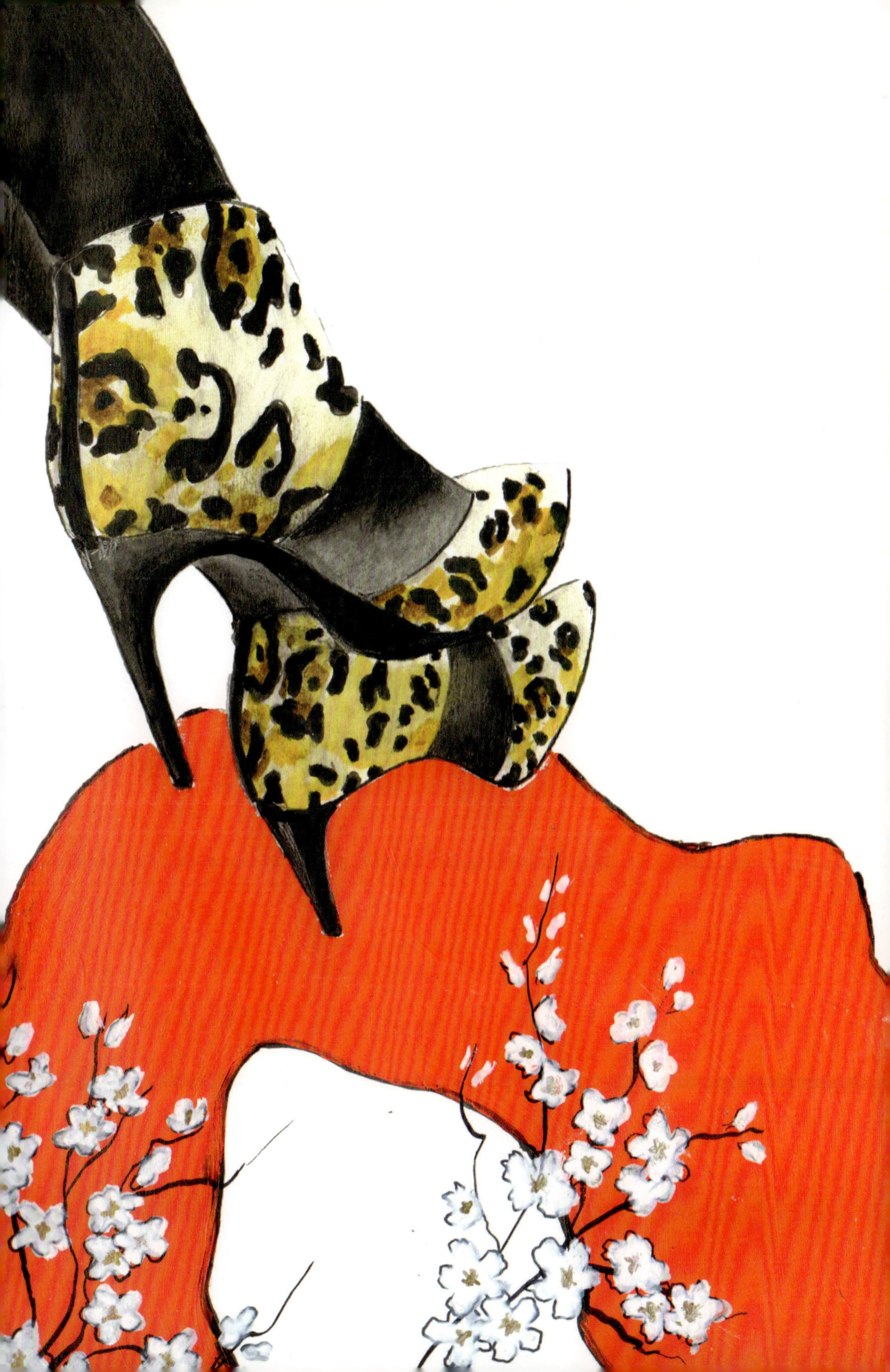

Thanks to all of you

Maggie and Fraser / without whom none of this was possible.

Barb / for whipping this project into shape and honestly believing I could do it.

Bernadine / for the endless coffees and laughter.

Marcelle and Lance / for always being there.

Ken and Carol / for their unflagging belief in me.

Laura / who fought for me all the way through. I miss you still.

Dymphny / whose advice was invaluable.

My family / my brother Jeff and his family, my sister Trudy and hers, the best cousins ever - Jeff and Janice.

Susan, Don, Kazim and the admin team / for all the support.

Peter and Linda / for having us as extended house guests.

Arlo / for doing the same.

My distance friends / Kim Lee and Kal, Joyce, Nadine, Jon and Cormac, Rob, who sent me something everyday to make me laugh, Murray, who has gone through his own hell.

My medical team / who I can't name ... my oncologist and his assistant, my surgeon, my radiation oncologist and the team at the homeopathic clinic. I am alive thanks to all of you.

My friends in NB / Lisa, John, Larissa and James, Candice W., Harry Michael, Donna, Jim, the "boys in the band" and all the hangers on.

My friends in Calgary / Marjan, Colin, Laurel, Dale, Donna, Brenda, Meike.

My GP friends and colleagues / Lyle and Shannon, Rena, for sharing her story of survival, Alan, Ali, Jocelyn, Pam, Frank, Eric, Val and Dwain, Murray and Chris, Candace H, Drennan, Christy and my dance girls.

The Art Gallery of Grande Prairie / for the exhibition and book launch.

Mom / Who when I tell her I love her always says ... I love you more.

And Doug / My über-talented designer husband without whose constant support I could not have made it thorough any of this. I have lost track of the hundreds of hours that made this final project possible. Amongst the many things you are ... awesome ... together we made a book. Which is way better than a bear ...

And lastly to all of who you might actually read this or better yet look at the pictures ... thank you.

Outtakes

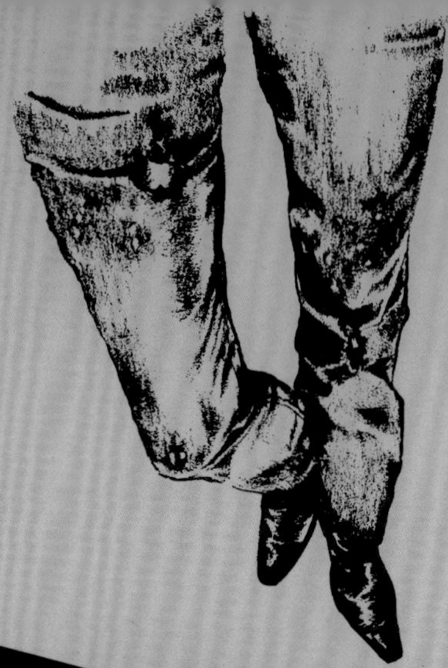

"Damn it Jim, I'm an artist not a writer."

I don't know how to have cancer. It is my first time.

My mother had her usual response, which, always left us confused as children – she laughed and told us not to do that."

Curled up on the couch with the cat, reading Dostoevsky, me, not the cat. I know I don't own a cat and if cats could read they wouldn't read him anyway, but it is my montage.

An ignoble and unjust end to a great pair of socks.

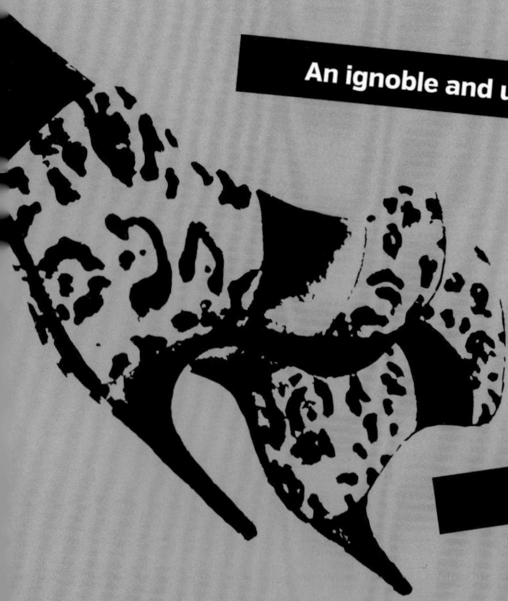

Emails and morphine don't mix …

It is possible I will survive for the simple reason I'm too stubborn to fail at anything. Death would be the ultimate failure and not acceptable to me.

Actually I count myself lucky at still having a sense of humour but it is a bit intermittent.

Admittedly I am an academic and prone to over-thinking a left-hand turn ...

... it's only 4 months, it's only 3 weeks, it's only a couple of scars, it's only complete breast reconstruction, it's only compression stockings, it's only 6 months until your nails grow back, it's only a bad sunburn, it's only hair, it's only ...

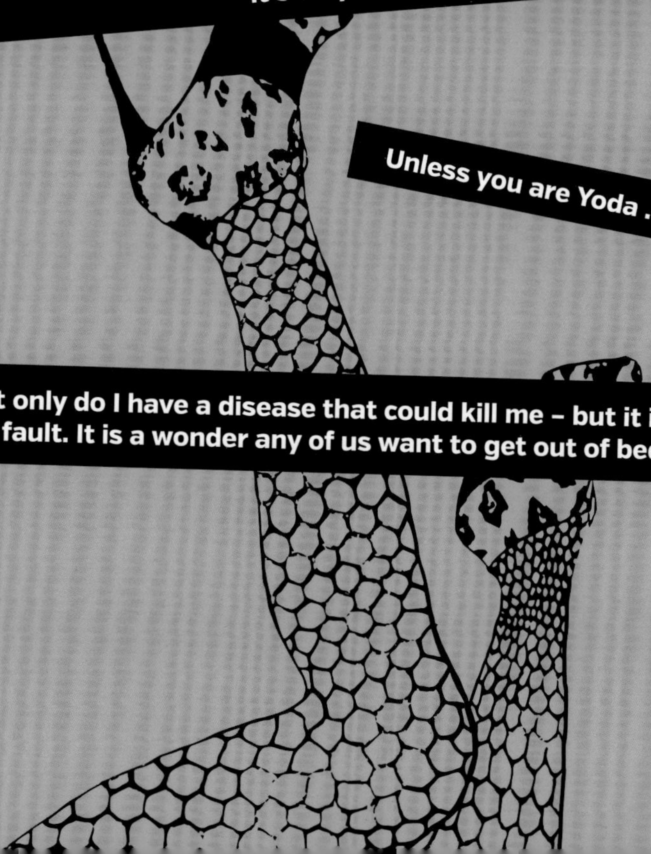

Unless you are Yoda ... advice give me not.

Not only do I have a disease that could kill me – but it is my fault. It is a wonder any of us want to get out of bed.